AMERICAN INDIAN HEALTH AND NURSING

Margaret P. Moss, PhD, JD, RN, FAAN, is an associate professor and assistant dean of Diversity and Inclusion at the University at Buffalo School of Nursing (State University of New York). Previously, she was associate professor, coordinator of the Nursing Management, Policy, and Leadership master's specialty, and the first director of the DNP program at the Yale University School of Nursing. She recently held a Fulbright Visiting Research Chair in Aboriginal/Indigenous Life and Culture in the North American Context at McGill University (2014). Dr. Moss earned her PhD in nursing from the University of Texas—Health Science Center at Houston, and her JD from Hamline University School of Law (St. Paul, Minnesota). She did a 2-year postdoctoral fellowship in aging at the University of Colorado Native Elder Research Center. Dr. Moss also spent 16 months as a health policy fellow staffing the U.S. Senate Special Committee on Aging—Robert Wood Johnson Foundation, Institute of Medicine, in Washington, DC (completed in 2009). From 2005 to 2008, Dr. Moss was the director of the Native Nurse Career Opportunity Program at the University of Minnesota School of Nursing. After being promoted to tenured associate professor there, she served as director of Inclusivity and Diversity (2006–2008), and she later became an associate director of the Minnesota Hartford Center and was appointed interim chair of the Leadership, Systems, and Informatics Policy Cooperative. Her clinical experience prior to teaching included serving as a staff nurse and then as house supervisor and patient education specialist at the U.S. Public Health Service, Indian Health Service/Santa Fe Indian Hospital (1991–1996). Dr. Moss has published 16 research papers, focusing primarily on American Indian elders; Zuni elders; and aging, migration, and remigration of American Indians and the impact on elders. She has written three book chapters, including one for *Complementary & Alternative Therapies in Nursing* (Springer Publishing Company). Dr. Moss has taught graduate courses in health policy leadership and cultural aspects of health care. She is a popular speaker and has delivered 35 invited papers since 2010, and has delivered a total of more than 60 invited papers internationally and nationally on health disparities, Indians and research, health policy, and healthy aging in American Indians. She is an enrolled member of the Mandan, Hidatsa, and Arikara Nation.

AMERICAN INDIAN HEALTH AND NURSING

Margaret P. Moss, PhD, JD, RN, FAAN

EDITOR

SPRINGER PUBLISHING COMPANY
NEW YORK

Springer Publishing Company, LLC
11 West 42nd Street
New York, NY 10036
www.springerpub.com

Acquisitions Editor: Margaret Zuccarini
Production Editor: Kris Parrish
Composition: S4Carlisle Publishing Services

ISBN: 978-0-8261-2984-0
e-book ISBN: 978-0-8261-2985-7

15 16 17 18 / 5 4 3 2 1

The author and the publisher of this Work have made every effort to use sources believed to be reliable to provide information that is accurate and compatible with the standards generally accepted at the time of publication. Because medical science is continually advancing, our knowledge base continues to expand. Therefore, as new information becomes available, changes in procedures become necessary. We recommend that the reader always consult current research and specific institutional policies before performing any clinical procedure. The author and publisher shall not be liable for any special, consequential, or exemplary damages resulting, in whole or in part, from the readers' use of, or reliance on, the information contained in this book. The publisher has no responsibility for the persistence or accuracy of URLs for external or third-party Internet websites referred to in this publication and does not guarantee that any content on such websites is, or will remain, accurate or appropriate.

Library of Congress Cataloging-in-Publication Data
Moss, Margaret P., author.
 American Indian health and nursing / Margaret P. Moss.
    p. ; cm.
 Includes bibliographical references and index.
 ISBN 978-0-8261-2984-0 — ISBN 978-0-8261-2985-7 (e-book ISBN)
 I. Title.
 [DNLM: 1. Indians, North American—United States. 2. Transcultural Nursing—United States. 3. Cultural Competency—United States. 4. Education, Nursing—United States. 5. Minority Health—United States. WY 107]
 RT86.54
 610.73089′97—dc23
                                                                      2015032103

Special discounts on bulk quantities of our books are available to corporations, professional associations, pharmaceutical companies, health care organizations, and other qualifying groups. If you are interested in a custom book, including chapters from more than one of our titles, we can provide that service as well.

For details, please contact:
Special Sales Department, Springer Publishing Company, LLC
11 West 42nd Street, 15th Floor, New York, NY 10036-8002
Phone: 877-687-7476 or 212-431-4370; Fax: 212-941-7842
E-mail: sales@springerpub.com

Printed in the United States of America by Bradford & Bigelow.

*I am dedicating this book to my two mothers, nature and nurture.
Both women went through nurse's training and each in her own way brought me
to where I am now, putting together this book. Viola Walks (born on the Fort Berthold
Indian Reservation/enrolled member, Three Affiliated Tribes of
North Dakota) and Norma K. Henke (Mom).*

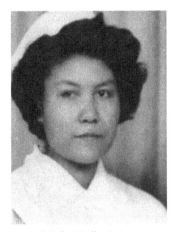

Viola Walks Lang
(1930–1999;
undated photo)

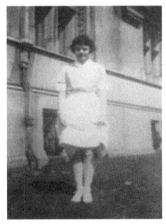

Norma K. Pegg (Henke),
(1924–2007; pictured at the
age of 19, in 1943)

Contents

Contributors

Nicolle L. Gonzales, MSN, RN, CNM
Diné—member of the Navajo Nation
Bridge Care for Women;
Changing Woman Initiative
San Ildefonso, New Mexico

Donna M. Grandbois, PhD, MSN, RN
Enrolled member of the Turtle Mountain
    Band of Chippewa Indians
Department of Nursing and Master of
    Public Health Program
North Dakota State University
Fargo, North Dakota

S. Neyooxet Greymorning, PhD
Southern Arapaho
Anthropology and Native American
    Studies
University of Montana
Missoula, Montana

Bette Jacobs, PhD, RN, FAAN
Cherokee
O'Neill Institute for Global and National
    Health Law
Georgetown University
Washington, DC

**Chief Mutáwi Mutáhash (Many Hearts)
Marilynn Malerba, DNP, RN**
Chief—Mohegan Tribe
Uncasville, Connecticut

Lisa Martin, PhD, RN
Member—Lac Du Flambeau Band of Lake
    Superior Chippewa Indians
Department of Nursing
St. Catherine University
Minneapolis, Minnesota

Ruth E. Meilstrup, RN (ret.)
Santa Fe Indian Hospital
Santa Fe, New Mexico

Margaret P. Moss, PhD, JD, RN, FAAN
Enrolled member of the Three Affiliated
    Tribes of North Dakota
School of Nursing
University at Buffalo–SUNY
Buffalo, New York

Christopher M. Nelson, MPH, BSN, RN
Public health nurse in Alaska
Community Health Nurse
Mendocino Coast Clinics
Fort Bragg, California

Lee Anne Nichols, PhD, RN
Citizen (tribal member) of Cherokee
    Nation of Oklahoma
School of Nursing
University of Tulsa
Tulsa, Oklahoma

C. June Strickland, PhD, RN
Cherokee
School of Nursing
University of Washington
Seattle, Washington

Lillian Tom-Orme, PhD, MPH, RN, FAAN
Navajo Nation
College of Nursing
University of Utah
Salt Lake City, Utah

Theodore C. Van Alst, Jr., PhD
Sihásapa Lakota
Department of Native American Studies
University of Montana
Missoula, Montana

Preface

When I conceived of this book, it was both as a nurse and an enrolled member of the Three Affiliated Tribes of North Dakota—that is, the *Mandan, Hidatsa, and Arikara Nation* on the Fort Berthold reservation. I have been a nurse for more than 25 years. And although I was born in Fargo, North Dakota, I have lived all over the country, mainly in urban areas. During that time, I experienced firsthand nursing both in Indian Country and in metropolitan areas with large American Indian populations, such as Portland, Oregon; Albuquerque, New Mexico; and Minneapolis, Minnesota.

I was only the 13th American Indian nurse to earn a doctorate in nursing, and I did so in 2000. In 2015, there are about two dozen American Indian nurses with nursing doctorates. As a nurse and as an educator, I have found materials related to American Indian health and nursing to be nonexistent. It also became apparent to me fairly quickly that regions, tribes, and cultural variations do matter when nursing in Indian Country. As a Plains Indian practicing at the Santa Fe Indian Hospital in the 1990s, I was struck by the huge cultural differences among this mostly Pueblo, Apache, and Navajo population. I had to learn what was culturally acceptable, relevant, and useful in the care of each of the patients at that hospital. The concepts I learned on the job, even as a Native American nurse, were never taught to me in any nursing program.

As Americans, we are presented with few opportunities to learn in depth about our Indigenous people. There is the cursory section or chapter in grade school, and maybe again in high school, and then nothing. The material, when it is presented, is always from the dominant culture's point of view. I myself have a degree in biology, three degrees in the field of nursing, as well as a degree in law. In none of these programs did I learn anything about American Indians, their health status, environment, issues, or outlook, with the exception of material taught in a targeted federal Indian law course. I have made it a mission to educate my students on each of these issues. For example, the vast majority of Americans do not understand that to be an American Indian in the United States is a political determination, not a racial one. In the eyes of the U.S. government, one is not an American Indian and will not have access to any services for American Indians, including access to Indian Health Services and Bureau of Indian Affairs Services, unless one is an enrolled member of a federally recognized tribe. These two government agencies, in large part, are the employers and educators of nurses caring for American Indians.

As we move into an era that promotes cultural competence, patient-centered care, and issues of consent and confidentiality, there are many moving parts that must be balanced. And when you add nursing to America's Indigenous people, the balance becomes even trickier when the backdrop of knowledge is missing. It is my hope that this book will be of interest to many groups beyond nurses and will provide a knowledge base from which to start. In Part I, contributors include two American Indian historians/anthropologists and nurses, both American Indian and non-Native, who have spent years nursing in Indian Country. In Part II, the contributors are all nurses, and all but one is American Indian, with the other currently working in and closely researching this population. Part III, written by myself and Chief Malerba, Mohegan, moves the reader through policy implications. I hope you will find the content both interesting on its own merits and useful in caring for this most underserved of U.S. populations.

Margaret P. Moss

Acknowledgments

*F*irst and foremost, I would like to thank all the people and patients in Indian Country, as well as the health care providers who work tirelessly to care for this most underserved of U.S. populations. I would especially like to thank all of those who have come in contact with the contributors of this text who provided the experience and insights from which they now draw.

Second, I am grateful to all of the contributors for their efforts on this first textbook on American Indian health and nursing. Without their willingness to share their specialized cultural knowledge, this effort could not have borne fruit.

Third, I thank my family, including my husband, Willie Moss; my sons, Hakeem Moss and Xavier Moss; and my daughters, Shakira Moss and Marique Moss, for the encouragement they gave me while composing this book. I would add a special nod to Xavier and his schoolmate Mariella Dragon, who drew out the cultural map and painstakingly listed all 567 federally recognized tribes for the appendix.

And finally, thanks to Teresa Abney, who copyedited for me with great care while I attended to content.

PART I

Indigenous America

*P*art I of *American Indian Health and Nursing* provides a national and historical look at the peoples of what is now the United States. (An appendix at the end of the book is provided with a complete listing of the 566 current federally recognized tribes.) This is followed by a view of pre- and postcontact indigenous America and the effects on health resulting from policies by the new dominant culture.

Next to be introduced is the idea that "nursing" has been occurring in indigenous America long before icons, such as Florence Nightingale, put a face to the profession. An introduction to nursing and the Indian Health Service (IHS) is then followed by health modalities outside of the IHS—that is, indigenous knowledge and traditional healing.

It is hoped that nurses will gain an understanding of the historical and political realities of American Indians and Alaska Natives. They will learn that both indigenous and Western modes of care are used. And finally, this new understanding will help deliver patient-centered care to today's indigenous people.

❖ ONE ❖

Overview

Margaret P. Moss

LEARNING OBJECTIVES

- ✦ The student will be able to identify the populations included in the terms *American Indians* and *Alaska Natives* (AI/ANs).
- ✦ The student will be able to integrate ideas of indigenous thought, such as the medicine wheel, into Western nursing ideas of mind/body/spirit and vice versa.
- ✦ The student will be able to discuss why separating AI/AN tribes into cultural groups will optimize nursing care in this population.

KEY TERMS

- ✦ American Indians and Alaska Natives or AI/ANs
- ✦ Metaparadigm (of nursing)
- ✦ Misidentification

KEY CONCEPTS

- ✦ Cultural groups
- ✦ Four directions
- ✦ Holism
- ✦ Medicine wheel

This book was written to include the subtext of "what you never learned in nursing school" about American Indians and health. This book takes the student beyond oversimplified ideas of "they don't look you in the eye" and "they want their hair back after brushing" to real context, background, and useful information about caring for American Indians in today's world.

American Indians and Alaska Natives (AI/ANs) have populated what is now the United States for at least the last 15,000 years (Goebel, Waters, & O'Rourke, 2008). Their numbers have fluctuated from estimates in the tens of millions precontact to an all-time low of 90,000, according to the 1900 Census, and back to a current count of around 2.8 million for persons reporting single-tribe membership/heritage, and over 5 million for persons reporting multiple tribal affiliations (U.S. Census Bureau, 2013). American Indians and Alaska Natives have some of the greatest gaps in care and health status in the United States as compared with any other group (Indian Health Service, 2003). These gaps, known as health disparities, have been largely attributed to consequences of contact (Jones, 2006). These health disparities will be discussed throughout the book by cultural regions.

Registered nurses (RNs) make up the largest segment of the health professions, at about 2.8 million (Health Resources and Services Administration, 2013). The oldest North American civilizations and the largest of the health professions have intersected for over 100 years, yet there has never been a book written about the interface of American Indians and nursing. Health care finds itself in a three-decade-long era of cultural competency (Brach & Fraserirector, 2000; Clark et al., 2011; Cross, Bazron, Dennis, & Isaacs, 1989), transcultural nursing (Leininger, 1988; Maier-Lorentz, 2008), and health equity approaches (Marmot et al., 2008), yet there has not been any formalized text on how these areas can be understood and operationalized within the field of nursing with AI/AN patients.

Box 1.1

The oldest North American civilizations have interesected with nurses for over 100 years, and yet there has never been a book written about the interface of American Indians and nursing.

Throughout this text, various authors will decide and define what terms to use to refer to the indigenous populations found in what is now the United States. This author will use the term *American Indian*, as *Indian* is still the legal term for the indigenous people in the United States. *Indigenous* will also be used throughout as a more generic, less politicized term. However, *Indian* is the term used in the U.S. Constitution and in the government entities—Bureau of Indian Affairs (BIA), IHS, and the Senate Committee on Indian Affairs, among others. There is a title in the U.S. Federal Code called "Indians"—Title 25. No other group has such a designation. Authors may use the more "popular culture" terms of *Native American* or *Native*, and/or the actual tribal nation's name. The seminal point here is that there are several terms used to describe this population. It is important to note that when speaking to AI/AN patients, the nurse should ask the person how *he* or *she* identifies. The consequences of misidentification are discussed in a following section. But for the purposes of this text, the authors will use various terms and give the rationale for use.

WHAT IS A TRIBE? FEDERAL AND STATE

In choosing nursing as a profession, it became clear to this author that there were several concepts prevalent in nursing that also held true in American Indian thought. Here, a caveat must be inserted that American Indians are not a racial, ethnic, or even political monolith. Illustrating this point, there are 566 federally recognized tribes—that is, tribal nations that the United States has deemed as partial sovereigns with which they have a nation-to-nation relationship (Bureau of Indian Affairs, 2015; see Appendix A). This relationship, referred to as the federal trust responsibility, is discussed in a later chapter.

The student is encouraged to review the list of the tribes and their names to gain a full picture of the number and variety of tribes in this country that nurses may encounter. Few people are able to answer correctly just how many tribes there are in the United States. Over 200 federally recognized tribes are found in Alaska alone. When visiting various states for speaking or other engagements, the author often asks the audience how many tribes are in their states. Anecdotally, in all my 15 years in academia, only one person answered correctly—this was in New York State in 2015. There are eight federally recognized tribes in New York State and three state-recognized tribes. This question was asked of nurses: If the nurse does not know who his or her patients are, how can she provide culturally competent care?

Did you know that American Indian nations are not found in every state? But tribes, as defined and acknowledged by the federal government, are found in 34 states: Alabama, Alaska, Arizona, California, Colorado, Connecticut, Florida, Idaho, Iowa, Kansas, Louisiana, Maine, Massachusetts, Michigan, Minnesota, Mississippi, Montana, Nebraska, Nevada, New Mexico, New York, North Carolina, North Dakota, Oklahoma, Oregon, Rhode Island, South Carolina, South Dakota, Texas, Utah, Virginia, Washington, Wisconsin, and Wyoming.

The names of tribes often give a clue or reference to history, language groups, or migration. As an example, the author's nation, the Three Affiliated Tribes of North Dakota, was named after the government assignment of the three different tribes, the Mandan, Hidatsa, and Arikara (Sahnish), on to the same reservation back in 1870 following the Fort Laramie Treaty (1868). Two of the tribes have a similar migration pattern from what are now the areas of Minnesota, South Dakota, and Iowa west to North Dakota and north up the Missouri River. They both belong to Siouan language groups, the Mandan and Hidatsa.

The Sahnish, as they call themselves, belong to a different language group and were found in eastern Nebraska. They migrated at a different time and in a different pattern from the other two tribes. Understanding history and patterns and language and cultural groups leads to a greater understanding of the AI/AN person who has presented to you for care.

Another example is the Rancherias, found in California. These tribes have a rich history and set of issues completely different from those found on the Plains, as explained in the chapter on California in Part II. When a patient identifies to the nurses as being a member, this should trigger the nurse to ask certain questions and invoke an understanding of trust issues, among other things.

STATE-RECOGNIZED TRIBES

There are several tribes that have been granted *state* recognition but not federal recognition. There are also tribes that have been granted both. Tribes with state recognition number 66 and are found in 14 states: Alabama, Connecticut, Delaware, Georgia, Louisiana, Maryland, Massachusetts, Montana, New Jersey, New York, North Carolina, Texas, Vermont, and Virginia (see Appendix B). Of these, Delaware, Georgia, Maryland, New Jersey, Vermont, and Virginia have state recognition only.

As a nurse and advocate, knowing the distinctions between membership in federal or state tribes involves understanding funding sources, government accountability, and access to care. State-only recognized tribal members will not have access to the U.S. PHS IHS, which is a federal health program specifically for enrolled members of federally recognized tribes. If there is no tribe–federal legal relationship, then no care will be provided or paid for as these programs are rooted in treaties and public laws with this specific group of tribes. The nurse will then know not to refer her patient to Indian Health Services or expect IHS contracted care to pay.

Some states, as listed previously, have taken it upon themselves to recognize certain tribes and have generated programs for health and welfare. They may advise and/or provide education through state-funded programming. For example, North Carolina has a well-established Commission of Indian Affairs with an Indian Child Welfare program (the federal Indian Child Welfare Act [1978] is unavailable to state-only tribes), which generates annual reports on Indian Health and other topics and offers a toolbox of resources (www .doa.state.nc.us/cia/resources.aspx#Reports). Most of North Carolina's eight tribes are state recognized, not federally recognized.

ETHNIC AMERICAN INDIANS

And finally, there are many disenfranchised indigenous people who, either by choice or circumstance, belong to no tribe. This could be through the breakup of families, fostering out children, adoption of children by non-Indians (which is now largely against federal law—the Indian Child Welfare Act, noted earlier), or through past federal policies of assimilation, as described in Chapter 3. These indigenous people have much of the same genetics, and biological tendencies toward diabetes, and so on, and will have epigenetic factors stemming from historical trauma. *Historical trauma* is trauma of ancestors affecting health in all domains today (BraveHeart & DeBruyn, 1998). They may feel disconnected, have identity issues, and guilt or shame regarding their dissociation.

The nurse should understand what issues may be behind the presenting health, mental health, emotional, or spiritual health of the ethnic Indian, and may share many of these with those who are tribal members. Tribal membership is a political determination, that is, one is a citizen of a nation but does not discount the shared health and other issues of the nonmember Indian.

Although there are tribal nations in only 33 states, nurses need to know that America's indigenous people are found in *every* state.

1: OVERVIEW ♦ 7

AMERICAN INDIANS AND NURSING—OVERLAPPING CONCEPTS

Although it is important to recognize the vast numbers of distinct tribes, there are certain threads of culture, beliefs, and thought that are woven throughout the many nations. And among these threads are two that are also shared with nursing: (1) holism (Smuts, 1926) and (2) the components of the *metaparadigm of nursing*—person, environment, health, and nursing (Fawcett, 1995).

HOLISM AND THE MEDICINE WHEEL

Nursing has, at its center, the treatment of the patient as a whole within a caring philosophy as distinguished from medicine's historical focus of "cure the disease" (Boschma, 1994). The body of literature around mind/body/spirit in nursing has grown along with the use of the term *holism* and its philosophy since the 1970s (Owen & Holmes, 1993). "[H]olistic health is usually defined in subjective, experiential terms including feelings of wellbeing, attitudes, a sense of purpose and spirituality" (Mark & Lyons, 2010, para. 4). This subjectivity incorporates the patient into the equation and brings in the "art" in nursing as in the "art and science" of nursing. It is this "art" aspect that intersects with AI/AN traditional ideas around healing and care. One scholar has defined "the art of nursing [a]s the intentional creative use of oneself, based upon skill and expertise, to transmit emotion and meaning to another. It is a process that is subjective and requires interpretation, sensitivity, imagination, and active participation" (Jenner, 1997, p. 5). It can be argued that this is some of what the traditional AI/AN healer does—transmit emotion and meaning to another—for the purpose of healing.

"Holistic health presumes to enlarge the traditional sphere of medical (read 'allopathic') concerns from a narrow, largely technical focus on symptomatology and disease to a broadened domain including such health salient foci as nutrition, psychological and spiritual well-being, interpersonal relations and influences emanating from the environment" (Lowenberg & Davis, 1994, p. 581). Although holism has been a concept largely acknowledged in nursing, it has had a slow start in solid incorporation into *practice* (Owen & Holmes, 1993). However, nursing, arguably more than any of the other health professions, embraces ideas of the whole person (mind/body/spirit) as the treatable entity, and in fact will see the family and community as the "patient" by extension in many settings. The term *holism* was coined by Smuts (1926) as an intersection of science and philosophy in noting that the whole results from interdependent parts in the universe, and does not exist in isolation of those parts (Smuts, 1926). This concept, then, has been applied in the field of nursing as to the body itself, and the person in the health environment.

Parallel to this concept lies the framework often referred to as the medicine wheel, which is found in many tribes. We have presented a generic medicine

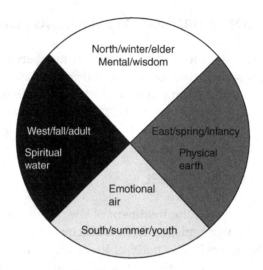

FIGURE 1.1 Medicine wheel.

wheel here (Figure 1.1). Different tribes may place different attributes in the four sections although, generally, the age attributes hold as presented here: The infant starts in the "east" and the life span continues around in a clockwise fashion, finishing in the "north."

The medicine wheel represents the four directions, that is, four dimensions, of the person—physical, emotional, spiritual, and mental—and attributes of the Earth, as well as the stages of life. Four is often one of the sacred numbers in tribes. These interconnecting parts can be seen as the interconnectedness of the concept of holism.

The four directions are an important constant concept running throughout Indian country. Indian country is an actual term used to describe trust lands, pueblos, reservations, and designated Indian communities and the people in them. Many dances, prayers, the medicine wheel, and other cultural instances can be found that honor all four directions. It is important to note that this book itself is organized in relation to the four directions, starting with areas in the east, heading south, west, and ending in the north. This pattern is discussed more fully in the section on cultural groups.

THE METAPARADIGM OF NURSING

The second area where ideas of both nursing and indigenous thought overlap is in the very metaparadigm of nursing. "A metaparadigm is the most general statement of a discipline and functions as a framework" (Metaparadigm, n.d., para. 1). It is interesting to note that the number four plays a part here as well. In the nursing metaparadigm, there are four global concepts: (1) health, (2) nursing, (3) person, and (4) environment (Fawcett, 1995). There is no such metaparadigm of medicine, for example.

Here, *health* concerns life processes, well-being, and optimal functioning in illness or wellness. *Nursing* is seen as those activities found within the *nursing process*—assessment, nursing diagnosis, planning, intervention, and evaluation in the delivery of care to the person. *Person* is the recipient of nursing care and can include, as previously mentioned, families and communities. And finally, the *environment* includes all of the physical surroundings, including agencies and organizations, as well as society at large (Fawcett, 1995).

These nursing concepts of holism with mind/body/spirit inclusion and the added environmental component are completely in line with much of the threads of indigenous knowledge and thought in health and health care. Therefore, nurses have not only physically intersected with AI/ANs for years, but can also be seen as having a deeper global thought connection. This text seeks to present this as a basis for understanding the nursing care that is optimal for AI/AN patients today. This basis should be familiar to the nurse.

PERSON AND MISIDENTIFICATION

Of central importance in nursing is understanding who the patient is in front of you, that is, the *person*. In this era of patient-centered care and cultural competency, misidentification of American Indians is an inestimable problem. Patient-centered care is a term of most recent importance in the Patient Protection and Affordable Care Act (2010), where it appears throughout. Patient-centered care includes input by both the patient and the caregiver, and comprises individualized plans of care. A hallmark of this type of care is to increase quality and safety.

It is unfortunate that one hallmark of care of AI/AN patients is in misidentification. This comes about largely when the nurse has little knowledge of the populations around his or her practice, and fails to ask patients how they identify when first doing an assessment. American Indians do not all look a certain way, and cannot always be identified through appearance.

As the reader will learn in Chapter 3, being American Indian in the United States is primarily a political designation over racial and ethnic identifications. Therefore, one cannot always "see" this political, national-origin characteristic.

The nurse who does not know that the patient before him or her identifies as American Indian will not be able to deliver the patient-centered or culturally competent care that is demanded today for optimum outcomes. Nor will the nurse know what to ask regarding the patient's spiritual needs, whether he or she is practicing other types of medicine, who his or her next of kin is (usually different than state next-of-kin designees), or what his or her first language is.

Data from the IHS show that recalculations of most data must be offered to incorporate this idea of misidentification. It runs not only throughout patient data, but also through research data, the census, and almost any arena in which demographic data are captured. Awareness and effort in this area alone in nursing would assist in better care and better data for AI/ANs.

IMPORTANCE OF CULTURAL GROUPS

Beyond the individual, this text offers the idea of cultural groups as an organizing principle in providing care. The depth and breadth of tribal nations presented (see Appendix A) reveals an overwhelming cultural competency exercise for nurses. It would be impossible to know what each tribe's cultural beliefs, practices, and traditions are, especially in an often hidden, indigenous health care arena. Toward optimizing care for AI/ANs, this text seeks to divide the dizzying array of tribes into 10 cultural groups. These groups are either geographically or culturally adjacent, or both.

The groups used in this text are:

1. Northeastern Woodlands
2. Southeastern Woodlands
3. Southwest
4. Great Basin
5. California
6. Pacific Northwest
7. Northwest Plateau
8. Alaska
9. Northern Great Plains
10. Urban

These groups are presented going from east to north in a clockwise fashion as is culturally understandable throughout Indian country.

The first nine cultural areas are accepted groups that can be found with slight variations as to names and inclusion, but, for the most part, can be understood throughout Indian country. The category "Urban" has been added as, for the first time in U.S. history since the reservation period of federal Indian policy in the 1800s, more AI/ANs live off reservation than on. Urban Indians too have a range of issues that need to be understood by nurses. They have fewer resources for culturally focused health care, less understanding of who they are, higher misidentification than those on reservations, and an added cultural isolation factor than those on the reservations.

It cannot be emphasized enough that tribes, regions, and cultural groups are also not fully aware of each other's cultures. There are huge differences among areas, which is another reason this text is being offered (please see the author's own example in Box 1.2). In another instance, a non-Native nurse was working in the emergency department in a large southwestern Indian hospital. An older woman was brought in as a patient, and was seemingly covered in dirt and disheveled. The nurse instantly thought it was elder abuse and neglect, and proceeded to wash the woman. As Native nurses arrived to help with the patient, they were aghast as this was ceremonial ash that should not have been disturbed.

Box 1.2

The author is a Plains Indian from a North Dakota tribe who was raised in urban areas. She arrived to work as a nurse at the Santa Fe Indian Hospital and was new to New Mexico, and was not familiar with many of the practices found there.

In one simple instance, as she checked her patient, who was being rolled on a gurney to surgery, to make sure jewelry had been removed and IV (intravenous) lines were in place, she noted an ear of corn lying next to the patient. What was this for? Surely it was intentional. Who put it there? Why?

As she later learned, in Pueblo thought, corn represents life and the individual. The husks are the clothes, and the silk is the hair. It is a physical representation of spiritual life.

Never had the author learned this in standard nursing programs. Nor was she familiar with it from the Plains or urban areas.

CONCLUSIONS

This text serves to help all cultures understand the 10 cultural groups of AI/ANs both within the indigenous population and outside it. Ideas found in this text have been brought by experts in each area, and are things nurses likely never learned in nursing school. Only a greater understanding of the indigenous person and patient presenting to the nurse can optimize the outcomes and experience for all. Of primary importance is the connection the profession of nursing has with the AI/AN population in terms of a holistic understanding of the person and, in addition, the community and environment. If these shared tenets can be recognized and optimized, then health goals can likely be reached to the greater satisfaction of both the nurse and the indigenous patient.

STUDY QUESTIONS

♦ Why is it best to treat American Indians and Alaska Natives by cultural groups over ideas assigned to the one large group? Think of an instance such as the one presented in the callout example.
♦ How does patient-centered care move forward with a better understanding of AI/AN populations?
♦ What steps would you, as the nurse, take to avoid misidentification as an AI/AN?
♦ How can nurses use ideas already at the center of nursing to relate to their AI/AN patients?

USEFUL WEBSITES

♦ Bureau of Indian Affairs, www.bia.gov
♦ National Library of Medicine—Native voices on healing and medicine, http://www .nlm.nih.gov/nativevoices/exhibition/healing-ways/medicine-ways/medicine-wheel.html
♦ The American Holistic Nurses Association, http://www.ahna.org/About-Us/What-is-Holistic-Nursing

REFERENCES

Boschma, G. (1994). The meaning of holism in nursing: Historical shifts in holistic nursing ideas. *Public Health Nursing, 11*, 324–330.

Brach, C., & Fraserirector, I. (2000). Can cultural competency reduce racial and ethnic health disparities? A review and conceptual model. *Medical Care Research and Review, 57*, 181–217.

BraveHeart, M., & DeBruyn, L. M. (1998). The American Indian holocaust: Healing historical unresolved grief. *American Indian and Alaska Native Mental Health Research, 8*, 56–78.

Bureau of Indian Affairs. (2015). *Indian affairs—Who we are*. Retrieved March 20, 2015, from http://www.bia.gov/WhoWeAre/index.htm

Clark, L., Calvillo, E., Dela Cruz, F., Fongwa, M., Kools, S., Lowe, J., & Mastel-Smith, B. (2011). Cultural competencies for graduate nursing education. *Journal of Professional Nursing, 27*, 133–139.

Cross, T., Bazron, B., Dennis, K., & Isaacs, M. (1989). *Towards a culturally competent system of care: A monograph on effective services for minority children who are severely emotionally disturbed*. Washington, DC: Georgetown University Child Development Center.

Fawcett, J. (1995). *Analysis and evaluation of conceptual models of nursing*. Philadelphia, PA: F. A. Davis.

Fort Laramie Treaty. (1868). Treaty with the Sioux-Brule, Oglala, Miniconjou, Yanktonai, Hunkpapa, Blackfeet, Cuthead, Two Kettle, San Arcs, and Santee-and Arapaho, 4/29/1868; General Records of the United States Government; Record Group 11; National Archives.

Goebel, T., Waters, M. R., & O'Rourke, D. H. (2008). The late Pleistocene dispersal of modern humans in the Americas. *Science, 319*, 1497–1502. doi:10.1126/science.1153569

Health Resources and Services Administration. (2013). *The U.S. nursing workforce: Trends in supply and education*. Retrieved March 2015, from http://bhpr.hrsa.gov/health-workforce/reports/nursingworkforce/nursingworkforcefullreport.pdf

Indian Child Welfare Act, 25 U.S.C. §§ 1901–1963 (1978).

Indian Health Service. (2003). *Program statistics—IHS HQ publications*. Retrieved March 26, 2015, from http://www.ihs.gov/dps/publications/trends03/

Jones, D. S. (2006). The persistence of American Indian health disparities. *American Journal of Public Health, 96*, 2122–2134.

Leininger, M. M. (1988). Leininger's theory of nursing: Cultural care diversity and universality. *Nursing Science Quarterly, 1*, 152–160.

Lowenberg, J. S., & Davis, F. (1994). Beyond medicalisation–demedicalisation: The case of holistic health. *Sociology of Health & Illness, 16*, 579–599.

Maier-Lorentz, M. M. (2008). Transcultural nursing: Its importance in nursing practice. *Journal of Cultural Diversity, 15*, 37–43.

Mark, G. T., & Lyons, A. C. (2010). Maori healers' views on wellbeing: The importance of mind, body, spirit, family and land. *Social Science & Medicine, 70*, 1756–1764.

Marmot, M., Friel, S., Bell, R., Houweling, T. A., Taylor, S., & Commission on Social Determinants of Health. (2008). Closing the gap in a generation: Health equity through action on the social determinants of health. *The Lancet, 372*, 1661–1669.

Metaparadigm. (2003). *Miller-Keane encyclopedia and dictionary of medicine, nursing, and allied health* (7th ed.). Retrieved from http://medical-dictionary.thefreedictionary.com/metaparadigm

Owen, M. J., & Holmes, C. A. (1993). 'Holism' in the discourse of nursing. *Journal of Advanced Nursing, 18*, 1688–1695.

Patient Protection and Affordable Care Act, 42 U.S.C. § 18001 (2010).

Smuts, J. C. (1926). *Holism and evolution*. New York, NY: Macmillan.

U.S. Census Bureau. (2013). *2010 census CPH-T-6. American Indian and Alaska native tribes in the United States and Puerto Rico: 2010*. Retrieved March 20, 2015, from https://www.census.gov/population/www/cen2010/cph-t/t-6tables/TABLE%20(1).pdf

TWO

Precontact Indigenous North America

Theodore C. Van Alst, Jr.

LEARNING OBJECTIVES
♦ To identify and define terms of use concerning American Indian people
♦ To assist in understanding the depth and breadth of precontact Native America
♦ To help the reader recognize the diversity of Native cultures

KEY TERMS
♦ *American Indian* versus *Native American*
♦ Bering Strait Theory
♦ Migration
♦ Tribes

KEY CONCEPTS
♦ Cultural awareness
♦ Historical knowledge
♦ Sensitivity to diversity

The history of the people of the Western Hemisphere (also known as the Americas) is long and rich. And although Western scientists have theorized that the people arrived via the Bering Strait, American Indian people themselves provide thousands of different origin stories, none of which includes crossing a land bridge of any kind.

The main idea of the origins of people indigenous to the Western Hemisphere, once generally held as more or less indisputable (although this has been challenged repeatedly and is increasingly falling out of favor) by Western science, is known as the Bering Strait Theory. This theory held, generally, that small-ish groups of people wandered over a land bridge that existed during the last glacial period between the far northwest reaches of what is now North America (Alaska) and the very northeastern edge of the continent of Asia, and then populated the vast continents of the Western Hemisphere, from the Arctic Circle in the north to Tierra del Fuego at the southern tip of what is now South America, developing thousands of distinct languages and cultures along the way. The earliest version of the theory held that the migration had happened

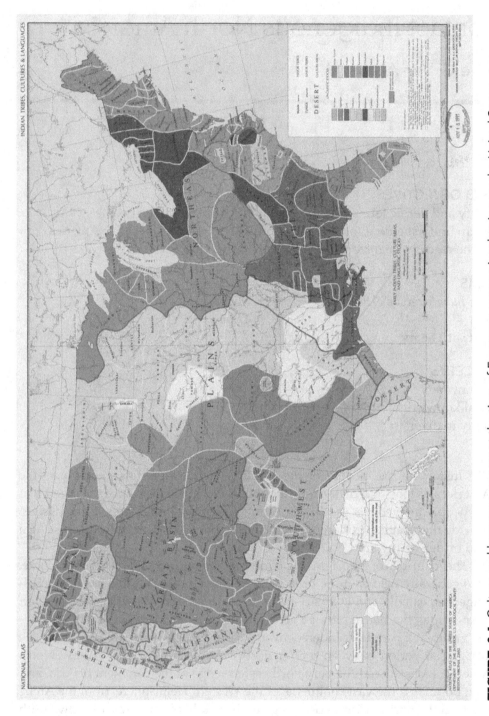

FIGURE 2.1 Culture and language groups at the time of European contact in what is now the United States.

Source: Library of Congress (n.d.).

a few thousand years ago, but that was revised in the 1940s to reflect a time of 10,000–12,000 years prior. (An excellent discussion of this theory and a list of additional readings is available in the "Bering Strait Theory" article [2011] cited at the end of this chapter.)

Today, the generally held timeline for the existence of people in the Americas seems to grow longer with each successive article and/or archaeological discovery. (See "When Did Humans Come to the Americas?" at Smithsonian.com as a good starting point in discussions on Clovis, which is part of the theory that the Americas were first settled by people who crossed the Bering Straits about 13,000 years ago, as well as other Western attempts to explain American Indian origins.) By way of example, recent recoveries show evidence of people living in the interior of what is now South America at least 14,000 years ago and longer. Other theories have held that although there were some migrations across the northern land bridge, there were also migrations by boat. It is posited that these migrations originated in Asia and Polynesia, with theorists citing linguistic, genetic, and even culinary evidence. (The presence of sweet potatoes and chickens in Peru is examined in "How the Sweet Potato Crossed the Pacific Way Before the Europeans Did" [Doucleff, 2013].)

HISTORICAL KNOWLEDGE AND DIVERSITY OF NATIVE CULTURES

In any instance, it is important to realize that by the time Europeans arrived in the Western Hemisphere, indigenous nations lived on vast continents filled with millions of people (middling estimates of North America are at 20 million people, and the Caribbean and Central and South America with over 120 million people at the time of contact) speaking thousands of languages, who all had intricate and highly developed technologies and social systems (imagine the social planning and civil engineering required to maintain the city of Tenochtitlan, which at European arrival had a population of well over 200,000 people, a city with over 1,000 civil servants alone maintaining the streets and recycling systems). Trade routes between the continents flourished (e.g., seashells from the Yucatan in Mexico being found during excavations of the 1,000+-year-old Cahokia Mounds in southern Illinois), and sophisticated political and diplomatic systems existed among various groups (think of the influence of the Iroquois Confederacy on the U.S. Articles of Confederation as well as the U.S. Constitution).

DEPTH AND BREADTH OF NATIVE CULTURES

At the time of contact with Europeans, indigenous nations in the Western Hemisphere had words and terms to describe both themselves as well as the other peoples around them. It is important to note that what we think of today as "tribes" were often confederated or allied groups of differing and independent people who would come together on occasion for a variety of reasons. Most tribal nations referred to themselves (in their own respective languages) as "The People," or something similar. For example, the Cherokee referred to themselves as *Ani-Yunwiya* (spelled **DhBӨ⬡** in their own syllabary), which means "Principal People." And although each of the *Očhéthi Šakówiŋ*, or "Seven Council Fires," had its own name (e.g., *Sihásapa* or "Blackfoot," *Oóhenuŋpa* or "Two Kettles"), the people known more broadly as "Sioux" (which is itself a European corruption of an Ojibwe pejorative) knew, and still know, themselves as *Lakȟóta* or "Allies."

At the point of contact, the land that we now know as North America was home to *millions* of people and *thousands* of tribal nations speaking *hundreds* of different languages (Figure 2.1). Even today, there are 304 separate federal Indian reservations for 566 federally acknowledged tribes in 34 of the United States, and a Bureau of Indian Affairs (BIA) that maintains 12 regional and 83 area offices that work with federal program services for American Indians. The Indian Health Service (or IHS, an agency that has its roots in the treaty obligations of the United States to provide medical assistance to American Indians) has 12 regional offices and a national headquarters in Rockville, Maryland, as well as 33 urban-centered, nonprofit urban Indian organizations providing health care services at 57 locations throughout the United States. There is also a Bureau of Indian Education (the BIE, which also has its roots in U.S. treaty obligations), that:

> oversees a total of 183 elementary, secondary, residential and peripheral dormitories across 23 states. 126 schools are tribally controlled under P.L. 93-638 Indian Self Determination Contracts or P.L. 100-297 Tribally Controlled Grant Schools Act. 57 schools are operated by the Bureau of Indian Education. The Bureau of Indian Education also oversees two (2) post-secondary schools: Haskell Indian Nations University and Southwestern Indian Polytechnic Institute. (Bureau of Indian Education, n.d.)

As we can see, the scope of American Indian populations and locations is extremely wide, and reflects a continuing rich history in the United States.

Recognizing this original and continuing diversity among American Indian people is extremely important both as a sign of respect to American Indian people and as something that is vital to their well-being. Recognition of the differences among American Indian people, which continue to endure despite centuries of attempts to lump them all into one category, is paramount in understanding concepts of sovereignty, nationhood, and modernity, all of which are vital to the health of American Indian people.

Therefore, in working with American Indian people both directly and indirectly, it is important to be aware of language, whether written or spoken. Let's define some terms.

DEFINING TERMS

For certain (usually older) generations, the term *American Indian* or *Indian* is actually preferred. For older populations, the term *Native American* is relatively new, and is often used in academic and government contexts. Many people shorten the term to *Native*, and that is an acceptable term for most. It is important to note that the treaties, which were made with the indigenous nations of this hemisphere, were signed between the United States and "Indians," and thus *Indian* is a legal term. That said, what people appreciate most, and what we would consider the very best course of action, would be to use the individual (or group) name. Thus, it is better to say, "a Lakota doctor," or "a Choctaw director," than "a Native American dentist." If the distinct tribal nation is not known, then "Native" should suffice in referring to individuals, should identifying them as such be necessary.

In review, Native North America was (and is) an incredibly rich, vibrant home to millions of people who have weathered great changes, including government-led wars and programs that attempted to assimilate them and their diverse cultures. After five centuries, American Indian people, their languages, cultures, and spiritual traditions endure and thrive in the face of immense pressures. In the end, it is this tremendous resilience and strength of spirit that helps Native people flourish in contemporary America.

CONCLUSIONS

In caring for American Indian and Alaska Native patients *today*, this understanding that there were people populating America before European contact is essential. They have an understanding of the environment and everything in it going back for millennia, not just a few hundred years. In this is an inherent appreciation of what would be optimum in terms of maintaining health in this very environment. What is known and understood by these first inhabitants needs to be heard and honored by nurses and incorporated wherever possible. All that has occurred since contact (to be discussed in Chapter 3) has greatly impacted the health of America's indigenous either by design or consequence. This must be taken into consideration in terms of trust between health care professional and patient.

STUDY QUESTIONS

◆ How long have America's indigenous people populated the continent?
◆ What estimates are there for how many indigenous people there were precontact? Can you compare that with how many there are today, and what was the lowest point?
◆ Why is it important for the nurse to understand this history?

RECOMMENDED READING

Aboriginal diabetes linked to loss of language. (2015, January 23). Retrieved January 29, 2015, from http://www.chathamdailynews.ca/2015/01/23/aboriginal-diabetes-epidemic-linked-to-loss-of-mother-tongue-study

Allen, L. (2014, July 30). *Navajo Nation turns to plant-based foods to reverse diabetes.* Retrieved February 2, 2015, from http://indiancountrytodaymedianetwork.com/2014/07/30/navajo-nation-turns-plant-based-foods-reverse-diabetes-156110

Burhansstipanov, L. (n.d.). *Traditional Indian medicine and Native American cancer patients*. Retrieved January 29, 2015, from http://www.litsite.org/index.cfm?section=Narrative-and-Healing&page=Perspectives&viewpost=2&ContentId=968

Gugliotta, G. (2013, February 1). *When did humans come to the Americas?* Retrieved February 1, 2015, from http://www.smithsonianmag.com/science-nature/when-did-humans-come-to-the-americas-4209273/?no-ist

Indian Health Service. (n.d.). *The federal health program for American Indians and Alaska Natives*. Retrieved February 1, 2015, from http://www.ihs.gov

Johnson, C. (1998, January 1). *The search for rain forest drugs*. Retrieved February 1, 2015, from http://www.uic.edu/classes/osci/osci590/12_2 The Search for Rain Forest Drugs.htm

Library of Congress. (n.d.). National atlas. Indian tribes, culture & languages. Retrieved from http://www.loc.gov/item/95682185/

Minority health: American Indian & Alaska Native populations. (2014, November 20). Retrieved February 1, 2015, from http://www.cdc.gov/minorityhealth/populations/REMP/aian.html

Quinn, A. (2007). Reflections on intergenerational trauma: Healing as a critical intervention. *First Peoples Child & Family Review, 3*(4), 72–82. Retrieved February 1, 2015, from http://journals.sfu.ca/fpcfr/index.php/FPCFR/article/view/62

Sturtevant, W. (1991). *National atlas. Indian tribes, cultures & languages: [United States]*. Reston, VA: Interior, Geological Survey. Retrieved January 31, 2015, from http://www.loc.gov/item/95682185/

Traditional Foods Project. (2014, September 26). Retrieved February 2, 2015, from http://www.cdc.gov/diabetes/projects/ndwp/traditional-foods.htm

U.S. Census Bureau. (n.d.). *2010 American Indians and Alaska Natives in the United States map*. Retrieved January 16, 2015, from http://www2.census.gov/geo/maps/special/AIANWall2010/AIAN_US_2010.pdf

U.S. National Park Service. (n.d.-a). *Indian reservations in the continental United States map index*. Retrieved January 16, 2015, from http://www.nps.gov/nagpra/DOCUMENTS/ResMapIndex.htm

U.S. National Park Service. (n.d.-b). *Indian reservations in the continental United States—Map*. Retrieved January 16, 2015, from http://www.nps.gov/nagpra/DOCUMENTS/RESERV.PDF

Warshauer, M. (n.d.). *Andrew Jackson and the Constitution*. Retrieved February 2, 2015, from http://www.gilderlehrman.org/history-by-era/age-jackson/essays/andrew-jackson-and-constitution

White, M. (n.d.). *Dr. Walt Hollow: A pioneer on the frontlines of Native American medicine*. Retrieved January 28, 2015, from http://www.tribalconnections.org/health_news/features/may2005p1.html

REFERENCES

Bering strait theory. (2011, January 1). Retrieved February 1, 2015, from http://www.historyandtheheadlines.abc-clio.com/ContentPages/ContentPage.aspx?entryId=1171632&currentSection=1161468&productid=5

Bureau of Indian Education. (n.d.). *Schools*. Retrieved February 1, 2015, from http://www.bie.edu/Schools/index.htm

Doucleff, M. (2013, January 23). *How the sweet potato crossed the Pacific way before the Europeans did*. Retrieved February 1, 2015, from http://www.npr.org/blogs/thesalt/2013/01/22/169980441/how-the-sweet-potato-crossed-the-pacific-before-columbus

❖ THREE ❖

Postcontact, Sovereignty, and Health[1]

Margaret P. Moss

The sovereignty that the Indian tribes retain is of a unique and limited character. It exists only at the sufferance of Congress and is subject to complete defeasance.
—(US v. Wheeler, 1978)

LEARNING OBJECTIVES

♦ Describe major changes postcontact.
♦ The student will be able to discuss sovereignty issues for American Indians and Alaska Natives as they relate to their populations' health status.

KEY TERMS

♦ Federal recognition
♦ Sovereignty

KEY CONCEPTS

♦ Contact
♦ Political designee versus racial

As presented in the overview chapter, the majority of health disparities seen in American Indians and Alaska Natives (AI/ANs) in 21st century America are the result of postcontact political histories that continue to be manifested today. The impact is either directly or indirectly from centuries of mistreatment. Federal policies calling for these actions are outlined later in this chapter. Although there have been some policies that support AI/ANs such as the intent of current overall policies of tribal *self-determination*, progress is slow in terms of reversing health outcomes, and obstacles are high.

---

[1] Much of the content in this chapter was first published in the *Hamline Journal of Public Law and Policy* as "American Indian Health Disparities: By the Sufferance of Congress" (Fall 2010).

DEFINING *POSTCONTACT*

Contact refers to the point in history during which a significant influx of Europeans came to what is now North America. Prior to contact, as discussed in the previous chapter, there were tens of millions of indigenous people almost solely populating this continent. Therefore, contact is generally thought to be marked by the arrival of Christopher Columbus in 1492. There have, of course, been various theories of Nordic, Asian, and other groups' earlier arrivals; however, here we are concerned with the arrival and sustained influx of Western Europeans.

SOVEREIGNTY

In the previous chapter, the student learned that upon contact, and for several 100 years, Indian nations were thought of as sovereign nations. Sovereignty refers to a nation having the final ability and authority to govern itself in all matters. At contact, Indian nations were treated as such and treaties between the United States and these nations were drawn up and executed. However, the last treaty between the United States and Indians was signed on March 3, 1871. After this, the United States decided that tribes were no longer sovereign nations. According to the U.S. Code, Title 25 § 71—*Future Treaties with Indian Tribes*:

> No Indian nation or tribe within the territory of the United States shall be acknowledged or recognized as an independent nation, tribe, or power with whom the United States may contract by treaty.

In postcolonial America, federally recognized American Indian tribes are partial or quasisovereign nations with the "power to self-govern" (Indian Civil Rights Act, 1968) and, as such, have certain structures in place such as "heads of state," police, courts, schools, and social services to varying extents (Wilkins & Lowawaima, 2002). These social/political structures often look like those found in the United States' dominant culture (Wilkins & Lowawaima, 2002).

It is important to recognize that individual tribes maintain hierarchies for religion, medicine, and cultural practice and maintenance that may not be apparent to the untrained eye or naïve visitor, including those in the federal government and in health care (Moss, 2000). Understanding this is significant for nurses. A particular tribe or community in Indian country may not have a Western clinic or hospital, so the assumption may be made that there is no health care. However, some tribes have a layered, specialist system of care—including mental health specialists, midwives, bone and muscle specialists, and others—that is unknown by those outside of the tribe. This is another reason nurses outside of the cultural group of interest should become familiar with the health needs and care, both traditional (here, meaning indigenous) and Western or allopathic.

Defeasance (loss of) versus maintaining and strengthening sovereignty is arguably the number one issue in Indian country (Deloria & Lytle, 1998). This partial sovereignty (tribes) within a sovereign nation (United States) is what distinguishes a tribal reality and existence that is unmatched in America's dominant culture or any of its minority or immigrant populations (Deloria & Lytle, 1998).

The political status of AI/ANs within the United States is unseen by most Americans. Indigenous people in the United States are viewed as a racial minority. There is little understanding that they are a political minority. This misunderstanding holds true with those in health care and health research. Rarely are studies presented in major health and research arenas that attend to issues and outcomes of AI/AN populations. It is amazing that even federal agencies, which should be knowledgeable about this political status and its implications, are not accommodating in their service (see Box 3.1).

Box 3.1

An example of how tribal sovereignty and health care research intersect, resulting in further delays and gaps in knowledge, follows:

The National Institutes of Health (NIH) is the largest federal agency that funds health research. There are 27 institutes and centers making up the NIH.

At times, there are "special calls" for proposals on a topic. The topic will be reviewed by experts particular to that special topic, for example, epigenetics. This is also true for the Centers for Disease Control and Prevention and other federal agencies.

The problem is in the turnaround time for proposals. Often, it is only a few short months—perhaps only 12 weeks. When doing health care research with a partially sovereign nation-tribe in this case, the nurse must approach the tribe's institutional review board, and/or the Tribal Council and/or the head of the tribe, and possibly the cultural head if different, and gain permissions above and beyond what normal permissions are sought by researchers in all other communities.

Seeking tribal permissions for research is quite time consuming. This could take up to a year and can rarely be done in the time allotted for these special calls for proposals. These calls often have particular connection to tribes, and yet the phenomenon will never be explored using this mechanism. This results in further gaps in understanding, care, and outcomes.

This political status of being "less than sovereign" (when formerly sovereign) may, in fact, be a significant factor in the health status of today's AI/ANs. American Indians/Alaska Natives, America's most regulated people (25 U.S.C. ch 1–44), intersecting with health care, one of the most complex systems of the United States (Mechanic, Rogut, Colby, & Knickman, 2005), enter a nexus that is a complex merging of federal, state, and tribal laws and programs. Navigating the health care system for anyone in the United States can be daunting, but even more so for its indigenous population, and for a variety of *unique* reasons.

Nurses must gain an understanding of this historical and political backdrop when treating AI/AN patients. History has affected trust levels, understanding of the dominant culture, including health care and, therefore, willingness to follow the dictates of health care professionals, and ultimately health outcomes.

WHO IS THE POSTCOLONIAL INDIAN/TODAY'S PATIENT?

Today, there are approximately 320,660,412 people in the United States (U.S. Census Bureau, 2015a). Of the over 320 million people, the U.S. Census Bureau 2015 projections available now for AI/AN populations show 4 to 6 million, depending on whether the individual is reporting one or more races (U.S. Census Bureau, 2015b). These numbers would indicate that 1.36% to 1.9% of the U.S. population is AI/AN.

This is another area where the political determination of AI/AN in the United States is of importance. There are several categories of AI/AN populations. There are federally recognized tribes, federally unrecognized tribes, state-recognized tribes, and individuals belonging to no tribe but with lineage that can either be proved or may just be suspected, but is claimed (Wilkins & Lowawaima, 2002). The importance for nurses lies in who is due services provided by various governmental agencies. Only federally recognized tribal members are able to access federally provided services. These services will be outlined in subsequent chapters. States may provide state-recognized tribes with certain programs or services. Disenfranchised, ethnic Indians, that is, racially AI/ANs who are not enrolled in a tribe, may have access to minority programs or nonprofit and grant programs targeting AI/ANs regardless of tribal enrollment.

The Census numbers are based on self-report (Ogunwole & U.S. Census Bureau, 2006; U.S. Census Bureau, 2011). Self-reporting of AI/AN heritage has been variously argued as being underreported or overreported (Harris, 1994). It is seen as underreported when either tribes or individuals feel that the United States has no automatic right to count their exact numbers (Harris, 1994; Passel, 1976). Census numbers are overreported when persons fall into the last of the aforementioned categories and are either mistaken or unable to demonstrate lineage (Harris, 1994). Further, the Census is describing racial heritage, and not political status (U.S. Census Bureau, 2011).

Neither the Constitution nor its draftsmen foresaw or provided for the continuing existence of Indian tribes. (Fixico, 1986, p. 604) It is important to note that Congress alone determines a tribe's status within the federal system and can recognize or terminate any tribe's status, and has done so over the decades (Fixico, 1986); from the U. S. Code—Termination of Federal Trust:

> Publication; termination of Federal services; application of Federal and State laws upon removal of Federal restrictions on the property of each tribe and individual members thereof, the Secretary shall publish in the Federal Register a proclamation declaring that the Federal trust relationship to the affairs of the tribe and its members has terminated. Thereafter individual members of the tribe shall not be entitled to any of the services performed by the United States for Indians because of their status as Indians, all statutes of the

United States which affect Indians because of their status as Indians, excluding statutes that specifically refer to the tribe and its members, shall no longer be applicable to the members of the tribe, and the laws of the several States shall apply to the tribe and its members in the same manner as they apply to other citizens or persons within their jurisdiction. (Termination of Federal Trust, Title 25, Chapter 14, Subchapter XXX, § 703)

The implication here for nurses to understand is that the federal trust responsibility was formed as a result of case law in the early 1800s, as an obligation to those tribes that had given over land and resources via treaty and/or law in exchange for services in perpetuity. Among those are health services. When Congress decides that a tribe is no longer recognized as such by the government, then services are no longer offered.

To become an enrolled member of a federally recognized tribe, the tribes themselves accept applications for enrollment based on tribal rules, and usually a vote by the tribal council (*Delaware Indians v. Cherokee Nation*, 1904; Harmon, 2001). Many tribes require one fourth American Indian "blood quantum" to be eligible for membership of the tribe (Harmon, 2001). Still others require that the lineage be in their own tribe alone and not a total of mixed tribes (Harmon, 2001). One must apply for membership, which is not automatic by virtue of birth (Harmon, 2001). Enrolled citizens receive the benefit of a tribal nation with a political relationship with the United States. Enrolled members of federally recognized tribes are then dual citizens within the borders of their nation of origin. This again is a feature unique to American Indians in the United States (Deloria & Lytle, 1998).

Federal Recognition

Tribes that are recognized by the U.S. Congress are the only tribes with a U.S. government-to-government relationship (*Cherokee Nation v. The State of Georgia*, 1831; *Worcester v. Georgia*, 1832). There are 566 distinct federally recognized tribes in the United States (Bureau of Indian Affairs, 2015). Because of a series of decisions recognized as the Marshall Trilogy, it was established that the U.S. government and not the states had a relationship with tribes—a federal trust responsibility was established between the U.S. government and the tribes, and Congress would control which entities were tribes (*Cherokee Nation v. The State of Georgia*, 1831, p. 17). Further, only the U.S. government could make treaties with the tribes, and these treaties were to be held as the "supreme law of the land" (*Cherokee Nation v. The State of Georgia*, 1831, p. 5; *Worcester v. Georgia*, 1832, p. 595, para. 2). Again, no other group in the United States is thus distinguished.

Marshall wrote, "the relation of the Indians to the United States is marked by peculiar and cardinal distinctions which exist nowhere else" (*Cherokee*

Nation v. The State of Georgia, p. 16, para. 5). Today, Title 25 of the U.S. Code is entitled "Indians" (Indians, 1969). No other subgroup of the U.S. population is so contradistinguished, the differentiating factor being that "Indian" in the United States is a political determination and not simply a racial category (Wilkins & Lomawaima, 2002, p. 250).

The federal policies that have rolled out over the last 200 years have moved back and forth between seemingly "pro-Indian" policies and those that tried to get rid of "the Indian problem" (Hays, 2007). The intersection of federal policies with state and tribal laws further complicates any interactions, including those around health (Jones, 2006). And finally, these issues all combine to produce some of the most staggering numbers in describing the American Indians' health and socioeconomic statuses among the tribes.

It is imperative that there is an understanding of the history of American Indian experience, especially through the lens of the major series of federal policies on American Indians that have greatly affected their circumstances since the 1700s (Miller, 2006, p. xviii).

Using Miller's time frames, federal policy periods in American Indian matters affected the Removal Era (1825–1850); the Reservation Era (1850–1887) (Trennert, 1975); the Allotment and Assimilation Era (1887–1934; Adams, 1995; Trennert, 1988); the Indian Reorganization Era (1934–1940s); the Termination Era (1940s–1961; Fixico, 1986; Wilkinson & Biggs, 1977), and, finally, the Self-Determination Era (1961–present; Castile, 1998). American Indian elders, especially, have been affected by many of these policies either personally or indirectly through their parents' and grandparents' experiences. American Indian elderly over age 85 may not have been born as U.S. citizens, as American Indians were not widely granted citizenship in their country of origin until 1924 through the passage of the Snyder Act (Indian Citizenship Act, 1924).

Many of the federal policy eras relating to American Indians are widely known, some less so. All have had an effect on the health and well-being of today's American Indian. The Removal Era policies sought to move tribes to the west of the Mississippi River (Cave, 2003, p. 1337; Indian Removal Act, 1830). The Reservation period further outlined which areas the tribes could occupy (Bougler, 1972; O'Neill, 2002; Wilkins & Lomawaima, 2002). The Allotment and Assimilation Era allowed individual American Indians to hold land, but the net result was less land held overall (Berthrong, 1979; Shoemaker, 2003). It was hoped they would become like suburban homeowners and blend in (Berthrong, 1979, p. 335; Wilkins & Lomawaima, 2002, p. 106). It was during this time and beyond that the Indian boarding schools were used to assimilate young children (Trennert, 1988, p. 5). The Indian Reorganization Act professed to protect Indian lands, and rather than seeking to assimilate American Indians, recognized that they should be an important population in the United States (Deloria, 2002). During the Termination Era, 100 tribes lost recognition by Congress, negating any further trust responsibility (Fixico, 1986). The current era of self-determination was shepherded in the early 1970s, with the termination called a failure (Fixico, 1986; Indian Self-Determination and Education Assistance Act, 1975; Wilkins & Lomawaima, 2002).

All of these political and historical factors have been affecting American Indians for centuries. Now, one's tribal enrollment; tribe's status, whether federally recognized or not, boarding school experiences; relocation program involvement; loss of language, religion, traditional medicine, culture, or family connection; repatriation experiences; and intercultural adoption/foster care have to some extent entered the experience of today's American Indians. These were all experiences unique to the U.S. indigenous population, and, more important have direct health implications for American Indians.

INHERENT SOVEREIGNTY

Inherent sovereignty refers to the sovereignty initially enjoyed by tribes prior to European contact (Wilkins & Lomawaima, 2002). Prior to contact, the indigenous citizens of the continent governed themselves as independent nations without any external designation to do so or not. The description as to what a tribe is and, by extension, who an American Indian is in this discussion has largely been as seen through the eyes of the Congress (Resnik, 1989). The Doctrine of Discovery (*Johnson v. M'Intosh*, 1823), which described "conquerors" taking the land of indigenous people under some legal theory, set the stage for a shift from American Indians self-describing their status and the United States allowing a certain status (Wilkins & Lomawaima, 2002). Many American Indians today adhere to the idea of precolonial or inherent sovereignty (Wilkins & Lomawaima, 2002, p. 252). This tension of several hundred years must certainly play into the 500 years of persistent health disparity between America and its indigenous citizens (Jones, 2006).

HEALTH DISPARITIES

American Indians continue to face egregious disparities in health, even as the end of the second decade of the 21st century comes to a close. One does not have to leave the borders of the United States to find people tied with the lowest life expectancy in the Western Hemisphere in the Oglala Lakota on the Pine Ridge Reservation in South Dakota (Kunesh, 2007), where tuberculosis deaths nationally for American Indians are 750% greater than for U.S. all races (U.S. Department of Health & Human Services, 2002–2003), where diabetes rates are the highest in the world as on the Pima Reservation (Johnson, Nowatzki & Coons, 1996; Ravussin, Valencia, Esparza, Bennett, & Schulz, 1994), or where sexual violence against American Indian women is among the highest in the country (Hart & Lowther, 2008). These problems run the gamut from life expectancy and chronic disease to public health issues.

LIFE EXPECTANCY

Life expectancy in the United States for all people has increased dramatically since the early 1900s with the introduction of antibiotics; decreases in infant death rates; and increased nutrition awareness, availability, and programming (Shi, Tsai, & Kao, 2009). Life expectancy increased from an average of 49 years nationally in 1900 to an average of 77.9 in 2007 (Centers for Disease Control, 2011). However, although great strides were made to combat infectious diseases, by the end of the 1900s, chronic diseases and their tendency toward comorbidities and related functional declines have led to new challenges (Omran, 1971; Shi et al., 2009). Omran (1971) proposed the theory of epidemiologic transition to explain this phenomenon in the 1970s. Racial and ethnic minority populations seem to have been hardest hit. Health disparities cripple these groups regardless of a variety of factors such as insurance status, severity of problem, age, and income (Smedley et al., 2003).

American Indians are among the individuals most affected. Death rates, as compared with all U.S. races, from the Indian Health Service's (IHS) report, "Trends in Indian Health 2002–2003," can be seen in Table 3.1 (U.S. Department of Health & Human Services, 2002–2003, p. 4).

In the infectious diseases category, pneumonia and influenza are 47% greater than for the U.S. all-races death rates (U.S. Department of Health & Human Services, 2002–2003).

What is important to note is that these are averages. Diabetes can be as high as 10 times the national average. Suicide, as a public health problem, is the highest among American Indians than of any other ethnic group (Olson & Wahab, 2006), and the resultant life expectancy for American Indians has actually declined in some areas. The Pine Ridge Reservation in South Dakota has reported that males born today have a life expectancy of less than 50 years, the lowest in America (Link Center Foundation, 2011; U.S. Department of Agriculture, Rural Development, 2011). This astounding number returns us to the year 1900, or to Haiti, where numbers are similar (Pickering, 2004). In the IHS's "Trends in Indian Health" report for 2002–2004, American Indian life

TABLE 3.1 American Indian and Alaska Native Death Rates as Compared With All U.S. Races

CHRONIC DISEASES (% GREATER THAN ALL U.S. RACES)	PUBLIC HEALTH PROBLEMS (% GREATER THAN ALL U.S. RACES)
Tuberculosis—750	Motor vehicle crashes—234.6
Alcoholism—524	Unintentional injuries—153
Diabetes mellitus—193	Homicide—103.3
	Suicide—66
	Firearm injury—28

expectancy was about 5 years less than for U.S. all races, at 72.5 years. However, when drilling down to reservations and to those affected most by chronic and public health difficulties, the numbers are eye-opening.

THE DISAPPEARING AMERICAN INDIAN ELDERLY

Probably nowhere is the gap between Indian and Western views of medicine greater than in the minds of Indian elders.

—National Indian Council on Aging (p. 8)

In the 21st century, AI elderly have arguably the poorest health outcomes—shortest life spans, most chronic diseases (which come earlier and with more severity) and functional decline—compared with all other elderly groups in the United States (Moss, Schell, & Goins, 2006). By percentage of population, (a) there are more AI youth as compared with Whites and "all races" in the United States in their respective categories until; (b) age 30, where there are more in the White and "all races" categories; (c) a significant reverse trend by age 45; (d) double the number of 70-year-olds in the White versus American Indian category; and (e) in the 85+ group, three times as many elderly in the White and "all races" group versus the American Indian population (U.S. Department of Health & Human Services, n.d.). As a country, we appear to tolerate the "disappearing American Indian elder." Many American Indian elderly remain on their reservations or return to their reservations in later life. Unfortunately, there are few services on the reservations in the realm of eldercare.

As of 20 years ago, there were only 10 nursing homes on the 300+ reservations in the United States, and today, they continue to be scarce (Jervis, Jackson & Manson, 2002; Manson, 1989). There are few home health care, adult day care, respite care, or assisted living facilities for American Indians on reservations (Jervis et al., 2002), and, for a variety of reasons, American Indian elderly do not seek care off the reservation. These reasons include perceived racism, loss of ability to continue with cultural and religious practices, as well as loss of familiarity and independence as with any older person (Moss, 2005). American Indians will seek care from the IHS (Langwell, Anagnopoulos, Ryan, Melson, & Iron Rope, 2009), but the IHS does not offer much long-term care (Jervis et al., 2002).

CONCLUSIONS

The U.S. Congress has had a long and storied history of interaction with American Indian tribes (Deloria, 1992; Fixico, 1986; Hays, 2007). The tribes and the individuals making up the tribes have suffered crippling health outcomes, which have persisted throughout the relationship (Jones, 2006). Congress has chosen what group is to be recognized as a tribe and, therefore, who is an "Indian," that is, one who is an enrollee of one of the federally recognized tribes (Termination of Federal Trust, 2011). It is unclear to what extent these policies have had an impact on the individuals who count themselves as American Indians. But for the Termination Era, when tribes lost the government-to-government relationship and are now no longer tribes and their people are no longer (legally) American Indians (Fixico, 1986; Wilkinson & Biggs, 1977); or the assimilation period, where eligible people may have not enrolled their children, or their children were taken away and suffered greatly (Trennert, 1988); or the relocation (Fixico, 1986); or reservation periods (Bougler, 1972, p. 410; Chapman, 1936, p. 366; Trennert, 1975), where isolation and desolation were hallmarks, what would the health of Indians look like today?

These are experiences based on political status, which is a unique distinction for this population as against all other designated U.S. *minority* populations (Wilkins & Lomawaima, 2002, p. 250). Furthermore, these types of experiences have been ongoing for the last 500 years, another distinction as compared with any other racial/ethnic group, first in pre-colonized America and then in the United States (Jones, 2006).

There are new provisions for Indian health, such as long-term care, that have never been provided other than through small, short-term grants (Jervis et al., 2002; Manson, 1989). However, the funding for the programming has not yet been authorized (Indian Health Long Term Health Care, 2010).

STUDY QUESTIONS

♦ What is meant by *inherent sovereignty*?
♦ Explain how federal policies over the past 200 years could have an effect on AI/AN patients today?
♦ Have you as nurses ever learned this history, and why do you think it would be important to understand?

USEFUL WEBSITES

♦ *Indian Country Today*, News. Health Section, http://indiancountrytodaymedianetwork .com/department/health-wellness
♦ National Indian Health Board on the Indian Health Care Improvement Act, http:// www.nihb.org/legislative/ihcia.php
♦ Indians, U.S. Code Title 25—Indians, https://www.law.cornell.edu/uscode/text/25

REFERENCES

Adams, D. W. (1995). *Education for extinction: American Indians and the boarding school experience*. Lawrence, KS: University Press of Kansas.

Berthrong, D. J. (1979). Legacies of the Dawes Act: Bureaucrats and land thieves at the Cheyenne–Arapaho Agencies of Oklahoma. *Arizona and the West, 21*, 335–354.

Bougler, J. V. (1972). Indians—Reservations—Effect of later congressional acts on act establishing reservation boundaries. *North Dakota Law Review, 49*, 410, 413.

Bureau of Indian Affairs. (2015). *Who we are*. Retrieved November 28, 2010, from http:// www.bia.gov/WhoWeAre/BIA/

Castile, G. P. (1998). *To show heart: Native American self-determination and federal Indian policy, 1960–1975*. Tucson, AZ: University of Arizona Press.

Cave, A. A. (2003). Abuse of power: Andrew Jackson and the Indian Removal Act of 1830. *Historian, 65*(6), 1330.

Centers for Disease Control and Prevention. (2011). *FastStats—Life expectancy.* Retrieved November 26, 2011, from http://www.cdc.gov/nchs/fastats/life-expectancy.htm

Chapman, B. B. (1936). Dissolution of the Iowa reservation. *Chronicles of Oklahoma, 14,* 467–477.

Cherokee Nation v. The State of Georgia, 30 U.S. 1 (1831).

Delaware Indians v. Cherokee Nation, 193 U.S. 127 (1904).

Deloria, V. (1992). *American Indian policy in the twentieth century.* Norman, OK: University of Oklahoma Press.

Deloria, V. (2002). *The Indian Reorganization Act: Congresses and bills.* Norman, OK: University of Oklahoma Press

Deloria, V., & Lytle, C. M. (1998). *The nations within: The past and future of American Indian sovereignty.* New York, NY: Pantheon Books.

Fixico, D. L. (1986). *Termination and relocation: Federal Indian policy, 1945–1960.* Albuquerque, NM: University of New Mexico Press.

Forquera, R. (2001). *Urban Indian health.* Washington, DC: U.S. Department of Health and Human Services.

Future Treaties With Indian Tribes, 25 U.S.C. ch 3, subch 1@ § 71. (1988).

Harmon, A. (2001). Tribal enrollment councils: Lessons on law and Indian identity. *The Western Historical Quarterly, 32,* 175–200.

Harris, D. (1994). The 1990 census count of American Indians: What do the numbers really mean? *Social Science Quarterly, 75,* 580–593.

Hart, R. A., & Lowther, M. A. (2008). Honoring sovereignty: Aiding tribal efforts to protect Native American women from domestic violence. *California Law Review, 96,* 185–233.

Hays, R. G. (2007). *Editorializing "the Indian problem": The New York Times on Native Americans, 1860–1900.* Carbondale, IL: Southern Illinois University Press.

Indian Citizenship Act, 43 Stat. 253 (codified at 8 USC § 1401(b) (2006)) (1924).

Indian Civil Rights Act, 25 U.S.C. ch 15, subch 1 @ §§ 1301–1303 (1968).

Indian Removal Act, 4 Stat. 411 (1830).

Indians, 25 U.S.C. § 1 (1969).

Indian Self-Determination and Education Assistance Act, Pub.L. No. 93-638, 88 Stat. 2203 (1975).

Jervis, L. L., Jackson, M. Y., & Manson, S. M. (2002). Need for, availability of, and barriers to the provision of long-term care services for older American Indians. *Journal of Cross-Cultural Gerontology, 17,* 295–311.

Johnson v. M'Intosh, 21 U.S. 543, 573 (1823).

Johnson, J. A., Nowatzki, T. E., & Coons, S. J. (1996). Health-related quality of life of diabetic Pima Indians. *Medical Care, 34,* 97–102.

Jones, D. S. (2006). The persistence of American Indian health disparities. *American Journal Public Health, 96,* 2122.

Kunesh, P. H. (2007). Call for an assessment of the welfare on Indian children in South Dakota. *South Dakota Law Review, 52,* 247.

Langwell, K., Anagnopoulos, C., Ryan, F., Melson, J., & Iron Rope, S. (2009). Financing American Indian health care: Impacts and options for improving access and quality. *Find Brief, 12,* 1–4.

Link Center Foundation. (2011). *Life and conditions on the Pine Ridge Oglala Lakota (Sioux) reservation of South Dakota.* Retrieved March 25, 2011, from http://mendotadakota.com/mn/life-and-conditions-on-the-pine-ridge-ogala-lakota/

Manson, S. M. (1989). Long-term care in American Indian communities: Issues for planning and research. *Gerontologist, 29*, 38–44.

Mechanic, D., Rogut, L., Colby, D., & Knickman, J. (Eds.). (2005). *Policy challenges in modern health care.* New Brunswick, NJ: Rutgers University Press.

Miller, R. J. (2006). *Native America, discovered and conquered: Thomas Jefferson, Lewis & Clark, and manifest destiny.* Westport, CT: Praeger.

Moss, M. P. (2000). *Zuni elders: Ethnography of American Indian aging* (unpublished doctoral dissertations). University of Texas, HSC, Texas Medical Center, Houston.

Moss, M. P. (2005). Tolerated illness concept and theory for chronically ill and elderly patients as exemplified in American Indians. *Journal of Cancer Education 20*, 17–22.

Moss, M. P., Schell, M. C., & Goins, R. T. (2006). Using GIS in a first national mapping of functional disability among older American Indians and Alaska Natives from the 2000 census. *International Journal of Health Geographics, 5*, 37.

National Indian Council on Aging. (1996). *THE NICOA report: Health and long-term care for Indian elders.* Washington DC: Author. Retrieved from http://moon.ouhsc.edu/rjohn/longterm.pdf

Ogunwole, S. U., & U.S. Census Bureau. (2006). *We the people: American Indians and Alaska Natives in the United States.* Washington, DC: U.S. Department of Commerce, Economics, and Statistics Administration, U.S. Census Bureau.

Olson, L. M., & Wahab, S. (2006). American Indians and suicide: A neglected area of research. *Trauma, Violence, & Abuse, 7*(1), 19–33.

Omran, A. R. (1971). The epidemiologic transition: A theory of the epidemiology of population change. *Milbank Memorial Fund Quarterly, 49*, 509–538.

O'Neill, T. (2002). *The Indian reservation system.* San Diego, CA: Greenhaven Press

Passel, J. S. (1976). Provisional evaluation of the 1970 census count of American Indians. *Demography, 13*, 397–409.

Pickering, K. (2004). Culture and reservation economies. In T. Biolsi (Ed.), *A companion to the anthropology of American Indians.* Oxford, UK: Blackwell. doi:10.1002/9780470996270.ch7

Ravussin, E., Valencia, M. E., Esparza, J., Bennett, P. H., & Schulz, L. O. (1994). Effects of a traditional lifestyle on obesity in Pima Indians. *Diabetes Care, 17*, 1067–1074.

Resnik, J. (1989). Dependent sovereigns: Indian tribes, states, and the federal courts. *University of Chicago Law Review, 56*, 671–759.

Shi, L., Tsai, J., & Kao, S. (2009). Public health, social determinants of health, and public policy. *Journal of Medical Sciences, 29*, 43–59.

Shoemaker, J. A. (2003). Like snow in the spring time: Allotment, fractionation, and the Indian land tenure problem. *Wisconsin Law Review, 2003*, 729–788.

Smedley, B. D., Stith, A. Y., Nelson, A. R., Committee on Understanding and Eliminating Racial and Ethnic Disparities in Health Care, Board on Health Sciences Policy, & Institute of Medicine. (2003). *Unequal treatment: Confronting racial and ethnic disparities in health care.* Washington, DC: National Academies Press.

Termination of Federal Trust, 25 U.S.C. ch 14, subch XXX @ § 703 (2011).

Trennert, R. A., Jr. (1975). *Alternative to extinction: Federal Indian policy and the beginnings of the reservation system, 1846–51.* Philadelphia, PA: Temple University Press.

Trennert, R. A., Jr. (1988). *The Phoenix Indian School: Forced assimilation in Arizona, 1891–1935.* Norman, OK: University of Oklahoma Press

U.S. Census Bureau. (2011). *United States—Race and ethnicity—American FactFinder.* Retrieved February 7, 2011, from http://factfinder.census.gov/faces/nav/jsf/pages/community_facts.xhtml

U.S. Census Bureau. (2015a). *Population clocks*. Retrieved April 3, 2015, from http://www.census.gov/

U.S. Census Bureau. (2015b). *Population projections—2009 National population projections: Summary tables*. Retrieved from http://www.census.gov/population/projections/data/national/2009.html

U.S. Department of Agriculture, Rural Development. (n.d.). *Oglala Souix tribe empowerment zone*. Retrieved March 20, 2011, from http://www.rurdev.usda.gov/rbs/ezec/Communit/oglala.html

U.S. Department of Health & Human Services. (n.d.). Code of federal regulations (CFR), at Title 42-Public Health, § 136.12.

U.S. Department of Health & Human Services. (2002–2003). *Trends in Indian health (2002–2003)*. Retrieved from http://www.ihs.gov/dps/includes/themes/newihstheme/display_objects/documents/Trends%20Part%204-General%20Mort.pdf

Wilkins, D. E., & Lomawaima, K. T. (2002). *Uneven ground: American Indian sovereignty and federal law*. Norman, OK: University of Oklahoma Press.

Wilkinson, C. F., & Biggs, E. R. (1977). The evolution of the termination policy. *American Indian Law Review, 5*, 139.

Worcester v. Georgia, 31 U.S. 515, 6 Pet. 515, 8 L.Ed. 483 (1832).

FOUR

The Roots of American Indian "Nursing"

Margaret P. Moss

LEARNING OBJECTIVES

♦ Identify differences between honoring old and new knowledge as it relates to nursing practice.
♦ Distinguish between ideas rooted in indigenous nursing and Western ideas of nursing.
♦ Adapt the metaparadigm of nursing and American Indian thought.
♦ Revisit key ideas, such as the circle, four directions, and medicine wheel, in integrating care of today's American Indians.

KEY TERMS

♦ Corn/cornmeal blessings
♦ Herbalism
♦ Holism
♦ Midwives

♦ Prayer stick
♦ Smudging
♦ Sweat lodge

KEY CONCEPTS

♦ As in other cultures, indigenous people were "nursing" before the word or profession existed.
♦ Storytelling was and is important in conveying cultural and even health information.

♦ "Old ways" are carried on today: In health care, the "old ways" may be termed *traditional medicine* or *healing*.
♦ Traditional nursing/health care may be "hidden" from the allopathic provider or casual observer.

This chapter introduces the reader to the roots of "nursing" in American Indian life. Many practices and beliefs that have developed over millennia are used even today, so it is important to understand that they have been around longer than the profession of nursing itself. Throughout this book, as the learner is introduced to indigenous cultural groups across different regions of the United States, new ideas related to health and nursing will emerge that are both overlapping and unique from tribe to tribe. This brief introduction to some terms will be useful throughout the text. Authors may repeat these ideas in their own areas.

The indigenous peoples of North America were given the name "Indians" by European explorers searching for new trade routes to India who mistakenly thought that they had found Asian Indians (Flanders, 1998). Today, in the United States, there are 566 federally recognized tribes that are distinct nations (Bureau of Indian Affairs, 2015). The title *Indian* has been used historically in the United States to refer, in general, to all indigenous peoples of the nation. Although America's indigenous people, American Indians and Alaska Natives (AI/ANs), preceded Europeans by 15,000 years, North American Indians were prohibited by federal law from obtaining citizenship on this soil until 1924 (Deloria & Lytle, 1984).

Many AI/AN tribes have within their "origin stories" the details of how they came to live in the place now known as the United States of America (Bunzel, 1932; Dorsey, 1904). They have within their cultural traditions a strong connection to their ancestors. Important for nursing, ancestors may be viewed as part of the extended family or community.

Box 4.1

Important for nursing, ancestors may be viewed as part of the extended family or community.

The four directions and the four seasons, as discussed in Chapter 1, hold great meaning for AI/ANs. Wintertime for tribes, both in the North and in the South, has traditionally been a time spent telling stories about tribal ancestors. These ancestral stories were told for many reasons, but most important, they were used for the transfer of cultural wisdom. The stories rarely changed over time, and were told only at certain times by selected people. Prayers, dance, or movement accompanied the stories. The dances and appropriate times of storytelling have rarely changed over many hundreds of years. One author writes that this unchanging type of memorized ritual or "formulaicness is valued when wisdom is seen as knowledge passed down through generations" (Tannen, 1982, p. 6). Indians have traditionally valued ancient, accepted wisdom, using storytelling and dance to transmit that wisdom, whereas contemporary societies value novelty and believe new information is the manifestation of wisdom. This is one area of variance that the nurse caring for an indigenous person should understand. The nurse would like to utilize best new practices and try new methods, concepts and procedures, whereas the AI/AN may be wary of "new" care ideas. The approach must then be inclusive of the patient's need, understanding, and input. The nurse's care goal may vary from the patient's goal.

American Indian elders have traditionally been charged with passing on "old" knowledge. The roots of the elders' knowledge, both male and female, emerged as a result of their intimate and historic awareness of their environment, and their understanding of the interaction and connection among the land, plants, and animals indigenous to a particular location. Listeners who were children were the main targets of the elders' teaching through storytelling. The elders' lessons included how to act in the tribe, what to do in certain life situations, how to relate to others, what proper language to use, what words to speak at a certain time, and the ways to build moral character. In some tribes, the lessons became part of a cultural tradition that did not change despite societal changes that occurred as a result of outside influences, such as European contact. It is through these stories, and the use of the spoken word, that one is able to understand the historical roles of people in tribal societies. It is within this traditional history that one finds the story of nurses, and how AI/ANs nursed their sick.

The word "nurse" did not exist in 19th-century American Indian language or healing tradition. However, it is known that in many tribes, there was a well-formed hierarchy of both men and women guided by tribal rules who were charged with taking care of others. American Indian women nursed their families and those in the wider community through a sense of duty and a "life of service" (Nerburn, 2010, p. 26).

One example of a life of service can be found among the Dakota people of Minnesota. The role of a daughter in a Dakota family was to "visit the unfortunate and the helpless, carry them food, comb their hair, and mend their garments" (Nerburn, 2010, p. 27). Parents were proud to offer their daughters' services to the community. The eldest daughter was called "Wenonah," meaning "bread giver" or "charitable one" (Nerburn, 2010, p. 27). Young women who nursed others were not necessarily related to those whom they helped.

In other tribes, in what is now known as the state of New Mexico, one's "nurse" was chosen according to kinship lines. The ill were often related specifically to their caregivers. Events, such as birth and clan placement, designated nursing responsibilities. For example, at the birth of her niece or nephew, a paternal aunt was given a specific ceremonial role by the parents of the child. Her role was to nurse the mother and child during the birth, and subsequently care for the child during his or her illnesses (Parezo, 1992; Eggan, 1950). This relationship, specified by but moving beyond mere kinship, cultivated a special connection between that child and the aunt forever. Of importance to nursing, state next-of-kin rules usually designate parents, siblings, and grandparents, moving out from parents. Usually, only if the previous group is incapacitated or unavailable does it move down the line. Aunts and uncles would be down the line. Culturally, aunts and uncles may be the first-line medical decision makers, depending on tribe and region. When caring for the AI/AN patient, it would be important to ask who should be in on care decisions and care conferences.

PURIFICATION AND PRAYER IN AMERICAN INDIAN HEALTH BELIEF

In the eighteenth century, Abigail Adams—wife of President John Adams— wrote to her husband about a woman who had washed her whole house with hot vinegar following her son's illness (McCullough, 2004). Since at least the

18th century, cleanliness has been associated with health. And since the 1800s, nursing care has included the maintenance of cleanliness of the body and the environment of the ill (Nightingale, 1912).

American Indians also made the connection between health and cleanliness. Daily washing of the body, especially of the feet, was thought to be purifying of both mind and body (Nerburn, 2010). The holy man of the tribe blessed people's homes, purifying them, before the new occupants entered for the first time. Purification through fasting and abstentions was also part of tribal life. Fasts were used to clear both the mind and the body, as well as increase the ability of a person to be open to "ingestion" of the spiritual. Abstentions varied from tribe to tribe and included the prohibition of meat, fats, alcohol, and sexual activity at certain times, and for varied lengths of time. For example, when the Zuni men perform a sacred offering to the ancestors known as "planting a prayer stick," they must abstain from sexual activity and foods, such as meat, fat, and alcohol, for 4 days (Bunzel, 1932; Moss, 2000). A prayer stick is made to represent the human being: The stick is the body, usually made of cottonwood and about 7 inches long, the feathers represent the clothes, a cotton cord is the belt, and the stick is directed toward certain gods in part as offerings (Bunzel, 1932). Prayer sticks are used in ceremonies during the year.

Nineteenth-century American Indian healers knew how to treat infectious diseases. For example, an old Indian woman living in Montana told stories of being cured of smallpox, known as the "bad-sickness," by a medicine man. However, this was unusual as many tribes found that the power of imbalance from the smallpox was greater than the power of the medicine man to recreate balance in the sick (Linderman, 1932). The concept of imbalance among the American Indian can best be defined as falling off or straying from one's path in life predetermined by the ancestors or god(s) (Moss, 2000). Staying on one's path is one way American Indians believe their health is optimized.

Although many cultural and geographic differences existed among 19th-century American Indian tribes, similar themes about health and illness existed. These themes included ideas of medicine/healing/helping, religion, magic, and duty, as demonstrated in the American Indians' belief that spirituality should be incorporated in the cleansing of their bodies, homes, and spirits. Additional themes included the belief that witchcraft, soul loss, taboo actions, bad deeds, and thoughts could take one off one's path and into imbalance or illness (Clarke, 1991; Moss, 2000). The Swinomish tribe of Washington, in particular, records the belief that "bad feelings, social conflict and unresolved tensions" (Clarke, 1991, p. 138) could make a person ill.

Ohiyesa, a Dakota man born in the mid-19th century, taught that, according to traditional American Indian teaching, everything that one did was a prayer. Ohiyesa, who later became Charles Alexander Eastman, earned an undergraduate degree at Dartmouth and a medical degree at Boston College. He wrote *Soul of an Indian* (Nerburn, 2010) based on his own life experiences and the teachings his elders passed to him. He demonstrated an Indian's perspective of the importance of a clean and healthy environment when he wrote that: "pestilence followed upon crowded and unsanitary dwellings resulted in a loss of spiritual power from too close contact with one's fellow men" (Nerburn, 2010, p. 11). He was speaking of White communities in crowded cities, not of American Indians of the time (Figure 4.1).

MAKING MEDICINE

Health and balance within Indian tribes was maintained by a variety of groups, such as priest societies, lay midwives, bone pressers, healers, and nurses. Magical medicine was performed usually by men in medical or priest societies within the tribe to counteract illness that was brought on by evil, bad thoughts such as jealousy, or witchcraft. Some tribes, such as the Nez Perce in the Plateau area, had medicine women believed to have magical powers to counteract illness (Axtell, 1997).

In other tribes, women held the role of "nurse." They did not possess the magical powers of medicine per se, but possessed great knowledge related to therapeutics, such as massage, sweating, bloodletting, and botanicals (Bunzel, 1932). The nurses often worked side by side with medicine men. They provided herbal remedies and caring for the ill, while the medicine man purified the affected person by removing evil from them (Moss, 2000). The nurses' role did not include engaging with the evil thought to be the cause of an illness. After the medicine man's work was complete, the nurse continued her work of caring for the ill.

The nurses' work included the "making of medicine." Plants were harvested, and the AI/AN nurses made specific remedies, such as teas and salves. But to the AI/ANs and their nurses, "making medicine" meant more than just

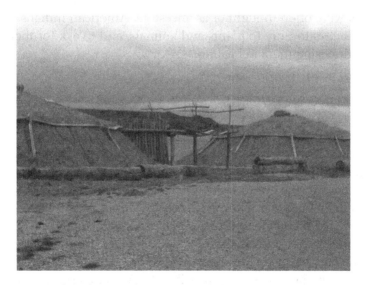

FIGURE 4.1 Earth lodges on the Mandan, Hidatsa, and Arikara Nation (Plains).
Photo: Moss (2012).

preparing oral remedies. The purpose of medicine was to nourish the spiritual and emotional balance within the ill person. This was achieved not only through remedy gathering and making, but also through group singing, offering blessings and prayers to the ancestors, and grinding corn.

Four plants hold particular significance in ceremonies: tobacco, sweet grass, sage, and cedar. One or more are used in the ritual of smudging. Smudging is a purification prayer using the smoke of these plants washed around the head and body using one's arms to move the smoke. The plants are often burned within a turtle shell to hold the medicine. Today, some hospitals and other facilities may have policies that allow the smudging ceremony for patients.

In the southwestern United States, cornmeal blessings were commonly used to maintain physical, mental, spiritual, or emotional health. A family matriarch typically made prayer cornmeal, which at times, had turquoise and coral added to it. This cornmeal was used throughout the year in blessings for her family members (Bunzel, 1932; Moss, 2000). Cornmeal blessings were typically offered daily. Elders advised younger people to go outside in the early morning when the spirits were out, offer their cornmeal, and "get a fresh wind into themselves" (Moss, 2000, p. 91). This daily ritual was believed to be the first step toward maintaining balance. Cornmeal also played an important part in the tribal nurses' preparation of the dead for their journey to the spirit world, as is described in this story told by one Indian of the time: "The young woman died. Her mothers and her brothers cried. They dressed her. They bathed her. Her aunt washed her hair. Her aunt dried her all over with prayer meal" (Bunzel, 1935, p. 412).

American Indian herb use has been well documented in the literature (Moerman, 2003). Some of the knowledge of healing plants, such as corn, was transmitted along the tribe's matrilineal lines. Many indigenous peoples' beliefs included the view that plants and animals were their brothers and sisters. Animals were often thought of as ancestors. American Indians believed that it was respectful to pray to plants and animals, and to ask for their wisdom and help before using them in healing.

WOMEN'S HEALING NETWORKS

In AI/AN cultures, indigenous women were integral to the healing network of the tribe. It was the women who carried out the therapeutic nursing measures needed in the tribes. In daily matters, the grandmother or matriarch in many tribes was the one to see to it that health in the household was maintained through daily blessings and offerings to the ancestors. It was the grandmother who provided medicine to the sick. She used medicines that she came to know about through her own lineage, or had obtained from another person in the tribe who had the medicine she wished to use.

A mother's healing role in the tribe was that of tending to her sick children. In caring for her children, she called on the advice of an aunt, the knowledge of the grandmother, and, when necessary, the knowledge, talents, and experiences of the network of healers in the villages.

Much as can be found today in the nursing literature on the metaparadigm of nursing (as discussed in Chapter 1; Fawcett, 1995), American Indian nurses were keenly aware of their connections to people (kinship, community), their environment (the Earth and sky and all the inhabitants), and health (all four domains including the physical, spiritual, mental, and emotional). They kept these concepts at the heart of their work while ministering to the sick person or community. This holistic way of viewing the person and her or his health is completely in synch with nursing.

CIRCLES AND THE NUMBER 4

The medicine wheel is a circle divided into quadrants that in part represent the ideas of physical, spiritual, mental, and emotional health, as well as the four directions. Combining these ideas again, prayers and dances may be performed in a circle starting in the east. With these basics as a foundation, tribes vary in their construction and meanings of the medicine wheel. Tribes speak of the four directions, four dimensions of the person; some have four worlds, and others fast for 4 days around holy times; still others wait 4 days to bury or dispose of the dead.

Sweat lodges are one mechanism for achieving either healing, purification, or balance with the integration of the circle. Sweats are used for various purposes, and differ from tribe to tribe. Some tribes traditionally never had a sweat, whereas others have adopted the practice from tribes that do. Some tribal customs did not allow the genders to mix, some were for prayer only, and some were for medicine and healing. Typically, a trained leader runs the sweat, and leads the prayer and direction of the sweat. Prayers are either spoken or sung, and medicine, possibly bear grease, and water figure in the proceedings. Large stones, called "the grandfathers," are heated to hundreds of degrees and placed in the middle of the lodge while participants sit in a circle around the pit that holds the stones. A doorkeeper watches the entrance (see Figure 4.2).

WELLNESS

American Indian women also participated in nursing care that was not related to illness but to the promotion of health. For example, some women were midwives. Midwives were either called to their role by supernatural forces or had it passed down through the family or had a special gift (Moss, 2000). A typical birth included the expectant mother lying on a bed of warm sand to deliver her baby. She was often given tea to help her relax, and other women from her clan then surrounded her while she gave birth (Bunzel, 1932). This description

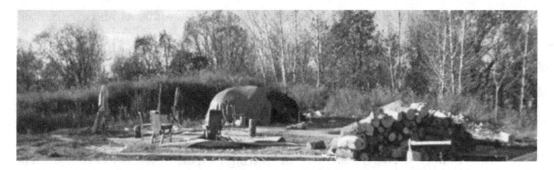

FIGURE 4.2 Annishinabe sweat lodge (woodlands/plains). *Photo:* Moss (2003).

from Southwestern tribal people of early birthing methods predates the natural childbirth methods that have emerged in contemporary society.

Prayer figured prominently in keeping one well—not only oneself but also others in the village and extending to the world. In the Zuni tribe, before eating one's meal, one should offer a portion of that meal to the ancestors/gods. The food is put into a spirit bowl and then offered to the river or burned. These bowls are in use today (see Figure 4.3).

In the late nineteenth century, an agent for the U.S. Department of the Interior published reports on the "primitive" nature of the Southwest American Indians in all spheres of their lives, including health and healing (United States Department of Interior, 1899). There are many who believe to this day that the time-honored methods of health care mentioned here are "primitive" (Cushing & Green, 1990), implying that they are in some way elementary and perhaps uncultured. In fact, the healing works performed by AI/AN nurses long before the formalization of nursing in the late 19th century, rather than being "primitive," might best be identified as "early expressions" of the concepts of community health nursing, nursing care, midwifery, herbalism, therapeutics, and hygienic practice in America. These time-honored healing practices have continued today in varying degrees of tribal life. For a variety of reasons, AI/ANs kept many of their practices hidden from view, partly because of the feelings expressed earlier, partly because they did not want their practices banned, and partly because culturally, often only those involved in the healing should know exactly what is taking place. This is important knowledge for today's nurses to understand.

CONCLUSIONS

Healing practices reflective of American Indian culture, such as herbalism, spiritual healing, the healing influence of the connection with the environment, and the healing concept of the connection among body, mind, and spirit, have not only survived the social changes in indigenous cultures of origin but have also gained popularity with the general American public and American nurses (Kreitzer, Mitten, Harris, & Shandeling, 2002).

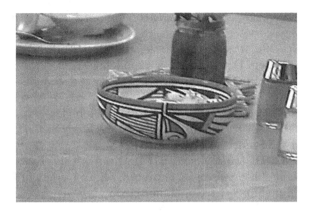

FIGURE 4.3 Spirit bowl Zuni (Southwest)
Photo: Moss (2000).

Even with the increasing interest in the healing practices and perspectives of American Indians, the health beliefs and traditional health practices of various tribes, especially the histories of AI/AN women and their nursing networks, have remained virtually unrecognized. The contribution of AI/AN nursing culture with its holistic focus can provide a foundation for the contemporary nurse who seeks a greater understanding of American Indian ancestral roots of spiritual nursing care.

STUDY QUESTIONS

♦ Discuss why American Indians and Alaska Natives may distrust Western medicine. Why would they prefer their traditional healing?
♦ Discuss how there is no "American Indian" way of nursing or achieving health (think tribes/regions).

REFERENCES

Axtell, H. P. (1997). *A little bit of wisdom: Conversations with a Nez Perce elder.* Norman, OK: University of Oklahoma Press.

Bunzel, R. L. (1932). *Introduction to Zuni ceremonialism.* Washington, DC: U.S. Government Printing Office.

Bunzel, R. L. (1935). *Zuni.* New York, NY: Columbia University Press.

Bureau of Indian Affairs. (2015). *Indian affairs—Who we are.* Retrieved March 20, 2015, from http://www.bia.gov/WhoWeAre/index.htm

Clarke, J. F. (1991). *A gathering of wisdoms—Tribal mental health: A cultural perspective.* (Swinomish tribal mental health project.) LaConner, WA: Swinomish Tribal Community.

Cushing, F. H., & Green, J. (1990). *Cushing at Zuni: The correspondence and journals of Frank Hamilton Cushing, 1879–1884.* Albuquerque, NM: University of New Mexico Press.

Deloria, V., & Lytle, C. M. (1984). *The nations within: The past and future of American Indian sovereignty.* Austin, TX: University of Texas Press.

Dorsey, G. A. (1904). *Traditions of the Arikara.* Baltimore, MD: Carnegie Institution for Science.

Eggan, F. (1950). *Social organization of the Western Pueblos.* Chicago, IL: University of Chicago Press.

Fawcett, J. (1995). *Analysis and evaluation of conceptual models of nursing*. Philadelphia, PA: F. A. Davis.

Flanders, S. A. (1998). *Atlas of American migration*. New York, NY: Facts on File.

Kreitzer, M. J., Mitten, D., Harris, I., & Shandeling, J. (2002). Attitudes toward CAM among medical, nursing, and pharmacy faculty and students: A comparative analysis. *Alternative Therapies in Health and Medicine, 8*, 44–47, 50–53.

Linderman, F. B. (1932). *Red mother*. New York, NY: John Day.

McCullough, D. (2004). *John Adams: The adventurous life-journey of John Adams*. New York, NY: Simon and Schuster.

Moerman, D. E. (2003). *Native American ethnobotany database: Foods, drugs, dyes, and fibers of native North American peoples*. Dearborn, MI: University of Michigan—Dearborn. Retrieved from http://herb.umd.umich.edu

Moss, M. P. (2000). *Zuni elders: Ethnography of American Indian aging*. Houston, TX: University of Texas Health Science Center at Houston.

Nerburn, K. (2010). *The wisdom of the Native Americans: Including the soul of an Indian and other writings from Ohiyesa and the great speeches of chief*. Novato, CA: New World Library.

Nightingale, F. (1912). *Notes on nursing: What it is, and what it is not*. New York, NY: D. Appleton and Company.

Tannen, D. (1982). *Spoken and written language: Exploring orality and literacy*. New York, NY: Ablex.

United States Department of the Interior. (1899). *Indian agent report in Albuquerque area*. Washington, DC: U.S. Government Printing Office.

❖ FIVE ❖

The Indian Health System[1] and Nursing

Ruth E. Meilstrup and Margaret P. Moss

LEARNING OBJECTIVES
The learner will be able to:
♦ Explain the history, structure, and funding of the Indian Health Service (IHS)
♦ Describe the employment systems and nursing opportunities in the IHS
♦ Differentiate the ways in which nursing care of American Indians and Alaska Natives differs from that of the general population
♦ Discern trends and challenges for nursing in the IHS

KEY TERMS
♦ Affordable Care Act
♦ Chronic kidney disease (CKD)
♦ Civil service
♦ Indian Health Service
♦ Indian preference

♦ PL 63-638
♦ Public Health Service Commissioned Corps
♦ Self-determination

KEY CONCEPTS
♦ Contract Health Services
♦ Cultural beliefs
♦ Direct care services
♦ Indian preference

♦ Multidisciplinary
♦ Patient-centered medical home
♦ Tribal self-determination

Health care in the United States that is *specific* to American Indian/Alaska Native (AI/AN) care is highly regulated, greatly underfunded, and not easily accessed by those AI/ANs who reside in cities. By *specific* we mean health care provision that is based on treaty or law offered only to those members of federally recognized tribes in consideration of the ceded lands and rights, and therefore, without additional fees.

Of course, AI/ANs, just as all Americans, can access other forms of health care and payment, such as private insurance, fee for service, or state-financed

[1] Much of the content in this chapter was first published in the *Hamline Journal of Public Law and Policy* as "American Indian Health Disparities: By the Sufferance of Congress" (Moss, M.P., Fall 2010).

and/or administered Medicaid/Medicare programs, or through other federal programs such as the Department of Veterans Affairs. However, in view of high poverty, employment-based insurance in the United States, and, in many cases, barriers to government programs, such as excessive rules and paperwork, and inaccessible offices, lack of computers, and language barriers, often the Indian Health System, though limited, is deemed the system of choice. The formal Indian Health System is known as the I/T/U or Indian Health Service, Tribal Health, and Urban Health Care.

THE INDIAN HEALTH SERVICE

The "I" in the I/T/U refers to the Indian Health Service—a federal agency under the U.S. Department of Health and Human Services—which is charged with care for American Indians and Alaska Natives (AI/ANs) based on treaties and law (IHS, 2015; IHS, n.d.-b). The IHS is a national health program, somewhat like the Veterans Affairs system for U.S. veterans. One must be an enrolled member of a federally recognized tribe in order to obtain services (U.S. Department of Health & Human Services, n.d.-a). This refers back to the federal trust responsibility and the government-to-government relationships established between tribes and the federal government.

History of the Indian Health Service

The origin of the IHS is rooted in the initial treaties forged between the U.S. government and indigenous peoples beginning in 1784. The obligation of the federal government to provide for the health care of AI/ANs evolved over time, and in 1955, the IHS was established under the jurisdiction of the surgeon general of the United States Public Health Service, within the Department of Health and Human Services.

In 1970, President Richard M. Nixon affirmed the relationship between the federal government and the sovereign Indian nations, advancing the concept of "tribal self-determination" and tribal management of health care programs, leading to the IHS as it is today.

Funding

The IHS is not an insurance program, but rather a system of health care facilities and services. Funding comes from congressionally authorized budget appropriations; revenue from third-party payers; including Medicare, Medicaid, and private insurance; and tribal subsidies.

The IHS encourages individuals using their facilities to obtain health insurance under the Patient Protection and Affordable Care Act (ACA; 2010). This provides coverage for contract health services, which are medical treatments and diagnostic services not provided within a particular Service Unit, and also provides third-party revenue for the local facility, which improves the ability of that facility to provide more services. Contract health departments oversee payment for those services that are not provided by the IHS facilities, which would be direct care services (Committee on Indian Affairs United States Senate, 2011; U.S. Department of Health & Human Services, n.d.-b). These can include surgeries, emergency care, and MRIs, among other services (Committee on Indian Affairs United States Senate, 2011).

Eligibility

Persons who are enrolled members of any of the federally recognized tribes are eligible for care at IHS facilities. Persons residing in urban areas or away from their own tribe who are seeking care in another Service Unit or area office may be eligible only for direct care services, which are services provided at that location.

Even though the ACA permits the insured to seek care at a broader choice of facilities, the IHS remains the only practical option for residents of remote reservations. But even when there is a choice, it is common for AI/ANs to prefer to obtain their care at IHS facilities. The cultural knowledge and sensitivity of providers at IHS facilities offers a greater sense of respect and safety.

However, the IHS has been woefully underfunded since its inception. In the field, there are reports of budgets at 40% of need, or 60% less per capita expenditures than for per capita health expenditures nationally (IHS, 2007, p. 270). One hears of "life or limb" requirements for services contracted out (Langwell et al., 2009; Petereit et al., 2008). And, finally, one hears that to get paid care you had better get sick by June (Committee on Indian Affairs United States Senate, 2011).

Annually, the IHS provides primary/outpatient care (11,778,527 visits; IHS Fact Sheets, 2010), some inpatient care (50,349 visits; IHS Fact Sheets, 2010), and public health services (420,778 visits; IHS, 2011). There are few critical care services and only limited long-term care grant programs (Jervis, Jackson, & Manson, 2002). There are 163 Service Units that are either federally or tribally run (IHS Fact Sheets, 2010). These units are found in 12 IHS geographic areas and serve 2 million AIs (IHS Fact Sheets, 2010). Direct services are provided through hospitals (45), health centers (296), Alaska village clinics (166), health stations (121), and school health centers (17); most of these are tribally run with federal funding (IHS Fact Sheets, 2010; Figure 5.1).

Hospital care may only offer medical units, and may not have surgical capabilities or complex care capability. Contract care is woefully underfunded. A comparison of federally funded programs can be seen in Figure 5.2.

The majority of these programs are based on public law. As previously stated, the IHS was rooted in *treaties* and public law. Article VI, paragraph 2, of the U.S. Constitution makes treaties *the supreme law of the land*, and yet the IHS has been critically underfunded for decades as compared with programs based solely on public laws.

Health Care staff includes physicians, nurse practitioners, nurse midwives, physician assistants, registered nurses, licensed practical nurses, nursing

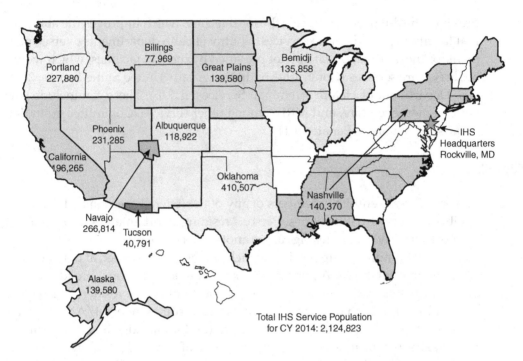

FIGURE 5.1 Indian Health Service population by administrative areas.

Source: U.S Department of Health and Human Services (2014).

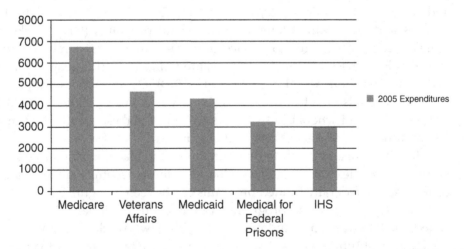

FIGURE 5.2 2005 IHS per capita expenditures as compared with other federal health expenditures.

Source: Indian Health Services (n.d.-b).

assistants, dietitians, and pharmacists, plus clerical support staff. Ancillary services include dentistry, optometry, behavioral health, social services, and environmental health services. The Office of Environmental Health consults and advises on provision of safe water, sewage, and solid waste for tribal communities.

Health Boards composed of tribal representatives provide consultation to the Service Units, and are a conduit for communicating information to tribal members.

Most important, for nurses entering the IHS, there are several hierarchical entities at work in the facilities. Many nurses will not be familiar with the distinctions among civil service, Public Health Service Commissioned Corps, and tribal hires. This will be discussed in the "Nursing in the International Health Service" section later in the chapter.

TRIBAL HEALTH

The "T" in I/T/U refers to tribal health provision. We are currently in the federal policy era of Indian self-determination (Indian Self-Determination and Education Assistance Act, 1975). Tribal health provision of care is one facet of Indian self-determination. Tribal health is entwined through a series of contracts and compacts with the federal system. *Self-determination* refers to allowing tribes greater control over how programming is run. They hire personnel and take care of day-to-day operations.

The IHS takes on a consultative, managerial, or funding role. For example, other than the hospitals, most of the direct service centers listed in the previous section are tribally run (IHS Fact Sheets, 2010). Through the Indian Self-Determination and Education Assistance Act of 1975, tribes are able to take control of programming with federal monies that would have gone to IHS-provided care (Indian Self-Determination and Education Assistance Act, 1975).

Public Law 63-638

In 1975, Congress passed the Indian Self-Determination and Education Assistance Act (PL 63-638), authorizing federal agencies, including the Department of Health and Human Services, to make grants directly to tribes and granting the tribes the authority to administer those funds. Basically, Congress encourages individual tribes to assume the responsibility for managing its own health care. Tribes have opted to take over portions of the programs in some cases, and entire programs in others. Implications for nurses are that more and more nursing jobs fall under tribal contracts, affecting salary, benefits, and job security.

The IHS is mandated to encourage and support tribal self-determination under "638." Where this has happened, there are varying degrees of success, largely based on the size of the tribe involved. Generally, the Navajo Nation is successfully implementing "638," although they still rely on assistance with staffing through contracts with the Public Health Service Commissioned Corps.

In the field, one will hear this being referred to as "going 638" (Reference to Pub. L. No. 93-638). However, funding shortfalls persist in the Indian Health System whether in an IHS-run facility or a program that is tribally run. These shortfalls play out as difficulty in discharging various functions, such as recruiting and maintaining an adequate health professional workforce, maintaining and updating equipment and facilities, maintaining adequate supplies, and the ability to cover care that is contracted out (Langwell et al., 2009). These difficulties translate into a transient workforce, notoriously long wait times, closure of facilities, and unpaid bills (Langwell et al., 2009). Thus, the American Indian health disparity continues into this newest century.

Box 5.1

A controversial 638 compact occurred with Santo Domingo (Kewa) Pueblo, formerly a part of the Santa Fe Service Unit (SFSU), in 2012. Some tribal members have rejected using the Kewa Health Center, and travel a short distance to neighboring clinics at Cochiti Pueblo and San Felipe Pueblo or the Santa Fe Indian Hospital facility for their care. The SFSU lost about 30% of its overall budget in this compact, but remains obligated to provide care to whoever presents themselves. Santo Domingo Pueblo contracts with SFSU for some service, but the SFSU was forced to severely cut back staffing to accommodate the budget cut, leading to the largest reduction in force in the history of the IHS. All parties, including nurses, are still trying to adapt to the changes.

URBAN HEALTH

The "U," which refers to the final arm of the I/T/U system, is likely the most crippling of the three to the health of American Indians. Urban health provision is almost nonexistent in that it is funded at only 22% of need when it *is* available, with 18 new urban areas having been identified that could support services where there are currently no services (IHS, n.d.-c). There are problems unique to urban American Indians who often suffer loss of culture, identity, disenfranchisement, and marginality, more so than their reservation-based relatives. Resulting from federal policies and related funding streams, only 1% of the IHS budget was going toward urban Indian programs at the turn of the 21st century, resulting in more access problems to health care than reservation-based Indians (Forquera, 2001). This 1% budget (in 2000) was especially troublesome as, from the 2000 Census, 2,698,724 American Indians lived inside metropolitan areas versus 1,420,577 who lived outside metropolitan areas (Forquera, 2001).

New York City (in all five boroughs) has nearly 90,000 American Indians, more than any other city in the United States (Forquera, 2001). If these AI/ANs were described in terms of tribes, they would represent the seventh largest tribe in the United States (Ogunwole, 2010). The American Indian Community

House (2011, para. 3), with some contracted IHS monies, describe themselves as "a multi-faceted social support agency and cultural center." They do not provide direct health care services.

As a result of the Indian relocation program of the mid-1900s, many American Indians moved to either coast to find jobs and homes, which in most cases fell short (Fixico, 1986). Cut off from family and culture, where no health programs for AI/ANs were available, health disparities once again persisted.

From 2000 Census figures, more AI/ANs lived off reservation for the first time since the reservation period was instituted in the mid-19th century (Forquera, 2001). As a result of this shift, there needs to be a concerted effort focused on urban health care. In fact, monies to urban programs have been cut drastically this decade. About 29.8 million IHS dollars were allotted to urban programs in 2001, and 28.8 million from other sources, making a total of $58.6 million available to urban programs (IHS, 2011b). By census, there were 4 million American Indians, with 60% living off reservation (Forquera, 2001; IHS, 2011b). There are approximately 2 million who are eligible for IHS services as determined by the government-to-government relationships (Forquera, 2001; IHS, 2011b). This translates to less than $30/person/year for health care in urban settings.

FUNDING THE AMERICAN INDIAN HEALTH IMPROVEMENT ACT

At the beginning of the Indian Self-Determination Era, the Indian Health Care Improvement Act was introduced in the Senate in February of 1975, and signed into law as Public Law 94-437 in 1976. The major provisions of this law can be found in Table 5.1.

The Indian Health Care Improvement Act was set for reauthorization in 1984, yet the last full reauthorization of the Act was in 1992 (Forquera, 2001; IHS, 2011b). There occurred an 18-year lapse in the U.S. Congress in any reauthorizations until the Act garnered permanent reauthorization with the signing of the ACA in March 2010 (Affordable Care Act, 2010). Now that American Indian health has been rolled into the broader national health law, it remains to be seen whether persistent underfunding and persistent health disparity will improve or remain the same.

NURSING IN THE INDIAN HEALTH SERVICE

There are three distinct employment systems in the IHS: civil service, Public Health Service Commissioned Corps, and tribal. Each system has a different salary structure, set of benefits, and some variation in job opportunities. Civil service refers to those employees directly hired by the federal government under either general service or executive service pay grades. As the name implies, these are civilians in government service. Civilians in these categories range from housekeeping staff through administrative personnel.

TABLE 5.1 Wording From the Summary of the Indian Health Care Improvement Act (1976)

TITLE	AREA	PROVISION
I	Indian Health Manpower	Authorizes the Secretary to offer grants and scholarships to public or private nonprofit health or educational entities to increase American Indians in the health professions.
II	Health Services	Authorizes expenditures over a 7-year period for patient care, field health, dental care, mental health, inpatient mental health services, ... and maintenance and repair.
III	Health Facilities	Authorizes expenditures ... for the construction and renovation of hospitals, health centers, health stations, and other facilities of the Service. Authorizes the equipping and staffing of such facilities. Requires consultation with affected Indian tribes before such funds are expended.
IV	Access to Health Services	Makes hospitals and skilled nursing facilities of the Indian Health Service, whether operated by the Service or a tribal organization, eligible for Medicare reimbursement payments ... Requires the Secretary to use such payments for making improvements in such hospitals and facilities to bring them into compliance.
V	Health Services for Urban Indians	Authorizes contracts with urban Indian organizations to assist them in establishing and administering programs to meet urban Indian health needs. Sets forth requirements of eligibility ... to ... aid in familiarization of Indians with available services, determine the size of the Indian populations served by such organizations, determine the extent of unmet health care needs of such populations.
VI	American Indian School of Medicine	Directs the Secretary to study the need for and feasibility of establishing a school of medicine to train Indians to provide health services to Indians.
VII	Reporting to Congress	Requires specific reviews and reports on programs under this Act to be submitted to Congress.

Those in the Public Health Service Commissioned Corps are members of uniformed but unarmed service. Much like those in the armed services, they sign up for tours of duty and bear the ranks of lieutenant, captain, and so on. Health care workers in the "Corps" hold bachelor and higher degrees, and can be nurses, physicians, and executives. The surgeon general of the United States is the head of the PHS Corps.

And finally, tribal members may be hired directly and may work within the hospitals and clinics. Uniquely, the IHS is mandated to use Indian preference (IP) in hiring. Under IP, an American Indian is the first preference in hiring. In IHS, 69% of all employees are American Indian; this percentage varies by job description. In some cases, the IP policy may limit the hiring or advancement opportunities for non-Natives. Generally, the applicants for a position are grouped as IP and non-IP. IP applicants are considered before any non-IP candidate is even presented to the nurse managers.

However, there *are* many types of opportunities for nurses in the IHS: direct patient care in clinics and hospital settings, community-based patient care through the Public Health Service nursing programs, management, and program support, such as infection control, discharge planning, utilization review, and compliance with federal and accreditation requirements.

The nursing vacancy rate is consistently high—between 15% and 25%. There are several reasons for the high vacancy rates: the hiring process is slow and managed regionally, facility sites are often remote and not seen as desirable, and individual sites may delay posting vacancies because of budgetary problems.

The benefit package for the civil service is generous, with a regular pay structure based on longevity, annual performance awards, generous annual leave, accumulative sick leave, health and life insurance, and retirement packages. In addition, there is tuition reimbursement, continuing education, relocation assistance, and, in more remote locations, low-cost housing.

The Public Health Service Commissioned Corps personnel are eligible for jobs not only with the IHS, but also with other agencies under the Public Health Service, including the Centers for Disease Control and Prevention (CDC), National Institutes of Health (NIH), and the Centers for Medicare & Medicaid Services (CMS). The benefit package is the same as for the other uniformed services, and advancement is through a military structure. Civil service nurses can transfer into the Commissioned Corps after hire, depending on hiring quotas within the PHS. Nurses employed by tribal facilities have salary and benefit packages through the tribe, and are not considered federal employees.

NURSING OPPORTUNITIES IN THE INDIAN HEALTH SERVICE

Newly graduated registered nurses may start out in ambulatory care clinics or on inpatient hospital units. Ask your prospective employer about the orientation process, whether preceptors are used, and what your work schedule and hours will look like. Community-based clinics may offer Monday-through-Friday workweeks, but hospital-based settings are typically open 7 days a week, including holidays, and for 12 to 24 hours daily. Compressed work schedules or 12-hour shifts are normal in hospital settings. In smaller facilities, floating among departments is common workforce management.

Depending on the facility, the ambulatory care clinics offer care to patients on an appointment or walk-in basis, and may have urgent care beds connected to the clinic. Larger facilities offer nurses an opportunity to specialize in the ambulatory care settings, but nurses should be prepared to be generalists, able to work with a variety of disease specialties and age ranges.

A new initiative to improve patient care continuity is in use at several IHS sites. Called the patient-centered medical home, the concept consists of a multidisciplinary patient care team comprising a primary care physician or midlevel provider, RNs, nursing assistants, and specialists related to the team's focus. These teams enhance nurses' ability to develop long-term relationships with patients and families, initiate interventions appropriate for the patient, and offer educational information about disease prevention and management.

Hospital sites include ambulatory care services, urgent care units, emergency departments, and inpatient specialty areas, including medical–surgical, intensive care, progressive care, pediatrics, obstetrics, and operating rooms.

There are many opportunities for clinical specialization and advancement in the management structure. Some of these roles are discharge planner, case manager, utilization review coordinator, point-of-care testing coordinator, quality-improvement manager, diabetes educator, as well as unit clinical supervisors, shift supervisors, and nurse executive. These roles are essential to meeting accreditation requirements and documenting progress toward care benchmarks established by Congress. Often, roles are combined in middle-management positions.

Public health nursing (PHN) is a specialty that is based in the community. PHNs interface with community-based programs, including Head Start, schools, and senior centers, as well as providing in-home care needs assessments and hospital follow-up care. At hospital discharge, nurses send a referral to the PHN describing the hospital course and posthospitalization concerns.

Supporting the PHNs are nonprofessional, tribally employed community health representatives (CHRs). CHRs take on a variety of community-based health responsibilities, including home visits, arranging transportation to clinics, and organizing community health events. Familiar with local dialects and unique cultural aspects, they are often advocates for the needs of individual patients.

PERSONAL STORIES

The reasons nurses choose to work for the IHS vary from the practical to the altruistic. Nurses who are AI/ANs have often grown up using IHS as their health care provider, and want to live in their communities, where IHS is the most practical employment choice. When IHS hospitals or clinics are close to private sector options, or when a nurse who has no personal connection to a remote reservation location but chooses to work in IHS, the reasons often become stories worth telling.

The following are some of the reasons why nurses join the IHS:

1. Native nurses who want to help their own people seek employment through the IHS. They are familiar with the particular problems in their community, and want to make a difference in their community. It is not uncommon, however, for Native nurses to choose not to work in their own community where they are too close to people they know. There are often other nearby options.
2. Non-Native nurses with personal ties to the Native community also seek out the IHS. For example, there was one non-Native nurse who was married to a Native and had children who were tribal members. After many years in the private sector, she came into the IHS because of her family.

3. Non-Native nurses who have no personal connections to Native communities also join the IHS. Some have lived in areas where there is a significant Native population, but others move across Country in pursuit of this opportunity.

For nurses who desire the rather unique experience of living and working close to AI/AN culture, the IHS is the choice. The opportunity to get to know Native families is very special. In the first author's experience, indigenous families are closely knit. The small size of the clinics and hospitals means that the nurse will interact with several generations of a family. One may have the opportunity to care for families prenatally, then see the children and his or her parents through well-child visits, and into adulthood. When a family member is hospitalized, it is normal for another family member to stay with the patient.

The first author, who is non-Native, came to the Santa Fe Indian Hospital in 1990, and worked there for 24 years, spending the majority of the time on the inpatient unit. In the light of my past experience in the private sector for 20 years in a variety of specialties, including medical, surgical, pediatrics, obstetrics, and psychiatry, I was ideally prepared to work in a small hospital where nurses were "jacks-of-all-trades." When we decided to relocate to New Mexico, I initially talked with several of the hospitals in the area, but when I discovered an opportunity at the Santa Fe Indian Hospital, it felt like a calling.

Initially, there was a romantic sense of adventure and discovery. With 20 years' nursing in the private sector as a basis for comparison, I found my Native American patients very friendly and highly appreciative of my efforts, and that helped to make my work rewarding. The benefits associated with federal employment kept me there until I retired.

The Santa Fe Indian Hospital is unique among IHS hospitals in that it is located in an urban area, but is the service point for several small Pueblo tribes. Most IHS facilities, in contrast, are located on reservations, and serve a single tribe. IHS hospitals in urban areas, such as the Alaska Native Medical Center in Anchorage and the Phoenix Indian Medical Center, may serve several tribes as well as urban Natives from tribes throughout the Country.

I found that the family structure of the Pueblos, as well as the other tribes, is very strong and central to the culture. Individuals within the extended family feel a sense of responsibility to their elders and to their offspring. The nuclear family is not an AI/AN concept. Grandmas, grandpas, aunties, uncles, sisters, and brothers help mothers and fathers with the children. Children, grandchildren, nieces, and nephews all help with the elders. In a much greater sense than in the general population, the village raises the children.

The opportunity to enjoy Pueblo hospitality on feast days is a very special experience for someone working with these tribes. Santo Domingo (Kewa) Pueblo's annual feast day is the largest Native ceremony in the Americas. Visitors are welcome to most feast-day celebrations. Coworkers and patients commonly invite IHS personnel to the dances and into their homes to enjoy the feast-day meal prepared by their families.

CULTURAL BELIEFS AND NURSING CONSIDERATIONS

There are specific traditional practices that one may encounter only in the hospital setting. Natives often wear or carry a fetish or medicine bag (usually a small leather pouch filled with cornmeal or corn pollen). In the hospital, these may be pinned to the hospital gown or tucked under a pillow, so care must be taken to preserve these items. Other items, such as feathers or bowls of cornmeal, may be on nightstands and should not be disturbed.

Mothers sometimes wish to take their placentas home for burial. Patients who have had amputations have wanted to bury the limb at home. Some believe that hair in their hairbrushes must be burned rather than discarded in the trash, and save it to take home. This is because many indigenous people feel that one's spirit resides in every piece of the person, making even hair sacred and therefore something that must be attended to properly. Traditional Native patients may believe drinking ice water is harmful, so ask before filling water pitchers with ice.

The practice of wearing socks to bed may be cultural or simply a result of not having central heating. If people do not change their socks, they are at increased risk for athlete's foot infections, which can lead to cellulitis. They may own only one or two thick pairs of socks. Some only have outhouses and incomplete plumbing, and keep the socks on all the time for warmth. Assessment of feet is extremely important, especially in a population with such high rates of diabetes mellitus.

There is a strong discomfort in having windows uncovered after dark; a belief that unsettled spirits roam at night and might be peering in the windows is discomfiting, so the conscientious nurse draws the curtains promptly.

Care of the dead varies among the tribes. Navajo (Dine) are not comfortable dealing directly with dead bodies, so are likely to use funeral homes. Among the Pueblos, burial is a family and tribal event, in which family members prepare the body for burial as opposed to using funeral homes and morticians. This even includes transporting the body from the hospital to the home, which usually occurs early in the day after the death. Four days of observances follow.

Spiritually, there is often an overlap between traditional beliefs and the Christian beliefs introduced by Europeans to the Americas. It is not uncommon to have a Catholic priest called to the bedside, followed by a medicine man at a later time. It is IHS policy to facilitate the use of traditional healing practices when desired. In the Navajo Nation, IHS hospitals have dedicated spaces for the use of traditional healers, and often also have a sweat lodge on site.

One still finds elderly patients who are not fluent in English. Younger family members are primarily English-language speakers, however, and are, although this is not optimal, they can provide an interpreter for clinic visits and hospital stays.

COMMON PATIENT DIAGNOSES IN THE HOSPITAL SETTING

When nursing in Indian Country, you will find several health issues are common, as stated in Chapter 3. Because diabetes is endemic in the Native population, it is common to find diabetes as a primary diagnosis or comorbidity in the hospitalized patient. Diabetes exacerbates infectious processes, and is the reason a simple cellulitis or an upper respiratory infection progresses to a severity requiring hospitalization.

The dry climate of the Southwest causes dry and cracked skin, and cellulitis is a common ailment, requiring a course of intravenous (IV) antibiotics. Respiratory infections require oxygen therapy during treatment, especially at the higher altitudes of the Rocky Mountain region tribes, as well as IV antibiotics. Indications for hospital admission include acute dehydration, low oxygen saturation levels, and treatment requiring cardiac monitoring and intravenous medications.

In hospitals with surgical services, many general surgeries require postoperative care. Obstetrics accounts for another type of hospital admission. These include antepartum complications, such as preeclampsia, normal labor and delivery and postpartum care, and cesarean deliveries, which have a longer postpartum stay. Unfortunately, few IHS hospitals offer all of these services.

Elderly or disabled patients who require care at extended care facilities (ECFs) need preadmission hospitalization for assessment and referral. Although Native families often prefer to provide care at home for their elders, increasing employment in Native communities, often a result of improved tribal economic development, makes providing that care more difficult. Very few tribes have their own ECFs.

Antibiotic-resistant superbugs, such as *methicillin-resistant Staphylococcus aureus*, require extended hospitalizations for IV antibiotic therapy. Osteomyelitis and gangrene, complications of diabetes, are also indications for long-term antibiotic therapy. Most tribes cannot afford to allocate funds from the limited monies available for contract health services for home-infusion therapy provided by private agencies, and lack adequate staff to provide this home care service. Hospitalization may be the most cost-effective route to provide long-term antibiotic therapy.

Because the funding for inpatient units is supported by the general budget of the Service Unit, rather than third-party reimbursements as in the private sector, and because of the distance patients may travel for care, hospital stays can be longer than in the private sector. The doctors have some latitude in determining readiness for discharge based on a patient's individual circumstances. This is an especially common practice in Alaska, where patients are transported from bush communities for hospitalization, even in private sector facilities. The Alaska Native Medical Center even has housing available on campus for posthospital care.

TRENDS IN INDIAN HEALTH CARE

The impact of the ACA and PL 63-638 on the IHS has yet to be fully appreciated. The IHS will remain the primary source of care for most reservation-based AI/ANs for the foreseeable future. The federal funding for the IHS is conservative compared with that for other federal agencies. IHS personnel have always joked about working for an underfunded federal agency, but it is the chronic state of affairs in the IHS. The comparison of dollars spent per capita for IHS users compared with the total U.S. population is telling: according to most current data, IHS per capita is $2,849; total U.S. population per capita is $7,713.

It is important to note that the IHS is having some significant successes in health care. Most notable, the rate of AI/AN diabetic patients with chronic kidney disease progressing to dialysis has declined and is only slightly higher than that in the Asian and Anglo populations, and half the rate of the African American population.

Second, the structure of the IHS facilitates promotion of preventative health initiatives such as immunizations and general health screenings. The IHS database for health care statistics is larger than any other health database in the Country.

A final, and most notable, point to consider is the dedication of the IHS workforce to the overall mission of the IHS. In the authors' experiences, stories of employees going "above and beyond" to serve their patients are commonplace. Understanding how to optimize the health care dollar is key. And a passion for caring for this population is palpable.

The limited budget, however, impacts the breadth of services provided in the IHS, and there have been transfers of care services from direct care services to contract health services. The limited monies for contract health services result in rationing of some treatments that would be commonplace in the private sector, such as knee and hip replacements or breast reconstruction after mastectomy.

Enrollment in ACA insurance plans should increase the availability of services not provided with direct care. The ACA may eventually lead to a decline in IHS facilities and services, particularly in urban areas.

Advances in health management have had a significant impact on the number and length of hospitalizations throughout the United States, not just the IHS. Immunizations for influenza, pneumococcal pneumonia, respiratory syncytial virus, and meningitis have reduced medical admissions for these diseases. Surgical advances have changed procedures so that, for example, cholecystectomy, a common surgery for IHS patients, is now a day surgery, unlike 30 years ago when it required a 4- to 5-day hospitalization. Improved access to home health services like IV infusion therapy and oxygen therapy through private insurance under the ACA will reduce the need for hospitalizations.

A FINAL WORD ON NURSING

The nurse choosing to work in an IHS or tribal facility should have appropriate expectations and an understanding of the culture and resources involved. This background will enhance your success and satisfaction as well as that of the AI/AN patient. The status and environment of the workplace is one matter, but another important consideration is the community in which you will be living. Some locations are very urban, some are small towns, and many are very remote. Cost of living will also vary. So doing research on these external considerations will lessen your own culture shock.

Working as a nurse completely out of culture within Indian Country may be stressful, but will also be rewarding and unlike any other experience. Every individual comes with his or her own background and experience. If the IHS is a fit for you, you can have a great career within it.

CONCLUSIONS

The federal responsibility set forth in the courts has through the years provided American Indian health care that has been critically underfunded and under-staffed, and that has not followed many of the original provisions set out by the Indian Health Care Improvement Act (1976). There has been no American Indian Medical School. There have been programs, such as INMED, the Indians into Medicine program, that have been successful; others, however, have shrunk or closed (UND School of Medicine, 2011). The same is true for other health professions. Facilities have closed, health professionals are hard to attract, and the overall outcome is that American Indians are dying earlier, hit harder by chronic disease, have less access to health care, and suffer more severely than many of their non-Native counterparts (Jones, 2006; Langwell et al., 2009; Mechanic, 2005; Smedley, Stith, & Nelson, 2003; Wilkins & Lomawaima, 2002; Zuckerman, Haley, Roubideaux, & Lillie-Blanton, 2004).

There are new provisions for Indian health, such as long-term care, that have never been provided other than through small, short-term grants (Jervis et al., 2002; Manson, 1989). However, the funding for the programming has not yet been authorized (Centers for Medicare & Medicaid Services, 2013).

Finally, in the U.S. Congress itself, there is a Senate Committee on Indian Affairs that oversees much of what the IHS is accomplishing (S. Res. 4, Sec. 105, 95th Congress, 1st Session [1977], as amended by S. Res. 127, 98th Congress, 2nd Session [1984]. This committee conducts the confirmation hearings for the director of the agency, among other duties. However, on the House side, there is no such committee. The affairs of Indians in Congress are divided up. The issue of an Indian Affairs committee was recently broached on the House side, but was rejected by Speaker Pelosi (Rave, 2007). By the sufferance of Congress, the tribes exist, at least in political terms. The tribes themselves, whether recognized or not, remain sovereign on their lands in their eyes and hearts. As nurses, whether AI/AN themselves or non-Native, the cohesion between thoughtful care of the person and the community bolsters what the Congress has not.

CRITICAL-THINKING EXERCISE

♦ Your patient has been given information about the ACA, and the patient benefit service representative has encouraged him to apply for an ACA health plan. He tells you he has no intention of doing so, that his health care is a treaty obligation to him, and he expects the IHS to fulfill its obligation to provide his care. How would you respond to him?

STUDY QUESTIONS

♦ What information do you need from or about an American Indian patient to provide culturally appropriate care?
♦ Your patient has died. What do you need to do to prepare the body?
♦ Discuss the potential impact of the Affordable Care Act on the Indian Health Service.

USEFUL WEBSITES

◆ Indian Health Service information, www.ihs.gov
◆ Indian preference, civil service, and other information, www.usajobs.gov
◆ National Institute of Diabetes and Digestive and Kidney Diseases, http://kidney
.niddk.nih.gov/kudiseases/pubs/kustats/#6 kidney statistics
◆ Public Health Service, www.usphs.gov

REFERENCES

Affordable Care Act, 25 U.S.C. § 1623 (2010).

American Indian Community House. (2011). Home page. Retrieved March 28, 2011, from http://www.aich.org

Centers for Medicare & Medicaid Services (2013). *Health care reform and long-term care: A study of impact on nursing homes in Indian Country.* Retrieved November 13, 2015, from https://www.cms.gov/Outreach-and-Education/American-Indian-Alaska-Native/AIAN/Downloads/Health-Care-Reform-and-Long-Term-Care.pdf

Committee on Indian Affairs United States Senate. (2011). *Access to contract health services in Indian Country.* Senate Congressional Hearing, 110th Congress 2007–2008. Washington, DC: U.S. Government Printing Office. Retrieved March 26, 2011, from http://frwebgate.access.gpo.gov/cgi-bin/getdoc.cgi?dbname=110_senate_hearings&docid=f:44489.pdf

Fixico, D. L. (1986). *Termination and relocation. Federal Indian policy, 1945–1960.* Albuquerque, NM: University of New Mexico Press.

Forquera, R. (2001). *Urban Indian health.* Washington, DC: U.S. Department of Health and Human Services.

Indian Health Care Improvement Act, Pub. L. No. 94-437 (1976).

Indian Health Service. (2007). *The IHS primary care provider.* Retrieved from https://www.ihs.gov/provider/includes/themes/newihstheme/display_objects/documents/2000_2009/PROV0907.pdf

Indian Health Service. (2011). *Program statistics—IHS HQ publications.* Retrieved March 25, 2011, from http://www.ihs.gov/NonMedicalPrograms/IHS_Stats/files/Trends%20Part%204-General%20Mort.pdf

Indian Health Service. (2015). *Basis for health services.* Retrieved from https://www.ihs.gov/newsroom/factsheets/basisforhealthservices/

Indian Health Services. (n.d.-a). *The gold book—First 50 years of the Indian Health Service.* Retrieved from http://www.ihs.gov/newsroom/factsheets/

Indian Health Services. (n.d.-b). *2005 IHS expenditures per capita compared to other federal health expenditure benchmarks 1.* Retrieved December 2, 2010, from http://www.ihs.gov/nonmedicalprograms/budgetformulation/documents/per%20capita%20hlth%20expend%20comparison%20charts%202-6-2006.pdf

Indian Health Services. (n.d.-c). *Office of urban Indian health programs.* Retrieved from http://www.ihs.gov/urban/

Indian Self-Determination and Education Assistance Act, Pub.L. No. 93-638, 88 Stat. 2203 (1975).

Jervis, L. L., Jackson, M. Y., & Manson, S. M. (2002). Need for, availability of, and barriers to the provision of long-term care services for older American Indians. *Journal of Cross-Cultural Gerontology, 17,* 295–311.

Jones, D. S. (2006). The persistence of American Indian health disparities. *American Journal of Public Health, 96,* 2122.

Langwell, K., Anagnopoulos, C., Ryan, F., Melson, J., & Iron Rope, S. (2009). Financing American Indian health care: Impacts and options for improving access and quality. *Findings Brief: Health Care Financing & Organization, 12*, 1–4.

Manson, S. M. (1989). Long-term care in American Indian communities: Issues for planning and research. *The Gerontologist, 29*, 38.

Mechanic, D. (2005). *Policy challenges in modern health care*. New Brunswick, NJ: Rutgers University Press.

Ogunwole, S. U. (2010). *American Indian and Alaska native population: 2000: Census 2000 brief*. Darby, PA: Diane Publishing.

Petereit, D. G., Molloy, K., Reiner, M. L., Helbig, P., Cina, K., Miner, R., ... & Roberts, C. R. (2008). Establishing a patient navigator program to reduce cancer disparities in the American Indian communities of Western South Dakota: Initial observations and results. *Cancer Control: Journal of the Moffitt Cancer Center, 15*, 254.

Rave, J. (January, 2007). Rehberg calls for the creation of House Indian Affairs panel. Retrieved November 13, 2015, from http://missoulian.com/jodirave/rehberg-calls-for-the-creation-of-house-indian-affairs-panel/article_16cdb2fc-1f61-532f-acd7-da7ed6ba68ef.html

Smedley, B. D., Stith, A. Y., & Nelson, A. R. (2003). *Unequal treatment: Confronting racial and ethnic disparities in health care*. Washington, DC: National Academies Press.

University of North Dakota School of Medicine & Health Sciences. (2011). *Indians into medicine*. Retrieved March 28, 2011, from http://www.med.und.edu/inmed/about.html

U.S. Department of Health and Human Services. (2014). *HHS FY2015 budget in brief*. http://www.hhs.gov/budget/fy2015-hhs-budget-in-brief/hhs-fy2015budget-in-brief-ihs.html

U.S. Department of Health & Human Services. (n.d.-a). Code of Federal Regulations (CFR), at Title 42—Public Health, § 136.12.

U.S. Department of Health & Human Services. (n.d.-b). Code of Federal Regulations (CFR), at Title 42—Public Health, Part 136—Indian Health, Subpart C—Contract Health Services, §§ 136.21–136.25.

Wilkins, D. E., & Lomawaima, K. T. (2002). *Uneven ground: American Indian sovereignty and federal law*. Norman, OK: University of Oklahoma Press.

Zuckerman, S., Haley, J., Roubideaux, Y., & Lillie-Blanton, M. (2004). Health service access, use, and insurance coverage among American Indians/Alaska Natives and Whites: What role does the Indian Health Service play? *American Journal of Public Health, 94*, 53–59.

SIX

Beyond the IHS: Indigenous Knowledge and Traditional Approaches to Health and Healing

S. Neyooxet Greymorning

What is herbal doctoring? Herbal doctoring is where we take the plants that God has put upon this earth for mankind to use. All the plants and trees and animals have something they can give that can cure something.

—Russell Willier, Cree Healer

LEARNING OBJECTIVE

♦ The goal of this chapter is to demonstrate the survival and continuity of Native healing knowledge despite threats from Western expansion and assimilation pressures imposed by missionaries and government officials.

KEY TERMS

♦ Ethnobotany
♦ Indigenous healers
♦ Medical anthropology

KEY CONCEPTS

♦ American Indian healers
♦ Botanical remedies
♦ Herbal doctoring
♦ Medicinal uses of plants

Indians of the Americas have had a long and successful tradition of dealing with health issues. Although Native traditions associated with health and healing have recently been seriously fragmented, this knowledge has not disappeared, as made evident by pharmaceutical pursuits to exploit Indigenous medicinal knowledge. This chapter examines ethnobotanical knowledge of select tribal groups of the Americas, discussing how this knowledge has been applied, historically threatened, and at times used as an alternative to Western society's "medicine men." This chapter also discusses the increasing number of hospitals allowing Native healers to apply their knowledge in the care of Native and, occasionally, non-Native patients.

INDIGENOUS KNOWLEDGE AND TRADITIONAL APPROACHES TO HEALTH AND HEALING

Although the impact of European expansion and colonization has changed the world and lifestyles of Indigenous North Americans, Indigenous peoples' cultural knowledge and practices, though endangered by historical efforts to eradicate Native cultures and traditions, have persisted into the 21st century. This chapter examines a compendium of Native ethnobotanical healing knowledge, as it generally existed historically, as well as discusses contemporary applications of this healing knowledge and practices by individuals within select Indian tribes of the Americas. This chapter also looks at how this traditional healing knowledge is slowly being returned to as an alternative to contemporary clinical medicine. It closes with a discussion on a small but growing acceptance among hospital administrators to allow Native healing practitioners within mainstream hospitals to apply their healing knowledge and practices with Native, and, on occasion non-Native, patients.

A Paucity of Literature

When a subject search was initiated for articles and/or research on American Indian healers and healing traditions through PubMed (one of the largest medical search engines available that accesses a database of over 19 million citations through the U.S. National Library of Medicine), only 52 articles were cited. Topics addressed by these articles included: quality of life, distress in Navajo healing, prevalence of arthritis, narratives of cancer survivors working with healers, Aboriginal women as caregivers of the elderly, prevalence of mental disorders and utilization of mental health services, ceremonial use of tobacco, health issues on the Pala Indian reservation from 1903 to 1920, care of Native women, Native Americans in medicine, the need for Indian healers, implications for healing with Navajo medicine, a lay theory of healing in Spain (I thought it odd this was listed), empowerment of minority communities, Navajo use of healers, and observations of a health and healing system in a Papago community.

Only two of the articles dealt with the topic of Indian healers, and those were from the perspective of the healers' experience as healers. Two articles of particular interest addressed the lack of research in the area of Native healing. In the first, "Traditional Native Healing: Alternative or Adjunct to Modern Medicine?" Zubrek (1994) concluded with a comment on the difficulty physicians had in forming a definition of traditional Native medicine. The other article, "An Overview of Aboriginal Health Research in the Social Sciences: Current Trends and Future Directions," by Wilson and Young (2008), found that of the

96 papers they reviewed, the majority dealt with health status and nonmedical determinants of health. In their conclusion, they pointed out the need for further research to address the gaps in the current body of literature. When I conducted a search under the subject heading of "American Indian healing," although 170 citations were identified, the majority were topically similar to those reported by Wilson and Young. An interesting observation about these articles is that although the search was conducted through the U.S. National Library of Medicine's search engine, over 90% of the articles listed were authored in Canada, perhaps an indication of how scarce research on this particular topic in the United States has been. One reason for this may lie in the history of Indian health care services in the United States.

TROUBLES WITH INDIAN HEALTH CARE SERVICES

Not long after its creation in 1824, the Federal Bureau of Indian Affairs (BIA) was charged with the responsibility of overseeing the health and well-being of Native Americans. In part, this grew out of clauses that found their way into numerous treaties between the U.S. government and Indian Nations, and Acts that the government legislated for the "good and welfare of Indian tribes." From its inception to the present, the government's responsibility of providing health services for Indians has been laden with problems of corruption and mismanagement, putting at risk the very people it was meant to serve. In 1955, the specific task of overseeing health care issues for over 500 Indian tribal groups was turned over to the federal government's Department of Health Service (DHS), in their newly created Indian Health Services (IHS). The change, however, did not necessarily create better services or conditions. "When the IHS was transferred from the Bureau of Indian Affairs to the Public Health Services in 1955, both its medical facilities and staffing were inadequate to meet the needs of Indians" (Association of Schools of Public Health, 1987, p. 354). Although U.S. officials had long been aware of poor health care services for Native Americans, this generally did not become public knowledge until some time after the release of the Meriam report (Meriam, 1928).

In *Healing Ways, Navajo Health Care in the Twentieth Century*, Davies (2001) summarized numerous Navajo complaints about the poor service they received at IHS Navajo:

> many felt as though they were sheep being put through the sheep dip . . . cultural barriers between Navajo and non-Indian healthcare workers made the IHS experience especially difficult . . . physicians . . . often appeared indecisive, incompetent, or rude. (Davies, 2001, pp. 118–119)

Over 80 years after the release of the Meriam report, the Indian Health Service continues to be plagued by issues of mismanagement in a number of areas, which led IHS to develop a website as a means of reporting mismanagement concerns. During the 1970s, physicians at IHS facilities were exposed as being responsible for the forced sterilization of hundreds of Indian women. One of the more dramatic examples included two 15-year-old Indian girls who went into a hospital in Montana for appendectomies and were sterilized without their knowledge:

> What happened to these . . . females was a common occurrence during the 1960s and 1970s. Native Americans accused the Indian Health Service of sterilizing at least 25 percent of Native American women who were between the ages of fifteen and forty-two during the 1970s. (Lawrence, 2000, p. 400)

As Davies (2001) noted about the emotional consequences of sterilization on women:

> "One of the results of the large numbers of forced sterilizations performed on Indian women is that . . . their identity as life givers had been severely undermined." The findings led many American Indians and concerned non-Indians to believe that the IHS may have been engaging in a program of "genocide" through population control. (p. 132)

During the summer of 1978, while working on the Rosebud Sioux reservation in South Dakota for a youth program, I conducted some preliminary investigations of health practices as part of my doctoral research interests in medical anthropology. One afternoon, a 16-year-old girl was thrown from a horse and broke her forearm. When she was admitted to IHS, I was stunned as I watched a doctor put a cast on her arm without setting it. When I tentatively inquired about the status of the girl's arm, the doctor was dismissive. In the end, I drove the girl to Cherry County Hospital in Valentine, Nebraska. Fortunately, the doctor was convinced to x-ray the girl's arm. The x-ray revealed that the girl's arm was not set; it was still broken in the cast. Although there are instances in which a break that has not been set can heal over, there nonetheless remains a real possibility that fatty material produced by the bone marrow could have been released into the bloodstream, putting the girl at risk of a fatal fat embolism (Hussain, 2003). This is just one example of the poor health care practices of the time. Concerns over IHS mismanagement led Senator Byron Dorgan, Chair of the Senate Indian Affairs Committee, to state that from 2006 through 2010,

> we have been aware of and attempted to force the IHS to deal with very serious cases of mismanagement, malfeasance, retaliation against whistleblowers as well as potential criminal behavior . . . I believe this type of mismanagement in the region over a long period of time has negatively affected health care provided to Native Americans. These problems must be remedied. (Dorgan, 2010)

Few people know that over 600 distinct tribal groups still exist in North America (Smithsonian *Handbooks* of American Indian Languages). Even fewer are aware that a large portion of today's pharmaceuticals are derived from medicinal plants, and in many cases are based on the knowledge that Indigenous peoples have regarding the utilization of such plants. Over the past 30 years, the scientific and pharmaceutical quest to profit from the ethnobotanical knowledge of Native healers has substantially increased. According to Marc Plotkin, a leading authority on ethnobotany and voted Environment Hero for the Planet by *Time* magazine in 2001:

> Industrialized countries still rely on nature for medicine to a much higher degree than almost anyone realizes. Almost half of all the best-selling pharmaceuticals in the early 1990s were natural products or their derivatives. A recent study of 150 major pharmaceuticals showed that 100 percent of drugs employed for dermatology, gynecology, or hematological purposes; 76 percent of those used for allergy, pulmonary and respiratory purposes; 76 percent used to treat infectious disease, and 75 percent employed for general medicine and analgesic purposes are derived from or based on natural products. (Plotkin, 2001, p. 26)

Many modern pharmaceutical discoveries have been made as a result of tapping into the knowledge of Indigenous healers (see Table 6.1, cited in the next section). In Vogel's (1990) introduction to *American Indian Medicine*, he states:

> Some people mistakenly believe that synthetic drugs have eliminated Indian and natural remedies . . . altogether about 220 substances used by the Indians were listed in the *USP* and *National Formulary* between 1820 and 1965.
>
> *USAN* and the *USP of Drug Names* through June 1981, lists thirty-two substances or derivatives from substances used medicinally by American Indians. Among others are atropine, derived from *datura* (jimson weed), used as a parasympatholytic; *cascara* . . . *cocaine*; *tubocurarine chloride* . . . incorporating elements of *curare* (arrow poison), a muscle relaxant; ipecac, a famous emetic . . . *podophyllum* . . . from may apple root . . . *kaolin*, an absorbant; *papain*, from papaya, an enzyme; *Peruvian balsam*, a rubefacient; and *balsam* of Tulu, an expectorant. (Vogel, 1990, p. ix)

Although a number of authors have written on Indian curative knowledge and traditions, perhaps one of the most widely read books on Native medicinal plants is *Indian Herbalogy of North American* by Hutchens (1991). In this well-researched study, Hutchens has documented over 200 plant names and medicinal uses. A problem with the majority of what has been written is that specific information on the tribal names or specific preparations is lacking. A possible explanation for this can be derived from the following.

> Many herbal medicines were, and still are, considered to be private property of a family. Secrecy was felt to be very important and in many instances the identity of the herb used was known only to the healer. Often even the patient didn't know what plant was being used. (Turner, Thomas, Carlson, & Ogilvie, 1983, p. 46)

Although traditions associated with health and healing have been seriously impacted by the onslaught of colonization, the healing knowledge of Indigenous peoples has not disappeared, and in some instances might be shared with people not only within a group, but with those of a different region. In *Tales of a Shaman's Apprentice*, Plotkin illustrated the ability to adapt medicinal knowledge to a new environment when he wrote of his experience in Suriname. Plotkin's interest in Suriname was peaked when he learned that descendants of slaves in Jamaica used rosy periwinkle (*Catharanthus roseus*) to treat "blood problems." Scientists from Canada and the Eli Lilly Company of Indianapolis, Indiana, became interested in this plant and eventually isolated 70 different alkaloids from it. One of the alkaloids, vincristine, has been used to treat Hodgkin's disease, in addition to childhood leukemia and other childhood cancers. Another example illustrating how Indigenous people can adapt medicinal knowledge to a different region, and also indicative of how this knowledge can spread, occurred in Australia in 2003. Members of the Big Day family from the Crow reservation in eastern Montana had traveled to Byron Bay, New South Wales Australia, to take part in an annual music festival. While at the festival, a young Australian woman was showing signs of going into shock after being bitten by a venomous spider. One of the senior members of the Big Day family was nearby and offered his help. He went off to find a plant he had noticed earlier that belonged to the same family of plants he used to treat spider bites back in Montana. He found the plant and used it to treat the bite victim. As a result of his knowledge and being present, the woman did not go into toxic shock, and her condition stabilized (H. Big Day, personal communication, March 29, 2010).

When Europeans began to settle throughout Indigenous North America, their knowledge of the medicinal properties of plants was quite limited, whereas the Indigenous people they encountered had honed their knowledge of plants for treating ailments to an appreciable level. In addition to knowing how to unlock the medicinal attributes of plants, Dr. Volney Steele wrote:

> The quality of medical practice of the Indian was at least comparable and perhaps even superior to that of the European. Native American men and women had identified scores of herbs to treat illnesses. They knew about cathartics, antifebriles, tonics, astringents, antiseptics, and numerous other natural remedies. Native healers also understood the value of massage, bandages, splints, suturing, applied heat, and

enemas. Sweat lodges and bathing in hot springs were used to treat lung disease, skin disorders and rheumatism.

Anthropologists have discovered . . . obsidian knives, copper forceps, suture material of human or animal hair, analgesic substances derived from . . . plants, fine mesh cotton gauze, and crude antiseptics, together with a knowledge of anatomy, allowed . . . aborigine surgeons to perform amputations, treat fractures, and remove arrows. (Steele, 2006, pp. 19–20)

Smith (1928) recorded more than 200 botanical remedies in use by the Meskwaki Indians alone, and in 1933, Dr. Brooks (1933) stated,

the Indian medicine man practiced successfully Cesarean section, symphisiotomy; he understood and applied the wide use of trephining; . . . he installed dental plates and bridgework; he even supplied his patients with artificial limbs . . . Indians of the days of Custer . . . well understood the treatment of fractures, dislocations, and his treatment of gunshot wounds . . . was efficient and in many respects admirable . . . I have also observed . . . the efficiency of pioneer medicine, which owed its origin mostly to the red medicine man. (pp. 16–17)

Sanapia, an Oklahoma Comanche medicine woman who began her training when she was 13 years old, was considered to have had a late start. The acquisition of knowledge—in this case healing knowledge—is labor intensive, admitting of no real short cuts. The skills of Native healers are layered, generations thick, and result from years of study, training, and guidance that often began in childhood. In his study of a Comanche medicine woman, Jones (1984) noted,

It was during summer vacation prior to her last year at school that Sanapia's mother offered to train her to become a doctor. Sanapia was reticent at first but combined pressure from her mother and maternal grandmother persuaded her to at least consent to the first phases of this training program, that of learning to identify in their natural habitat the various floral medicines which her mother used in doctoring. (p. 24)

For many, the knowledge of plants used by Indians extends only as far as knowing that sage (*Artemisia* spp.) and cedar (*Juniperus* spp.) were used for smudging. ("Cedar" is a name applied to a number of different trees; in this context, it pertains to juniper species, *Juniperus* spp.)

Few know that the berries of a cedar (juniper) tree are still used by Indians in the American Southwest to cure eye infections, whereas the twigs of cedar when beaten into a mash and steeped in boiling water can be applied as a poultice on the chest for heart pain. When White medical practitioners discovered how Indian healers made use of cedar, they became intrigued to the point of investigating cedar for its medicinal value. This led to the medical use of cedar for diaphoretic and antispasmodic purposes. Medical exploration of cedar's value resulted in the plant being listed between 1942 and 1950 in the pharmacopoeia of the United States as a stimulant for the heart and uterine muscle.

Perhaps one of the best works on the life and role of a Native health practitioner was written about a Comanche medicine woman, referred to by the Comanche as an Eagle Doctor. David Jones spent 3 years, from 1967 to 1970, researching and documenting Sanapia's work as a medicine woman. His account of Sanapia as a Comanche Eagle Doctor stands as one of the most in-depth studies written about the training and underlying philosophy of an individual Indian healer. Although Jones's work is specific to the Comanche, it is worth examining the plants Sanapia used for a couple of reasons. First, the bulk of what has been written on Native herbology, or ethnobotany, although identifying plants and their uses, rarely identify the tribes that used the plants, choosing instead to make the general statements that the plants identified were used by "Indians." Second, few have written on the process of how an individual was trained to become a healer. Third, it is rare for a Native healer to allow an outsider to know the contents of her or his medicine kit as Sanapia did with David Jones. In this regard, Dr. Brooks (1993) noted:

> Indian guides have supplied us with very effective preparations . . . I am fully convinced that most . . . medicine men also employ a good many valuable drugs of which we know nothing, and I am certain that scientific study of some of their preparations would be of great benefit to us . . . but it is extremely difficult to get them to tell us what these preparations were. (pp. 18–19)

In *Medicinal Uses of Plants by Indian Tribes of Nevada* (1957), Train and colleagues wrote,

> To walk up to an Indian and ask for his medicinal plant lore handed down from his ancestors would most certainly meet with a blank stare. . . . This information is zealously guarded, not only from the white man but sometimes from Indian neighbors as well. (Train, Henrichs, & Archer, 1957, pp. 3–4)

Turner et al. (1983) also write, "the same traditions of inheritance and secrecy of herbal knowledge were practiced by the Makah and Nootka [Nuu-chah-nulth]." Dr. Steele (2006) states, "Modern medicine is skeptical of some stories of Indian healing methods but we can't be sure. Scientists continue to search for the answers to the mysteries of Native American medicine, but many tribes have guarded specific details from outsiders." This is not surprising, especially

with such ethnocentric ideas as "The so-called medicine man of today is simply an individual just two jumps ahead of his fellow tribesmen and alert to the
opportunity presented to make money by acquiring medicinal plant knowledge
handed down to him from generations past" (Train et al., 1957, p. 2). Only to
follow this sentence with

> several of the latter, notably, Ike Shaw (Shoshone) of Beatty, Bronco
> Charlie (Shoshone) of Ruby Valley, and Dan Voorhees (Paiute) of
> Walker River Reservation, had a wide knowledge of medicinal plants
> and a substantial record of effective cures behind them. (Train et al.,
> 1957, p. 2)

This type of discourse is problematic and leaves one wondering not only about
the individual making the comment, but also about his views of the people who
worked with him. Was this said because of what he personally gained from
them, possibly at no cost to himself, or was it because he truly recognized the
knowledge they had? The damage that can arise from statements like Train's,
along with pursuits for capital gain, should make it easy to understand why
Indians would guard their knowledge of medicinal plants. It is because of such
concerns that one should also realize the significance of Sanapia revealing the
contents of her medicine kit to Jones, and how this offers insight into an area
that might otherwise have remained unknown.

An aspect that is quite consistent among Native healers in North America,
and to a high degree among other Indigenous cultures outside of North America,
is the integration of physical and spiritual realms when healing. Turner
writes, "Many illnesses are treated by both herbal and spiritual means; often the
treatments are inseparable. . . . Many medicines are taken in complete secrecy"
(Turner, Bouchard, & Kennedy, 1980, p. 150). Plotkin (1993) described the integration of these realms as supporting a belief:

> that a continuum exists between the natural and the supernatural,
> and that the forces of the physical world and spirit world exist in
> equilibrium. The shaman—a combination healer–priest—is at home in
> both worlds and is responsible for maintaining the balance between the
> two . . . the very survival of a tribe or village depends on the shaman's
> prowess at communicating with the other world and . . . guidance
> on proper spiritual conduct. But perhaps most important of all, the
> shaman is a powerful medicine man.
>
> The medicine man contacted the spirit world to diagnose an
> affliction and to determine what special plants might be used needed
> to treat it. The typical . . . shaman thus served not only as physician
> but also as priest, pharmacist, psychiatrist, and even psychopomp—
> one who conducts souls to the afterworld. (p. 203)

SANAPIA'S MEDICINE KIT

Similar to Marc Plotkin's description of a medicine man, Sanapia's medicine kit contained a combination of botanical and nonbotanical items that could address the physical, psychological, and spiritual needs of a patient (Jones, 1984, pp. 48–64). Table 6.1 shows a partial list of the types of plants Sanapia utilized in her practice as an Eagle Doctor.

Although tallow is most commonly used ceremonially by a number of Indian tribes, Richard Dunlop described a Cheyenne doctor who used tallow in something of a surgical maneuver on William Bent when a throat infection became life threatening. "The medicine man strung a sinew with sandburs and dipped it into hot buffalo tallow. This he forced down Bent's throat . . . When the tallow melted, he jerked the string out, pulling the infected membrane with it. Bent survived" (Dunlop, 1965, p. 14). An item that Sanapia used in concert with tallow was red paint, which she prepared from the dark red clay found around Geary, Oklahoma. The paint was always used as part of her blessing ceremonies, especially at the end of ghost sickness treatments when she would paint the faces and lower arms and legs of her patients. This particular aspect of using red clay and tallow to paint the face, and sometimes hands, of individuals is common among many Indian tribes in the United States when a ceremony has reached

TABLE 6.1 A Partial List of the Types of Plants Sanapia Utilized in Her Practice as an Eagle Doctor

NAME	USES/TREATMENTS	TYPE
Bone medicine	Wounds, infections, boils, painsa	Nonbotanical item
Broom weed	Eczema and rashes	Botanical item
Wild caraway	Tuberculosis	Botanical item
Iris	Colds, upset stomach, sore throat	Botanical item
It's gray	Sedative and seizure victims	Botanical item
Itse	Rattlesnake, scorpion, spider bites	Botanical item
Juniper	Menstrual cramps, vertigo, and headaches	Botanical item
Looks-like-feathers	Stomach ailments, tuberculosis, and postnatal hemorrhaging	Botanical item
Peyote	Sedative, colds, pneumonia, internal disorders, arthritis, severe headaches, and heart pains	Botanical item
Porcupine quills	Infant loneliness	Nonbotanical item
Prickly ash	Toothaches and burns	Botanical item
Red mescal beans	Ear infections and deep ear sores	Botanical item
Rye grass	Cataracts	Botanical item
Sneezeweed	Nasal congestion	Botanical item
Tallow	Severe burns and constipation	Nonbotanical
White otter fur	Melancholy	Nonbotanical item
White sage	Insect and spider bites	Botanical item

its end. Rye grass, although a plant (possibly *Leymus cinereus*), had an innovative and specialized use for treating cataracts (see http://www.bluestem.ca/elymus-cinereus.htm). Sanapia would take a single blade and use it to surgically scrape the afflicted eyes of patients until their cataracts were removed.

When medicinal plants were harvested, they were collected almost exclusively around early fall, after the plants had reached their fullest potency from the sun's exposure. The roots and tops of plants were of particular interest to Sanapia because of the power of earth and sun. Cedar and *peyote* are the exceptions to this. In examining the plants that made up Sanapia's kit, it should be noted that some were obtained from Indian doctors of other tribes, *dooltsa* being one such plant. Sanapia learned the medicinal properties of this plant from the Shoshone of the Wind River reservation in Wyoming.

Sanapia believed that the curative properties of peyote could heal most anything, and in addition to being her most utilized botanical medicine, it was also used for treating ghost sickness. Richard Schultes (1938), considered the father of ethnobotany, wrote that many Natives believed peyote to be a cure-all for most ailments. Peyote could be taken in different ways: in its natural or green state, dried, as a tea, and rolled into a cigarette and smoked; it has widespread use within the Native American Church (La Barre, 1969; Slotkin, 1975; Stuart, 1987). Of its uses within the Native American Church, William Lyon notes, "It has been used to treat fevers, rheumatism, and paralysis and as a poultice for fractures, open wounds, toothaches and snakebites" (Lyon, 1998, p. 191). It is interesting to note that although peyote contains over 50 different alkaloids, modern science knows little about the bulk of these. In 1995, I witnessed a ceremony in Maranda City in which a young girl with several food allergies, mostly dairy, but wheat, oats, and tomatoes as well, was treated. The girl has been free of these allergies to date.

In the *Shaman's Apprentice*, Plotkin (1993) wrote:

> Early on I realized that I would never be able to record more than a fraction of the ethnobotanical information possessed by the shamans. . . . Moreover, it soon became increasingly obvious to me that it was at least as important that the ethnobotanical wisdom be perpetuated within the tribes themselves. To accomplish this, the Indians and I developed a methodology we call the Shaman's Apprentice Program, a process by which my notes . . . are translated back into the local language and studied. . . . The individual then teaches the accumulated wisdom to other young members of the tribe. (p. 18)

In a similar vein, well-illustrated books, like Hutchens's (1992) *A Handbook of American Herbs*, which details the uses of some 125 medicinal plants, and the *Encyclopedia of Native American Healing*, which examines 350 years of shamanistic healing practices of Indians throughout North America, can function similarly to an apprentice program when in the hands of Indian health practitioners and learners, who may explore these and discover plant uses and possible new applications. Native healers not only utilize such resources but are also engaging in outreach efforts, as has been seen with Russell Willier, a Cree healer, and Alma Schnell of the Crow Nation in Montana, who on April 20, 2000, delivered a public talk at the University of Montana on medicinal plants and healing knowledge that dated back to her great-grandmother. Such outreach efforts can result in others answering the shaman's call.

COOPERATIVE EFFORTS, AND UNEASY ALIGNMENTS

Marc Plotkin was frustrated and at an impasse. Having gone in search of new treatments for diabetes among the Tirio Indians, he learned they had neither heard of the disease nor seen its symptoms. Dejected, he was ready to pack it in and leave for home when Akoi, a Sikiyana Indian, stopped to talk. Relating his disappointment that the Tirio knew nothing of diabetes, Akoi asked him to describe the disease. After hearing the symptoms, he stated,

> Maybe the Tirio don't know that sickness but I do. . . . First he used his machete to peel long strips of white bark off a towering tree. Then he added the crushed waxy leaves of a trailside herb. Next he sliced off the stems of a twisted gray vine . . . and collected the sap. We brought it all back to the village . . . the old shaman began boiling it all together over a wood fire. (Plotkin, 2001, pp. xii–xiii)

Uncertain, Plotkin asked the shaman to describe when and how it was used. "You wash with it when you're unable to urinate . . . and you drink it when your feet are sore. I was stunned. Clearly this was not a treatment for diabetes" (Plotkin, 2001, pp. xii–xiii). That night, Plotkin was rushed to assist a physician with a patient whose blood-sugar level was over 500. She was dying of type-2 diabetes, and there was nothing either could do to save her.

> The Sikiyana healer appeared . . . looked over the patient . . . and turned to me saying, "that is the disease I was telling you about. What are you going to give her?" We admitted that we had no medicine that could effectively treat her condition. (Plotkin, 2001, pp. xii–xiii)

Asking for the potion he made earlier, he gave her two teaspoons. "By the next morning her blood-sugar level was almost normal. . . . By the end of the week, her blood-sugar level was normal and the gangrenous sores . . . had started to heal" (Plotkin, 2001, pp. xii–xiii).

In September of 2010, a Native man walked into my office and ceremonially asked for my assistance. His son-in-law was in prison and had bowel cancer. Chemotherapy had caused his lower intestines to swell, all efforts to reduce this had failed, his health and well-being had become critical, and the general thought was that he had very little time left to live. I was told that the man did not want to die in the prison, but for reasons unclear to me, the warden would not allow him early release. This struck me as odd since he was scheduled to go before a parole board in 3 to 4 weeks. I wondered what horrible crime he had committed. The crime, for which he had served 3 years, was for domestic violence. After unsuccessfully trying to contact law professors at the university, I then turned to the Indian liaison at the state capital building. She suggested I contact the warden, which I did. After a somewhat long conversation, the warden agreed not only to allow the man's son-in-law to be admitted to Missoula St. Patrick's Hospital, but also cleared it with hospital administrators that a Native "doctor" could see him. I was present for this and observed how the officer in charge and hospital attendants were respectful when the patient was being "doctored." The patient was administered a mix of several different plants that were prepared as a tea that he drank twice a day. Surprisingly, neither hospital staff nor the officer in charge ever questioned the tea. After 3 days, the swelling subsided, and as of April 2011, doctors have not fully understood what caused his cancer to disappear. Although cooperative efforts between hospitals and Native healers are not a new occurrence, at one time this collaboration was infrequent, but over the past 25 years has shown signs of increased acceptance and cooperation have begun.

David Young, lead author of *Cry of the Eagle*, knew Russell Willier as a Cree medicine man and associate, and also as the man who kept his wife alive when doctors at an Edmonton hospital did not seem to know how to. David was first exposed to Russell's knowledge of medicinal plants one day in June 1985:

> [W]e walked with Russell through the woods at the western shores of Lesser Slave Lake, and Russell pointed out the various plants and trees he uses in his doctoring. . . . He knelt before a plant, prayed in Cree and placed a handful of tobacco in the ground. He was now allowed to take some of the plants of that species for medicine. . . . Periodically, when Russell was reluctant to disclose the specific use of a plant, he would simply tell us that "it goes in a combination" (Young, Ingram, & Schwartz, 1989, pp. 56–57)

Native doctors like Russell represent a changing perspective among a small group of Indian healers who are stepping forward to work in cooperation with health clinics and hospitals in the interest of healing. Dr. Mehl-Madrona (2008), of the University of Saskatchewan's College of Medicine, noted,

> Native American healing practices are being requested by Native Americans and non-Natives alike. A series of meetings among traditional Native American healers . . . resulted in a dialogue . . . how treatment could proceed . . . to introduce interested non-Natives to Native American healing practices.

Dr. Mehl-Madrona (2008) also stated, "Recent years have shown a surge of interest in the therapies of traditional cultures. . . . Some hospitals have included traditional Native American healers as part of their staff. Harvard University has created a Center to study alternative medicine." There are those who would view this as a risky route to take, yet taking such risks has brought a level of respect to an ancient practice in a modern era of Indian healing.

CONCLUSIONS

In reexamining the present status of Native people's traditional healing knowledge through plants, I am reminded of a grade-school question: "If a tree falls in the forest, is there a sound even though no one hears it?" I remember when asked this in fourth grade. When a few children ventured a yes, the teacher's response was that a sound could only exist if a person were in the forest to hear it. I was puzzled how the teacher could dismiss the fact that animals would hear the sound. When I brought this up, I was dismissed. This is often the arrogance of Western science: if it has not been observed, studied, and validated by their "experts," then it is either insignificant, does not exist, or is not true until it has been validated. Nevertheless, it is worth noting how long "science" was mystified by the flight of the bumblebee, and how the inability to scientifically explain this, which has finally been understood, never stopped or even slowed the flight of bumblebees. The point is that although Indians' knowledge of medicinal plants may not be where it was 80 years ago, it cannot be said that because science is not aware of the extent of that knowledge, it does not exist, or might even be experiencing a comeback. It further remains of interest that those people who hold biased perspectives, believing Native people's knowledge and use of medicinal plants must be acknowledged by Western science to be valid, invalidate a body of literature that has existed for well over 80 years by Western scientists and doctors whose research has not only been acknowledged by the scientific world, but has also been instrumental in synthesizing alkaloids from Native medicinal plants for use by pharmaceutical companies and the medical industry. Table 6.2 shows but a small list of pharmaceutical compounds derived from plants, with their therapeutic standing within the medical sciences, that have resulted through researching how these plants have been used medicinally by Native peoples. Moerman (2000), who discusses over 2,500 plant species in his book *Native American Ethnobotany*, states, "The first thing people usually ask about American Indian medicinal plants is, Do they work? . . . The short answer is yes" (p. 12).

Pharmaceutical companies, well aware of the financial benefits that can be gained by acquiring this knowledge from Native peoples, state without hesitation that it could mean billions of dollars to their companies. The process through which this knowledge is acquired, which people see as bringing credibility to the value of these plants, allows the explorers, researchers, and industries to remove Native people from the equation as the source from which it was first discovered. Over time, these acts, as history has shown through other alienating acts, can diminish and endanger the transmission of a Native tradition

TABLE 6.2 Clinically Useful Drugs From Tropical Rain Forest Plants

COMPOUND NAME	PLANT SOURCE	THERAPEUTIC CATEGORY IN MEDICAL SCIENCES
Ajmalicine	*Rauvolfia serpentina* (L.) Benth. ex Kurz (Apocynaceae) (Indian snakeroot)	Circulatory stimulant
Andrographolide	*Andrographis paniculata* Nees (Acanthaceae) (Karyat)	Antibacterial
Arecoline	*Areca catechu* L. (Arecaceae; Betel-nut palm)	Anthelmintic
Asiaticoside	*Centella asiatica* (L.) Urban (Apiaceae; Indian pennywort)	Vulnerary
Atropine[a]	*Duboisia myoporoides* R. Br. (Solanaceae) (Australian cork tree)	Anticholinergic
Bromelain[a]	*Ananas comosus* (L.) Merrill (Bromeliaceae) (Pineapple)	Antiinflammatory/ Proteolytic
Camphor[a]	*Cinnamomum camphora* (L.) Nees & Eberm. (Lauraceae; Camphor tree)	Rubefacient
Chymopapain[a]	*Carica papaya* L. (Caricaceae; Papaya)	Proteolytic/ Mucolytic
Cocaine[a]	*Erythroxylum coca* Lam. (Erythroxlaceae) (Coca)	Local anesthetic
Curcumin	*Curcuma longa* L. (Zingiberaceae; Turmeric)	Choleretic
Deserpidine[a]	*Rauvolfia tetraphylla* L. (Apocynaceae) (Snakeroot)	Antihypertensive/ Tranquilizer
L-Dopa[a,b]	*Mucuna deeringiana* (Bort.) Merrill (Fabaceae; Velvet Bean)	Antiparkinsonism
Emetine[a]	*Cephaelis ipecacuanha* (Brot.) A. Richard (Rubiaceae; Ipecac)	Amebicide/ Emetic
Glaucarubin	*Simarouba glauca* DC. (Simaroubaceae) (Paradise tree)	Amebicide
Glaziovine	*Ocotea glaziovii* Mez. (Lauraceae) (Yellow cinnamon)	Antidepressant
Gossypol	*Gossypium* spp. (Malvaceae; Cotton)	Male contraceptive
Hyoscyamine[a]	*Duboisia myoporoides* R.Br. (Solanaceae) (Australian cork tree)	Anticholinergic
Kawaina	*Piper methysticum* Forst. f. (Piperaceae) (Kava-kava)	Tranquilizer
Monocrotaline	*Crotalaria spectabilis* Roth (Fabaceae) (Rattlebox)	Antitumor agent (topical)
Neoandrographolide	*Andrographis paniculata* Nees (Acanthaceae)	Dysentery
Nicotine	*Nicotiana tabacum* L. (Solanaceae) (Tobacco)	Insecticide

(continued)

TABLE 6.2 Clinically Useful Drugs From Tropical Rain Forest Plants (*continued*)

COMPOUND NAME	PLANT SOURCE	THERAPEUTIC CATEGORY IN MEDICAL SCIENCES
Ouabain[a]	*Strophanthus gratus* (Hook.) Baill. (Apocynaceae; Twisted flower)	Cardiotonic
Papain[a]	*Carica papaya* L. (Caricaceae) (Papaya)	Proteolytic/Mucolytic
Physostigmine[a]	*Physostigma venenosum* Balf. (Leguminosae) (Ordeal Bean)	Anticholinesterase
Picrotoxin	*Anamirta cocculus* (L.) Wright & Arn. (Fish berry)	Analeptic
Pilocarpine[a]	*Pilocarpus jaborandi* Holmes (Rutaceae) (Jaborandi)	Parasympathomimetic
Quinidine[a]	*Cinchona ledgeriana* Moens ex Trimen (Rubiaceae; Yellow cinchona)	Antiarrhythmic
Quinine[a]	*Cinchona ledgeriana* Moens ex Trimen (Rubiaceae; Yellow cinchona)	Antimalarial/ Antipyretic
Quisqualic acid	*Quisqualis indica* L. (Combretaceae) (Rangoon creeper)	Anthelmintic
Rescinnami[a]	*Rauvolfia serpentina* (L.) Benth. ex Kurz (Apocynaceae; Indian snakeroot)	Anthypertensive/ Tranquilizer
Reserpine[a]	*Rauvolfia serpentina* (L.) Benth. ex Kurz (Apocynaceae; Indian snakeroot)	Antihypertensive/ Tranquilizer
Rorifone	*Rorippa indica* (L.) Hiern (Brassicaceae) (Nasturtium)	Antitussive
Rotenone	*Lonchocarpus nicou* (Aubl.) DC. (Fabaceae; Cube root)	Piscicide
Scopolamine[a]	*Datura metel* L. (Solanaceae) (Recurved thorapple)	Sedative
Stevioside	*Stevia rebaudiana* Hemsley (Compositae) (Sweet herb; Ka'a He'e)	Sweetener
Strychnine	*Strychnos nux-vomica* L. (Loganiaceae) (Nux vomica)	Central nervous system stimulant
Theobromine	*Theobroma cacao* L. (Sterculiaceae) (Cocoa, cacao)	Diuretic/Vasodilator
Tubocurarine[a]	*Chondrodendron tomentosum* R. & P. (Menispermaceae; Curare)	Skeletal muscle
Vasicine (Peganine)	*Adhatoda vasica* Nees (Acanthaceae)	Oxytocic
Vinblastine[a]	*Catharanthus roseus* (L.) G.Don (Apocynaceae; rosy periwinkle)	Antitumor agent
Yohimbine	*Pausinystalia yohimbe* (K.Schum.) Pierre ex Beille (Rubiaceae)	Adrenergic blocker Aphrodisiac

[a]Currently used in the United States.
[b]Now also synthesized commercially.
Source: Farnsworth (1988), Soejarto and Farnsworth (1989).

of healing through plants to successive generations. It is the hope, however, that through the published research of those scholars who have worked with and acknowledged tribal elders' medicinal plant knowledge, and those Native "doctors" who have engendered cooperative alliances with hospital administrators who have allowed them to extend their care to hospitalized patients, that this knowledge will remain to serve not only Native people's health needs, but non-Native people's as well.

STUDY QUESTIONS

♦ Pharmaceutical companies openly state that learning curative knowledge of Indigenous healers can result in a billion-dollar market for them. Yet the people from whom this knowledge comes often gain little to nothing. Are there ethical problems that this raises?

♦ Many Native people are very closed to having outsiders learn their knowledge of medicinal plants. In the face of centuries of dispossession, religious and cultural persecution, why should Indians change this attitude when corporations are the ones that profit (this is not restricted to monetary gain)?

REFERENCES

Association of Schools of Public Health. (1987, July–August). *Public Health Reports* 102(4), 352–356.

Brooks, H. (1933). The medicine of the American Indian. *Journal of Laboratory and Clinical Medicine, XIX*(1), 16–17.

Davies, W. (2001). *Healing ways, Navajo health care in the twentieth century.* Albuquerque, NM: University of New Mexico Press.

Dorgan, B. (2010). *2010 Senate Committee on Indian Affairs.* Retrieved from http://www.indian.senate.gov/news/press-release/dorgan-investigates-allegations-gross-mismanagement-within-indian-health-service

Dunlop, R. (1965). *Doctors of the American frontier.* New York, NY: Doubleday Press.

Farnsworth, N. R. (1988). Screening plants for new medicines. In Wilson (Ed.), *Biodiversity* (pp. 83–97). Washington, DC: National Academies Press.

Hutchens, A. R. (1991). *Indian herbalogy of North American.* Boston, MA: Shambhala Publications.

Hutchens, A. R. (1992). *A handbook of American herbs.* Boston, MA: Shambhala Publications.

Hussain, A. (2003). A fatal fat embolism. *Internet Journal of Anesthesiology, 8*(2). Retrieved from http://ispub.com/IJA/8/2/8579

Jones, D. E. (1984). *Sanapia: Comanche medicine woman.* Prospect Heights, IL: Waveland Press.

La Barre, W. (1969). *The peyote cult.* New York, NY: Schocken Books.

Lawrence, J. (2000). The Indian Health Service and the sterilization of Native American women. *American Indian Quarterly, 24*(3), 400–419.

Lyon, W. S. (1998). *Encyclopedia of Native American healing.* New York, NY: W. W. Norton.

Mehl-Madrona, L. E. (2008). Development of an integrated program with conventional American medicine and evaluation of effectiveness. In *Traditional (Native American) Indian medicine treatment of chronic illness.* Retrieved from www.healing-arts.org/mehl-madrona/mmtraditionalpaper.htm

Meriam, L. (1928). *The problem of Indian administration.* Baltimore, MD: The Johns Hopkins Press.

Moerman, D. E. (2000). *Native American ethnobotany.* Portland, OR: Timber Press.

Plotkin, M. (1993). *Tales of a Shaman's apprentice.* New York, NY: Penguin Books.

Plotkin, M. (2001). *Medicine quest.* New York, NY: Penguin Books.

Schultes, R. E. (1938). The appeal of peyote (*Lophophora williamsii*) as a medicine. *American Anthropologist, 40*(4), 698–715.

Slotkin, J. S. (1975). *The peyote religion: A study in Indian–White relations.* New York, NY: Octagon Books.

Smith, H. (1928). *Ethnobotany of the Meskwaki Indians.* Milwaukee, WI: Bulletin of the Public Museum of the City of Milwaukee.

Soejarto, D. D., & Farnsworth, N. R. (1989). Tropical rain forests: potential source of new drugs? *Perspectives in Biology and Medicine, 32*(2), 244–256.

Steele, V. (2006). *Bleed, blister and purge: A history of medicine on the American Frontier.* Missoula, MT: Mountain Press.

Stuart, O. (1987). *Peyote religion: A history.* Norman, OK: University of Oklahoma Press.

Train, P., Henrichs, J. R., & Archer, W. A. (1957). *Medicinal uses of plants by Indian tribes of Nevada.* Lawrence, MA: Quarterman Publications.

Turner, N. J., Thomas, J., Carlson, B. F., & Ogilvie, R. T. (1983). *Ethnobotony of the Nitinaht Indians of Vancouver Island* (Occasional Paper No. 24). Prince George, BC: British Columbia Provincial Museum.

Turner, N. J., Bouchard, R., & Kennedy, D. I. D. (1980). *Ethnobotony of the Okanagan-Colville Indians of British Columbia and Washington* (Occasional Paper No. 21). Prince George, BC, Canada: British Columbia Provincial Museum.

Vogel, V. J. (1990). *American Indian medicine.* Norman, OK: University of Oklahoma Press.

Wilson, K., & Young, T. K. (2008). An overview of Aboriginal health research in the social sciences: Current trends and future directions. *Finland: International Journal of Circumpolar Health, 67,* 179–189.

Young, D., Ingram, G., & Schwartz, L. (1989). *Cry of the eagle: Encounters with a Cree healer.* Toronto, Canada: University of Toronto Press.

Zubrek, E. M. (1994). Traditional native healing: Alternative or adjunct to modern medicine? *College of Family Physicians of Canada, 40,* 1923–1931.

PART II

Nursing in the 10 Cultural Areas: Regional and Tribal Issues for Nurses

*I*n Part I of this text, we provided an overview of Indigenous America in terms of intersecting ideas in American Indian/Alaska Native (AI/AN) thought and the tenets of nursing. We looked at national and historical pre- and post-contact influences and outcomes, especially on health. And we explored the roots of nursing before there *was* a profession. A description of the Indian Health Service, Tribal Health, and Urban Health Care (I/T/U) system for Indian health and what nursing looks like within the system were provided. And the final chapter in Part I gave a description with examples of some of the indigenous healing practices a nurse may encounter when caring for the AI/AN patient.

The beginning of the text was meant to introduce the reader to a *national* picture and understanding of shared experiences and beliefs. Part II shows how these experiences are/were played out in the various cultural regions of the United States. It is unlikely any nurse, AI/AN or not, would be able to innately offer culturally appropriate care to people of 566 distinct federally recognized tribes and 66 state tribes. Nurses who are indigenous do not know the practices and beliefs of all groups. Nurses who are non-Native do not know the practices and beliefs of all groups. Nurses in the rural or reservation areas, AI/AN or not, do not necessarily understand the urban AI/AN, and vice versa for urban nurses. Therefore, the body of this section breaks AI/AN care into 10 cultural groups where languages, beliefs, history, and geography will be similar even though differences do exist.

Note that the Northwest and the Plateau areas are offered as one unit but recognized as two of the 10 cultural groups. Urban has been added to the regional groups found in the 48 contiguous states and Alaska.

In breaking the nation up into these groups, the intent is to make Indigenous America and its populations, potential and actual patients, more understood, and care more targeted. Geography, environment, history, and circumstances are all a part of the AI/AN patient profile as much as the HbA1c, blood pressure, or body mass index. Following a traditional approach, the chapters will begin with the cultural groups starting in the East and moving clockwise to the north followed by the urban area (Figure II.1).

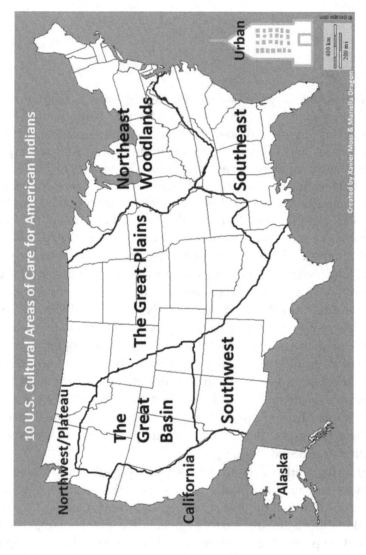

FIGURE II.1 The 10 U.S. cultural areas of care for American Indians and Alaska Natives.

Source: Courtesy of Xavier Moss and Mariella Dragon.

SEVEN

AI/AN Elders: Mapping Cultural Areas and Regional Variances in Health[1]

Margaret P. Moss

LEARNING OBJECTIVES
♦ To explain why maps are useful in describing a population that is 1% of the nation
♦ To identify health and function issues in American Indian elders
♦ To examine geographic information systems (GIS) as a viable research methodology in American Indian health
♦ To be able to distinguish functional disability variances by region in American Indians

KEY TERMS
♦ ADLs—activities of daily living
♦ GIS—geographic information systems

♦ IADLs—instrumental activities of daily living
♦ Mapping/cartography

KEY CONCEPTS
♦ Functional disability
♦ Health disparities

♦ Regional variations
♦ Underrepresented populations

Several concepts are presented in this chapter. First, it was important to add a research article into this nursing text. There is a dearth of research by American Indian nurses on American Indian populations in the literature, and even less on the elderly American Indian population. Second, a thread that runs throughout most AI/AN tribes is that elders are a source of history, caring, and teaching. They are culturally to be revered, and yet they suffer from extreme poverty, high functional disability, few resources, including health, and shorter life spans than all other U.S. races (Moss, 2006).

---

[1] This article was first published as Moss, M. P., Schell, M. C., & Goins, R. T. (2006). Using GIS in a first national mapping of functional disability among older American Indians and Alaska natives from the 2000 census. *International Journal of Health Geographics, 5*, 37. (Used with permission.)

Third, this chapter introduces the idea of looking at American Indian health beyond the idea of a monolithic race, and instead considers regional variances. Although a national database is used—the United States Census Bureau—results differ regionally, which is easily shown using geography and maps. Maps are useful when there are only 4 million or so (depending on data used) American Indians in a country of 320 million individuals (U.S. Census, 2015). One can "see" data on maps representing these often "invisible on the charts" people.

BACKGROUND

This study used geographical information systems (GIS) in the examination of functional disability in AI/ANs. GIS have not been used in nursing research "as a tool in the fight against disease" (Graham, Atkinson, & Danson, 2004, p. 219). Mapping and spatial analysis have largely remained tools used in the realm of public health. The largest area for GIS and chronic disease mapping, for instance, lies in cancer reporting (Brown, Eccles, & Wallis, 2001; Mullee, De Stavola, Romanengo, & Coleman, 2004). Most of these reports appear to originate out-side of the United States. In Hungary, one study was conducted that used the National Public Health Service to establish monitoring in primary care facilities on selected chronic diseases (Szeles et al., 2005). Another study from the United Kingdom points to GIS as an important tool with which to "join up" government and geographical data between agencies in tackling health issues (Higgs, Smith, & Gould, 2005). These resources are lacking in the United States. The Centers for Disease Control and Prevention (CDC) do track certain infectious diseases deemed reportable and rely on health agencies to supply the data. However, there is no national health system or coordination among health facilities in the United States, and, therefore, no ready database to track noninfectious, nonreportable chronic diseases. In fact, the GIS and health field internationally are largely filled with infectious disease studies and those on the effects of environmental pollut-ants (Briggs, 2005; Weinberg, 2005).

However, in the United States, where the public health focus has shifted from infectious diseases to chronic diseases (CDC, 2003), it will be important to trans-late this new technology for use in the chronic disease arena. American Indians, as a subpopulation of the United States, often suffer from chronic diseases at rates often two to three times higher than that of any other U.S. group. Although much is known about the high levels of chronic disease rates among AI/ANs (Administration on Aging, 1996; CDC, 2003; Indian Health Services [IHS], 1998; U.S. Department of Health and Human Services, 2001), little is known about functional disability among older AI/ANs. Chronic diseases affect AI/ANs at younger ages compared with the overall population, and with some diseases, at higher rates. For example, young adults age 25 to 44 years had an adjusted mortality rate of 26 per 100,000 for heart disease compared with 18 among same-aged Whites, and 8 per 100,000 died of diabetes compared with 3 among Whites (IHS, 1998). One tribe, the Pimas of Arizona, have the highest known prevalence of diabetes in the world (CDC, 2003). Arthritis, one of the primary causes of disability, is also high among older AI/ANs ("Prevalence and Impact," 1996).

In addition, the high prevalence of risk factors for chronic disease, such as obesity, alcohol, and tobacco use, has been well documented in AI/AN populations (IHS, 1998). Functional disability can be seen as an indication of the *impact* of chronic disease (Kelly-Hayes, Jette, Wolf, D'Agostino, & Odell, 1992). Measures of disability most widely used include limitations in activities of daily living and instrumental activities of daily living (Katz, Ford, Moskowitz, Jackson, & Jaffe, 1963). Functional status has been demonstrated as the single most important indicator for long-term care use (Kane & Kane, 1981). One factor that has made it difficult to develop a national profile of functional disability both for the population at large and for AI/ANs is the heterogeneity of the population. As of December 2003, there were 562 federally recognized tribes, speaking over 200 languages (Bureau of Indian Affairs, 2003), a number that does not include state tribes, federally unrecognized tribes, as well as urban populations. American Indian communities are largely unlinked by any comprehensive data source around functional disability.

In examining function and disability, this study employed the U.S. 2000 Census as the link to locate and describe the prevalence of functional limitation in AI/ANs at the turn of the 21st century. To date, relatively few studies have examined functional disability among older AI/ANs (Chapleski & Dwyer, 1995; Chapleski, Lichtenberg, Dwyer, Youngblade, & Tsai, 1997; Goins, Spencer, Roubideaux, & Manson, 2005; Hayward & Heron, 1999; Hennessy, John, & Roy, 1999; Kramer, 1999; Moss, Roubideaux, Jacobsen, Buchwald, & Manson, 2004; Waidmann & Liu, 2000). Prevalence estimates indicate that older AI/ANs experience some of the highest disability rates compared with other U.S. racial groups. Data from the Medicare Current Beneficiary Survey found that 30.1% of AI/ANs had a limitation in at least one ADL compared with 17.0% of their White counterparts (Waidmann & Liu, 2000). A study of 294 AI/AN elders in Los Angeles reported much lower percentages of functional disability, with toileting (4.9%) as the least frequent limitation and mobility (13.1%) as the highest (Kramer, 1999). In an attempt to gather national information on ADL limitations experienced by older AI/ANs, a survey was initiated by the National Resource Center on Native American Aging (NRCNAA). Moss and colleagues used the NRCNAA survey to conduct a secondary analysis focused on 90 older members of the Zuni tribe (Moss, Roubideaux, Jacobsen, Buchwald, & Manson, 2004). In this study, the mean number of ADL limitations was 1.4, with the most frequent ADL limitation in bathing (40%) and the least frequent in eating (11%). The results of this study indicated that the rates of disability were two to three times higher than those found in the Kramer study.

The problem addressed by this chapter is the lack of a national picture of the nature or extent of functional disability among older AI/ANs or whether there are differences by area of residence with regard to functional status. Mapping the occurrence and severity of functional disability among older AI/ANs can provide valuable information that can guide further inquiry.

The CDC does have a state-by-state database on behavioral health, the Behavioral Risk Factor Surveillance System (BRFSS). The BRFSS is a telephone survey that gathers largely state-level data related to chronic care (CDC, n.d.). The difficulty with this type of survey for AI/AN elderly is in the method itself. More AI/ANs in Indian country do *not* have a telephone than those who do (U.S. Census, n.d.-d). When considering the elderly, the percentage who have telephones drops. There are several tribes where elders either do not speak English or it is not their first language. For example, Navajo has almost 300,000 members 75% of whom still speak their language. Therefore, lack of phones, communication problems, and conceptual differences, that is, orality versus literacy, all point away from telephone use as an effective method for data gathering on AI/AN elders, particularly in Indian country. The census data are collected in person and in the mail with targeted efforts in Indian country.

There has been one attempt to gather national information on ADLs on AI/AN elderly specifically, namely, a survey initiated by the NRCNAA. The primary author used their survey to conduct a secondary analysis focused on just one tribe (Moss, Roubideaux, Jacobsen, Buchwald, & Manson, 2004). In this study of 90 Zuni elders, the mean number of ADL limitations was 1.4, with bathing (40%) the most frequent ADL limitation in and eating (11%) the least frequent. Therefore, these elders should be considered disabled, with rates from two to three times higher than those found in the Kramer study. These widely divergent results point to the need to understand spatial, tribal, and other differences in disability rates for AI/ANs. There were severe limitations in the NRCNAA survey for use in research. First, it was conceived for administrative purposes. The other survey problems included its use of convenience sampling, scaling errors in not providing a way to answer "no" to having limitations or chronic conditions, and a long-term care question that provided only two options—nursing home or assisted living. Along with survey construction issues, there were methodological issues such as bias in forming the questions. For example, the survey asks about sweat lodge use and church attendance. Many tribes do neither; these are largely Plains Indian activities. Therefore, the challenge is to use more creative methods to get at a national inclusive picture of functional disability in AI/ANs, and their current long-term care options. When the author retooled the instrument and used random sampling, the functional disability numbers dropped dramatically.

The purpose of this study was to create a first-national map of functional disability for AI/ANs aged 65 years and older. It is imperative to gain a picture of the nature and extent of functional disability among older adults so that access points to care, long-term care options, and availability data will inform policy and health care decisions and funding will correspond with need. The specific aims of the current study were to use census data to identify how many AI/ANs over age 65 report functional disability, and map spatial patterns of disability to assess any regional and rural/urban differences in functional disability.

METHOD

Geographical sampling and analyses were used in "traditional" location-based methods (Briggs, 2005) to provide visual analyses, that is, mapped evidence (Rytkonen, 2004) for functional disability patterns in AI/ANs from the U.S. 2000 Census. The utility of basic mapping is presented in this chapter. Simple overlays of the census data onto geography provide the basis for this study's methodology.

Sample

The United States performs a census of its population every 10 years, counting total population and asking detailed questions about demographics, housing, and income. This study was a secondary data analysis of the 2000 Census. Persons included for this analysis were age 65 years and older and self-identified as one race, "American Indian or Alaska Native." The 2000 Census was the first to allow the respondent to choose more than one race in identifying oneself. So as not to confound the results, the analysis included only those who chose one race. Further, as this was a "first look" we wanted to understand the picture of those who identify as American Indian "more than any other group." The rationale for this was that someone may have had a great-grandmother who was Indian and so checks the box for American Indian, although the risk factors and geographical and cultural differences may not exist or may not be prominent. These disparities are what we are attempting to map for this article. In 2000, 138,439 persons older than 65 years identified themselves as AI/ANs and no other race. Institutional review board approval was given by the University of Minnesota.

Measures

Data on disability status were derived from the Census "long form," which was sent to approximately one in six households in 2000. The Census distributes long forms randomly within geographic areas at rates that differ by population density. Rural areas are surveyed at rates higher than the nationwide average of one in six, and urban areas are sampled at rates lower than one in six (U.S. Census, n.d.-a). These data are extrapolated by the Census Bureau to create data for the entire population, and the extrapolated data were used in the analysis. According to tables on the U.S. Census website, there were only 11,578 males and 22,466 females over 65 years who identified as one race, AI/ANs, who lived alone. This is out of a total of almost 140,000 households with 65-year-olds and over who identified as one race: AI/ANs (U.S. Census, n.d.-c). Over 75% of all of these elders live with others. We would reasonably expect that the one in six households with AI/AN elders representing both genders answered these questions, or about 23,070.

In the Census questionnaire, ADL-targeted queries are worded differently than are standard ADL and IADL items. Standard ADL items often ask whether the participant needs no assistance, some assistance, or complete assistance with the standard measures of walking, bathing, and so on. The U.S. Census uses "yes" and "no" as the choices for whether one experiences functional limitations.

According to McBride, one or more ADL limitations are disabling, and two or more are severely disabling (McBride, 1989). One limitation of census disability data is that it reports counts of each disability within a unit of geography, so it is not possible to determine whether the same individual is appearing in the same counts. It is therefore not possible to address issues related to more than one disability. However, the census data do include one derived disability count, which is the total number of individuals responding affirmatively to any one or more of the disability questions. This derived count is utilized in Figures 7.2 and 7.5 of the analysis.

Impairment

The items in the U.S. Census used to define impairments included affirmative answers to question 16a ("Does this person have any of the following long-lasting conditions: Blindness, deafness, or a severe vision or hearing impairment?") and 17a ("Because of a physical, mental, or emotional condition lasting 6 months or more, does this person have any difficulty in doing the following activities: Learning, remembering, or concentrating?").

IADL Loss

Answering "yes" to question 17 ("Because of a physical, mental, or emotional condition lasting 6 months or more, does this person have any difficulty in doing the following activities?"), part c ("Going outside the home alone to shop or visit a doctor's office"), and part d ("Working at a job or business") was used to define IADL loss.

ADL Loss

Answering "yes" to question 16b ("Does this person have any of the following long-lasting conditions: A condition that substantially limits one or more basic physical activities such as walking, climbing stairs, reaching, lifting, or carrying?") and 17b ("Because of a physical, mental, or emotional condition lasting 6 months or more, does this person have any difficulty in doing the following activities: Dressing, bathing, or getting around inside the home?") was used to define ADL loss.

PROCEDURE

County-level data were extracted from Summary File 4 of the Census using a compact disc dataset issued by the Census Bureau. The data extracted were for tables PCT69 through PCT75 for AI/ANs older than age 65, which is the dataset for AI/ANs answering "yes" to any question falling under number 16 or 17 on the long form pertaining to impairment, IADL loss, and ADL loss. The resulting tabular data were imported into the GIS software program ArcView (Version 9, ERSI, 2005). The geographical data in a GIS, such as a file containing counties of the United States, commonly have attribute data associated with them. The table of disability data extracted from the Census contains one record per county, and the full dataset was brought into the GIS by joining each record to a county in the GIS. The resulting GIS dataset is richer than the original extracted data because, in addition to race, age, and disability information, the records have a spatial component that can be used in further analysis (i.e., cartographic visualization). Using the ADL/IADL data from the U.S. Census, spatial patterns of disability were mapped using varying levels of geographic overlays such as country, region, state, and urban/rural and reservation. (For a more comprehensive description of GIS use, see Moss and Schell [2004].)

Several of the maps are reproduced in the results reported here. Because the aim of the study was to create a preliminary nationwide picture of elder AI/AN disability levels, the maps attempt to present as much nationwide detail as possible, while at the same time not becoming so cluttered as to be unreadable. Counties were chosen as the unit of analysis for two reasons. First, in most cases it remains possible to distinguish individual counties at the scale reproduced in a typical journal article. Any greater level of detail, such as census tracts, would be unreadable. Second, counties were chosen to avoid constraints placed on census data to protect confidentiality. If the number of American Indians (or any race, respectively) is below 50 for a unit of analysis, no data are reported. The vast majority of the total AI/AN elder population (89%) can be found in counties with over 50 AI/ANs. However, at any smaller unit of analysis, the number of elder AI/ANs included in the results falls precipitously. Three thematic map types are employed to visualize nationwide levels of impairment in AI/AN elders. Figures 7.1 and 7.4 are known as proportional symbol maps, where the size of the symbol, in this case a square, is proportional to a quantity, in this case AI/AN elders. Proportional-symbol maps are most appropriate for visualizing counts of data, especially when the size of the data being mapped does not correspond to the spatial unit of analysis. In this case, small counties that are difficult to see may have large numbers of the variable being mapped. The second type of map, used in Figure 7.2, is a choropleth map in which the color of the county corresponds to the percentage of the variable being mapped. Choropleth maps are most appropriate for normalized data, such as rates of disability. The third map type, employed in Figure 7.3, is a dot map. Dot maps

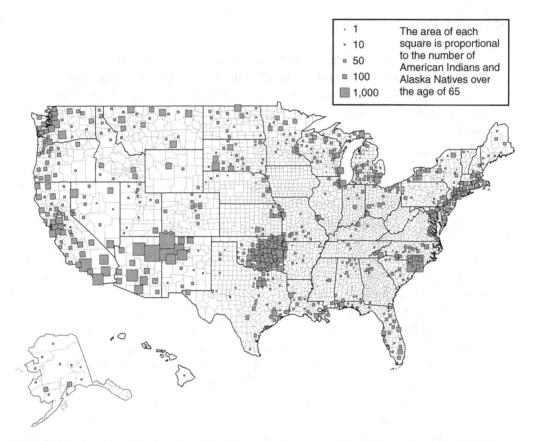

FIGURE 7.1 National distribution of AI/ANs age 65 years and older from the U.S. 2000 Census. *Source:* U.S. Census Bureau (2000).

create an impression of density and are most appropriate for showing distribution of a discrete population over space.

Raw counts of the number of AI/ANs age 65 and older, by county, are mapped in Figure 7.1 in order to give a general overview of the population distribution. The percentage of AI/AN elders who responded affirmatively to either of the functional disability questions—16 or 17—in the census questionnaire is depicted in Figure 7.2. This is a derived quantity, and does not provide detail on differences among impairment, IADL loss, and ADL loss. In Figure 7.3, we attempt to provide more detail. Part A of Figure 7.3 maps the ADL loss corresponding to census question 16b ("Does this person have any of the following long-lasting conditions: A condition that substantially limits one or more basic physical activities such as walking, climbing stairs, reaching, lifting, or carrying?"). Part B maps a second ADL loss, corresponding to census question 17b ("Because of a physical, mental, or emotional condition lasting 6 months or more, does this person have any difficulty in doing the following

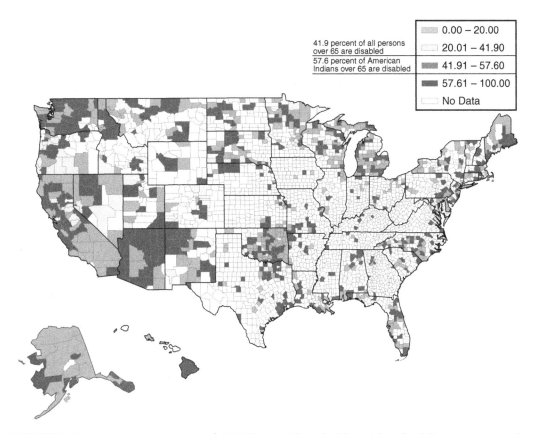

FIGURE 7.2 National distribution of AI/ANs age 65 and older with a disability as compared to all persons over 65 with a disability from the U.S. 2000 Census.
Source: U.S. Census Bureau (2000).

activities: Dressing, bathing, or getting around inside the home?"). Lastly, part C maps the IADL loss corresponding to Census question 17c ("Going outside the home alone to shop or visit a doctor's office").

Cartographic (mapping) visualization, in turn, suggests spatial patterns that can be explored further using other forms of quantitative analysis. Two clear patterns of functional disability that appear are differences between regions of the country, and differences between rural and urban areas. In the numbers reported on regional differences, the disability rates are further aggregated into four regions, Northeast, South, Midwest, and West, as defined by the Census Bureau (U.S. Census, n.d.-b). When reporting differences between urban and rural counties, urban counties were defined as those that are a part of a metropolitan statistical area, and rural counties as those that are not. The U.S. Office of Management and Budget makes determinations on which areas qualify as metropolitan statistical areas (U.S. Census, 2000).

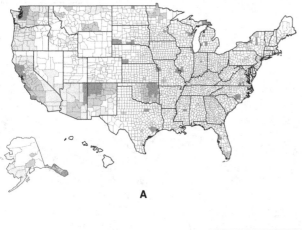

A

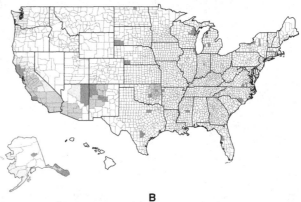

B

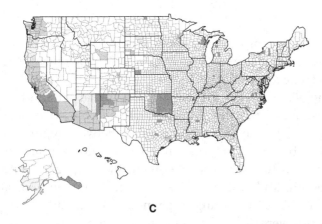

C

FIGURE 7.3 National distribution of disability in AI/ANs 65 and over for seleceted ADLs/
IADLs from the U.S. 2000 Census: (A) basic physical disability (e.g., walking),
(B) self-care disability (e.g., bathing), and (C) getting out and about.

Source: U.S. Census Bureau (2000).

RESULTS

The number and location of AI/ANs older than age 65 are mapped in Figure 7.1. According to the U.S. 2000 Census, there were 138,439 people who reported solely AI/AN race and were aged 65 years and over. This number comes from the regular, nonsample, Census short form. However, this is an approximation; in the analysis of county-level data, there were 122,994 AI/ANs aged 65 and over because counties with fewer than 50 AI/ANs were not included. The sample used in the current study received the long form to include data on disability, resulting in a final sample size of n = 23,073. As illustrated in Figure 7.1, older AI/ANs reside largely in the central corridor of the United States and in western states. However, they can also be seen on the maps in large numbers, in Michigan, for example, and along the eastern and southern coasts. Figure 7.2 shows a comparison of disability for all persons older than age 65 with otherwise similar AI/ANs. For all persons in the United States older than age 65, 41.9% have one or more disabilities, whereas in the case of same-aged AI/ANs, 57.6% have a disability ($p \leq .0001$). As shown on the map, the greater the proportion of AI/ANs in a particular county with a disability, the darker the shading on the map. It can be seen, for instance, that the island of Hawaii, the coastal and island regions of Alaska, northern Idaho, and California, Washington, New Mexico, Arizona, and Nevada have large percentages of disabled AI/ANs.

Different levels and kinds of disability are found in different regions. One ADL limitation, the ability to walk, shows a noticeable concentration in the Southwest (Figure 7.3A). Forty-three percent of AI/AN elders in the West and South answered "yes" to this item, 42% in the Midwest, and 39% in the Northeast ($p \leq .0001$). The ADL limitation of bathing, although noticeably less represented than the problem of walking, continues to be seen as a problem again in the Southwest and variously across the country (Figure 7.3B). Although there appear to be subregional differences, this ADL limitation does not vary significantly by region, with 16% in the South and Northeast, 15% in the West, and 12% in the Midwest ($p \leq .0001$). Finally, an example of an IADL limitation, getting out and about, is represented in Figure 7.3C. Twenty-nine percent of older AI/ANs report this limitation in the Northeast, 28% in the West, 26% in the South, and 24% in the Midwest ($p \leq .0001$; Figure 7.4).

The final map, Figure 7.5, is a comparison of disability between urban and rural areas. Most reservations in the United States lie in rural areas. There are, however, a few in or near metropolitan centers. Figure 7.5 shows the number of AI/ANs over the age of 65 with at least one disability mapped by county. The size of each square is proportional to the number of AI/ANs with a disability, and the shade used for the squares distinguishes urban from rural areas. Urban counties are defined as those that are part of a metropolitan statistical area, whereas rural counties are not. Nationwide, our analysis finds that 60.9% of AI/AN elders in rural areas, compared with 55.3% in urban areas, report at least one disability ($p \leq .0001$). Urban areas of disability exist along the Californian and eastern coasts. The largest percentages of rural disability are found in the

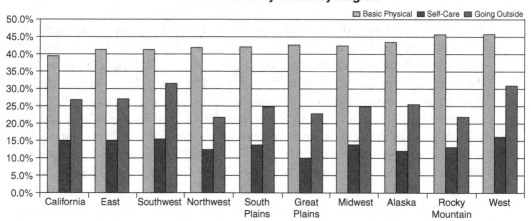

FIGURE 7.4 Distribution of older AI/AN by region from the U.S. 2000 Census.

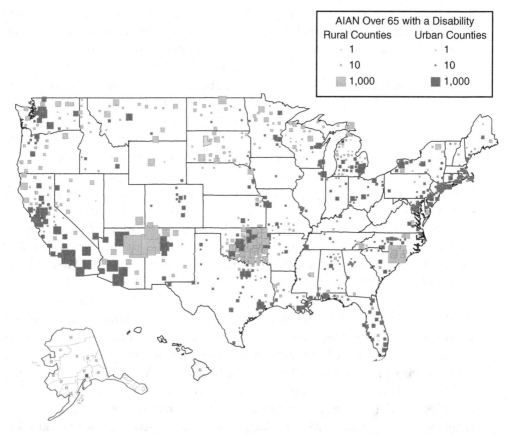

FIGURE 7.5 Geographic distribution of disability among AI/ANs 65 years and older showing urban versus rural differences.

Source: U.S. Census Bureau (2000).

Carolinas, Oklahoma, New Mexico, and Arizona. Texas, which has almost no rural representation for AI/AN disability, shows disability in Houston, Dallas, San Antonio, and El Paso.

DISCUSSION

Maps Help Visualize Those Who Might Otherwise Be "Lost" From the Data

Although mapping the location and population density of all AI/ANs over age 65 provides important demographic information, it fails to direct attention to areas where disability rates are disproportionately high. The current study yielded several maps, which show complex spatial and occurrence information from AI/ANs across all 50 states, including those that are home to the 560 tribes. These maps will be useful for understanding functional disability because they can be viewed instantly for trends and areas in need of services. For example, Texas has vast rural areas and relatively few older AI/ANs. However, when functional disability is mapped by area of residence, there are large urban areas in Texas, which contain AI/AN populations that have a high prevalence of functional disability. Furthermore, services, which focus on the special needs of AI/AN elders, are limited in some large cities, such as Houston. In another example, the lack of numbers of older AI/ANs in northern Idaho would not lead decision makers to allocate funding streams into the area for disability programs, yet these maps show that there is a disproportionate amount of AI/AN disability for those who are living there. Maps help visualize those who might otherwise be "lost" from the data.

This study was important in linking geospatial/population data that might influence the placement of services that are specific to the density and type of disability in a certain geographic area. A New Zealand study found that more attention must be paid to spatial information based on primary care in order to plan services for disadvantaged populations more effectively (Brabyn & Barnett, 2004). A U.S. study on marginalized populations found GIS an important tool in understanding the dynamics of population diversity and as a means of assessing marginal situations (Alexander, Kinman, Miller, & Patrick, 2003). There are 4.1 million AI/ANs according to the 2000 Census (Ogunwole, 2002). Although they represent only 1.5% of the total U.S. population, this number is greater than the population of Los Angeles, California, by half a million. Previous research has shown that AI/ANs develop chronic diseases at earlier ages and die from them at earlier ages (IHS, 1998). Thus, the tension between long-term care need and the inability of the health care system to deliver care where and when it is needed remains largely unresolved. The Indian Health Service (IHS), charged with providing care for AI/ANs, does not provide institutional long-term care, such as nursing home care, assisted living or adult day care, and does not report statistics on functional status. AI/AN families largely carry the burden of providing care for disabled elders although they themselves have few resources.

There are some tribal grant opportunities offered by the IHS to develop solutions to the elder care problem. However, these are relatively new and have only addressed a few tribes that have been successful in the granting process. Without detailed national data on functional disability, such as the information provided in the current study, the extent of long-term care needs among older AI/ANs will remain largely unknown.

Limitations of the current study include issues related to the data available from the U.S. Census such as inability to fully access some AI/AN communities, misidentification and related over- or underrepresentation, mobility of the group, and potential difficulty in answering the Census forms. Overrepresentation may occur when respondents incorrectly choose AI/AN as their race on the forms; there is no verification of being AI/AN. Anyone could in theory identify on the form as AI/AN whether or not there was a genetic basis to do so. Yet there are legal definitions that include being an enrolled member of a federally recognized tribe and not just having some degree of heritage (Title 25, U.S. Code). The legal definition would apply to those who are eligible for care under IHS criteria. A related problem is in deciding whether to use one race or any that include American Indians. It was hypothesized that many elders would choose AI/AN as their category, that is, one race. Therefore, in an attempt to make as clean a map as possible for a first look, we settled on this category. Another problem is underrepresentation, which occurs when access, mobility, and cultural problems preclude AI/ANs from successfully completing forms.

Further, the questions about disability are not standard ADL/IADL items. Nevertheless, as a baseline from which to work, the Census data do allow a preliminary picture of some aspects of functional disability in this group. More than 90 million Americans live with a chronic disease, and of these, 25 million suffer from major limitations in activity caused by chronic diseases (CDC, 2003). The looming burden of chronic disease and disability among AI/ANs (CDC, 2003; IHS, 1998) must become a priority in the U.S. health policy agenda. Although the life span of AI/ANs has increased over the last century, although still several years behind that of U.S. Whites (IHS, 1998), AI/ANs are now living longer with functional disability.

CONCLUSIONS

The significance of this study is that gerontologic programs and policies are data driven, yet there are a lack of reliable national-level data from U.S. health systems on functional disability among AI/ANs. This study provides a first look at function in a largely vulnerable, underserved, and marginalized U.S. population. A seminal recommendation arising from this study is for the U.S. Census to incorporate the accepted research and practice wording for ADLs and IADLs into the long form.

In doing so, the United States can begin to develop a comprehensive, linked database with which to monitor functional disability patterns temporally as well as spatially. This information could be translated and applied directly in gerontology toward meeting the needs of any slice of the population. Additionally, the White House Conference on Aging also meets every decade (mid decade), and would be able to incorporate such usable information in the formation of future gerontologic policy. Future studies are needed to extend this information into modeling causative factors for functional disability linked to disease and environment, spatial relationships to relevant health care services, and policy implications.

STUDY QUESTIONS
♦ What other health issues can you identify that would lend themselves to GIS methods?
♦ If an ADL is problematic for an American Indian elder, what would be the consequence? Pick one and discuss.
♦ If an IADL is identified as a problem regionally, how would you go about addressing this?

USEFUL WEBSITES
♦ Government census, www.Census.gov
♦ GIS information, http://www.gislounge.com/what-is-gis
♦ National Indian Council on Aging, http://nicoa.org

REFERENCES
Administration on Aging. (1996). *Home and community-based long-term care for Native Americans: Final report.* Washington, DC: U.S. Department of Human & Health Services.

Alexander, G. L., Kinman, E. L., Miller, L. C., & Patrick, T. B. (2003). Marginalization and health geomatics. *Journal of Biomedical Informatics, 36*(4–5), 400–407.

Brabyn, L., & Barnett, R. (2004). Population need and geographical access to general practitioners in rural New Zealand. *New Zealand Medical Journal, 117*(1199), U996.

Briggs, D. (2005). The role of GIS: Coping with space (and time) in air pollution exposure assessment. *Journal of Toxicology Environmental Health, 68*(13–14), 1243–1261.

Brown, M., Eccles, C., & Wallis, M. G. (2001). Geographical distribution of breast cancers on the mammogram: An interval cancer database. *British Journal of Radiology, 74,* 317–322.

Bureau of Indian Affairs. (2003 December 5). Indian entities recognized and eligible to receive services from the United States Bureau of Indian Affairs. *Federal Register, 68*(234), 68180–68184.

Centers for Disease Control and Prevention. (n.d.). *Frequently asked questions. Chronic disease prevention.* Retrieved from http://www.cdc.gov/brfss/faqs.htm#1

Centers for Disease Control and Prevention. (2003). *Chronic disease overview. Chronic disease prevention.* Atlanta, GA: National Center for Chronic Disease Prevention and Health Promotion.

Chapleski, E. E., & Dwyer, J. W. (1995). The effects of on-and off-reservation residence on in-home service use among Great Lakes American Indians. *Journal of Rural Health, 11*(3), 204–216.

Chapleski, E. E., Lichtenberg, P. A., Dwyer, J. W., Youngblade, L. M., & Tsai P. F. (1997). Morbidity and comorbidity among Great Lake American Indians: Predictors of functional ability. *The Gerontologist, 37,* 588–597.

Goins, R. T., Spencer, S. M., Roubideaux, Y. D., & Manson, S. M. (2005). Differences in functional disability of rural American Indian and White older adults with comorbid diabetes. *Research on Aging, 27*(6), 643–658.

Graham, A. J., Atkinson, P. M., & Danson, F. M. (2004). Spatial analysis for epidemiology. *Acta Tropica, 91*(3), 219–225.

Hayward, M. D., & Heron, M. (1999). Racial inequality in active life among adult American Indians. *Demography, 36,* 77–91.

Hennessy, C. H., John, R., & Roy, L. C. (1999). *Long-term care service needs of American Indian elders: The Indian Health Service Santa Fe unit.* Atlanta, GA: Centers for Disease Control and Prevention.

Higgs, G., Smith, D. P., & Gould, M. I. (2005). Findings from a survey on GIS use in the UK National Health Services: Organisational challenges and opportunities. *Health Policy, 72*(1), 105–117.

Indian Health Services. (1998). *Trends in Indian health.* Washington, DC: U.S. Government Printing Office.

Kane R. A., & Kane, R. L. (1981). *Measuring the elderly.* Lexington, MA: Lexington Books.

Katz, S., Ford, A. B., Moskowitz, R. W., Jackson, B. A., & Jaffe, M. W. (1963). Studies of illness in the aged. The Index of ADL: A standardized measure of biological and psychosocial function. *Journal of the American Medical Association, 185,* 914–919.

Kelly-Hayes, M., Jette, A. M., Wolf, P. A., D'Agostino, R. B., & Odell, P. M. (1992). Functional limitations and disability among elders in the Framingham Study. *American Journal of Public Health, 82*(6), 841–845.

Kramer, J. B. (1999). The health status of urban Indian elders. *HIS Primary Care Provider, 24*(5), 69–73.

McBride, T. D. (1989). *Measuring the disability of the elderly: Empirical analysis and projections into the 21st century.* Washington, DC: The Urban Institute.

Moss, M. P., Roubideaux, Y. D., Jacobsen, C., Buchwald, D., & Manson, S. M. (2004). Functional disability and associated factors among older American Indians. *Journal of Cross Cultural Gerontology, 19*(1), 1–12.

Moss, M. P., Schell, M., Goins, R. (2006) Using GIS in a first national mapping of functional disability in older American Indian and Alaska natives from the 2000 census. *International Journal of Health Geographics, 5*(37). doi:10.1186/1476-072X-5-37

Moss, M. P., & Schell, M. C. (2004). GIS(c): A scientific framework and methodological tool for nursing research. *Advances in Nursing Science, 27*(2), 150–159.

Mullee, M. A., De Stavola, B., Romanengo, M., & Coleman, M. P. (2004). Geographical variation in breast cancer survival rates for women diagnosed in England between 1992 and 1994. *British Journal of Cancer, 90*(11), 2153–2156.

Ogunwole, S. U. (2002). The American Indian and Alaska Native Population: 2000. *Census 2000 Brief.* Washington, DC: U.S. Department of Commerce.

Prevalence and impact of arthritis by race and ethnicity—United States, 1989–1991. (1996). *Morbidity and Mortality Weekly Report, 45*(18), 373–378.

Rytkonen, M. J. (2004). Not all maps are equal: GIS and spatial analysis in epidemiology. *International Journal of Circumpolar Health, 63*(1), 9–24.

Szeles, G., Voko, Z., Jenei, T., Kardos, L., Pocsai, Z., Bajtay, A., Papp, E., . . . Adany, R. (2005). A preliminary evaluation of a health monitoring programme in Hungary. *European Journal of Public Health. 15*(1), 26–32.

U.S. Census. (2000). *Urban area criteria for Census 2000—Proposed criteria: Notice.*

U.S. Census (2015). Population clock. Retrieved from http://www.census.gov.

U.S. Census. (n.d.-a). *Census 2000 basics.* Retrieved from http://www.census.gov/mso/www/c2000basics/00Basics.pdf

U.S. Census. (n.d.-b). *Census Bureau region and division codes, state and county federal information processing system (FIPS) codes, and minor civil divisions (MCD) and places with Census and FIPS codes.* Retrieved from http://www.census.gov/popest/geographic/codes02.html

U.S. Census. (n.d.-c). *Detailed tables.* Retrieved from http://http:factfinder.census.gorvleDDTable?_bm=y&geo_id=01000US&reg=Dec_2000SFAIAN_PCT014:01A&-ds_name=DEC2000SFAIAN&_lang=en&-redo=false&-fort=&mt_name=Dec2000_SFAIAN_PCT014&-CONTEXT=dt

U.S. Census. (n.d.-d). *Housing of American Indians on reservations: Equipment and fuels.* Retrieved from http://www.census.gov/apsd/www/statbrief/sb95_11.pdf

U.S. Department of Health and Human Services. (2001). *Trends in Indian health 1998–1999.* Rockville, MD: Indian Health Service, Division of Program Statistics.

Waidmann, T. A., & Liu, K. (2000). Disability trends among elderly persons and implications for the future. *Journal of Gerontology: Social Sciences, 55*(5), S298–S307.

Weinberg, J. (2005). Surveillance and control of infectious diseases at local, national and international levels. *Clinical Microbiology and Infection, 11*(Suppl. 1), 12–14.

EIGHT

Northeastern Woodlands

Marilynn Malerba

LEARNING OBJECTIVES

♦ Understand the changes that Northeastern Woodlands tribes experienced once contact with the European immigrants was sustained, and how that impacted traditional ways of life.
♦ Discuss the various health beliefs of Eastern Woodlands tribes, and how those beliefs are assimilated in the present day.
♦ Articulate the major health challenges that Eastern Woodlands Indians face, and how they are being addressed within their communities.
♦ Describe the geographic location of Eastern Woodlands Indians, and the various health facilities available to them.
♦ Discuss the structure of Indian Health Services, its limitations, and funding challenges.
♦ Discuss how traditional medicine is integrative in nature.

KEY TERMS

♦ American Indian/Alaska Native (AI/AN)
♦ Indian Health Service (IHS)
♦ Indian Health Program/Tribal Health Program/Urban Health Program (I/T/U)
♦ United South and Eastern Tribes (USET)
♦ Wampum

KEY CONCEPTS

♦ Sweats
♦ Heirloom seeds

Throughout Indian country, many different cultural beliefs and practices have been in continuous existence, both before and after European contact. It is important for any nurse caring for an American Indian/Alaska Native to approach the care of the AI/AN citizen with one simple belief: that health is more than just physical health. Here, *AI/AN* is used to describe the indigenous people found in what is now the contiguous 48 United States and Alaska, and points to the more legally driven aspect of the term for this population. Health is holistic in nature and encompasses physical, mental, spiritual, and cultural well-being. It reflects the state of harmony with the external and internal world. Much of the information contained in this chapter is gained through personal interviews with cultural leaders who kindly agreed to be interviewed. In keeping with oral tradition, these interviews share the past with the goal of informing subsequent generations.

This chapter is by no means inclusive of all Eastern Woodlands' Indians. The interviews provided are by individuals who agreed to participate, and are therefore not reflective of all tribes. Eastern Woodlands' tribes encompass New England, New York, and the Great Lakes Region in eight different states totaling 50 unique and individual tribes, which is discussed further in this chapter (see Table 8.1). Although there are shared practices and beliefs related to health, there are differences among the tribes as well, which nurses need to understand as they seek to provide care sensitive to the long-standing traditions of these AI/ANs. Another important point is to realize that the individual tribal members do not necessarily reside on their reservations or indigenous homelands. It is likely that a nurse residing in a particular area, such as Eastern Woodlands, will encounter a tribal member from the Pacific Northwest or Southwest, so it will be helpful to ask what practices and beliefs are important to this individual rather than assuming tribal identity based on location of service.

HISTORY OF THE AREA

As we think about all the tribes in this area, one unifying theme is that of change. Once contact occurred with the European immigrants, rapid change took place with regard to land use; encroachment on tribal lands; language; exposure to diseases that indigenous people had no immunity to, nor traditional medicines to combat; attempts at religious conversion; and changes to what had typically been a subsistence lifestyle. Tribes needed to be resilient, as well as strategic, as they adapted to an unfamiliar world now surrounding them.

One of these tribes—the Mohegan tribe—chronicled these changes in some of their documents. The most poignant representation of how life changed for Mohegan people once European immigration occurred is contained in a petition to the Connecticut General Assembly of Connecticut. The Mohegan Tribal Historian and Medicine Woman, Melissa Tantaquidgeon Zobel, believes that this petition was romanticized to properly capture the hearts of the intended audience and move them to action.

> We beg leave to lay our concerns and burdens at Your Excellencys Feet. The times are exceedingly alter'd. Yea the Times have Turn'd

TABLE 8.1 Programs Offered in New England and New York

Federal Direct Care Service Facilities

Lockport Service Unit
6507 Wheeler Road
Lockport, NY 14094

Mashpee Wampanoag Health Service Unit
483 Great Neck Road South
Mashpee, MA 02649

Micmac Service Unit
8 Northern Road
Preque Isle, ME 04769

Unity Healing Center
Regional Youth Treatment Center
448 Sequoyah Trail Drive
Cherokee, NC 28719

Contract Health Service Operations (Referred and Purchased Care)

Onandaga Contract Health Service
122 E. Seneca Street
Manlius, NY 13104

Tuscarora Contract Health Service
6507 Wheeler Road
Lockport, NY 14094

Tribally Administered Programs

Cayuga Nation
P.O. Box 11
Versailles, NY 14168

Houlton Band of Maliseet Indians
3 Clover Circle
Houlton, ME 04730

Mashantucket Pequot Tribal Nation
c/o Mashantucket Health Clinic
2 Matt's Path; P.O. Box 3060
Mashantucket, CT 06338

Mohegan Tribe of Indians of Connecticut
13 Crow Hill Road
Uncasville, CT 06382

Narrangansett Indian Tribe
4533 South Country Trail
Charlestown, RI 02831

Oneida Indian Nation Health Service
2 Territory Road
Oneida, NY 13421

Passamaquoddy Tribe Indian Township
P.O. Box 97
Princeton, ME 04688

Passamaquoddy Tribe Pleasant Point
P.O. Box 351
Perry, ME 04667

Penobscot Indian Nation
23 Wabanaki Way
Indian Island, ME 04468

Seneca Nation of Indians
Lionel R. John Health Center
P.O. Box 500
Salamanca, NY 14779

St. Regis Mohawk Tribe
412 State Highway 37
Hogansburg, NY 13655

Tonawanda Seneca Nation
P.O. Box 795
Basom, NY 14013

Wampanoag Tribe of Gay Head
20 Black Brook Road
Aquinnah, MA 02535

Urban Indian Health Programs

American Indian Community House
134 W. 29th Street 4th Floor
New York, NY 10001

Native American Lifeline Foundations, Inc. of Boston
2977 Centre Street
West Roxbury, MA 02132

ever thing Up side down, or rather we have Chang's the good Times, Chiefly by the help of the White People; For in Times past, our Fore-fathers live in Peace, Love and great harmony; and had everything in Great Plenty. When they wanted meat, they wou'd just run into the Bush a little ways with their Weapons and wou'd Soon bring home good Venison, Racoon, Bear and Fowl, if they Choose to have Fish, they wou'd only go the River or a long the Sea Shore and they wou'd presently fill their cannoous with Variety of Fish, both Scaled and Shell Fish,- and they had abundance of Nuts, Wild Fruit, Ground Nuts and Ground Beans, and they planted but little Corn and Beans. – and they kept no Cattle or Horses, for they needed none.-and they had no Contention about their lands. It lay in Common to them all, and they had but one large Dish, and they Cou'd al eat together in peace and love. – But alas, it is not So now. All our Fishing, Hunting and Fowling is entirely gone. And we have now begun to Work on our Land, keep Cattle, Horses and Hogs; and we Build Houses, and fence in Lots. And now We plainly See that One Dish and One Fire will not do any longer for us. Poor widows and Orphans must be pushed one side and there they must Set a Crying, Starving and Die. And So We are now Come tour Good Bretheren of the Asembly, With Hearts Full of Sorrow and Grief for immediate help. And therefore, our must humble and Earnest Request and Petition is that our Dish of Suckuttush may be equally divided amongst us, that everyone may have his own little Dish by himself, that He may eat Quietly, and do with his Dish as he pleases and let everyone have his own Fire. (Quaquaquid & Ashpo, 1789)

As described in this passage, the American Indians living in this region underwent a change from a hunter/gatherer society in which all land was communally used to a farming, cash-based economy in which land was individually owned and allotted. Joanna Brooks, quoting Jean O'Brien, notes this dilemma in her introduction to the writings of Samson Occum:

The impacts of colonization on traditional subsistence and trade economies made Native individuals and families especially vulnerable to the pressure to sell lands for money. Land sales, in turn contributed to the dissolution of the place-based kinship and intertribal networks that economically, culturally, spiritually and politically sustained tribal communities. . . . Limited access to traditional hunting and planting grounds changed the way Mohegans worked, worshipped, celebrated, dressed and ate. (O'Brien, 1997, pp. 9, 11)

If one thinks about traditional plant-based medicines, how did the fencing off and allotment of land affect the access to and purity of traditional medicines? How did this affect the nutrition of the indigenous people when access to the traditional hunting and growing fields was now limited by the encroachment of settlers? Mohegan Medicine Woman Gladys Tantaquidgeon (1899–2005) describes a similar experience on the Gay Head Territory of Martha's Vineyard, traditional territory of Wampanoag:

> In 1681, the old sachem Metarrk, in his will bequeathed to his children of Aquinnuh the rights which he and his forbears had enjoyed—the freedom to enjoy that beautiful land as long as they lived and to continue to live in peace and harmony. After the death of the old chief, his son Joseph sold the entire peninsula to Matthew Mayhew who in turn granted leases to other English settlers. The Indians were greatly disturbed because they had not agreed to sell the land which their old chief had given them. They appealed to the "Society for Propogating the Gospel" which purchased certain land rights and restored them to the Indians. The encroaching whites were so troublesome that in 1714, the Society was obliged to have a ditch dug across the neck, four feet wide and two feet deep and a heavy gate put up to keep the whites on their own land. (Tantaquidgeon, 1934)

Neighboring Mashpee Wampanoag, by her estimate, controlled 2,374 acres in the 1930s compared with the approximately 10,500 acres that was their territory in 1658.

The Akwesasne Mohawk people, or people of the flint, are the keepers of the Eastern Door of the Iroquois Confederacy. Their tribal government consists of the traditional longhouse government with chieftainships, clan mothers, and faith keepers in addition to the more modern form of governing through an elected tribal council. The Mohawk had a very early treaty with the immigrants illustrated in the Two-Row Wampum Treaty Belt that called for the two nations (Native and European) to have the right to travel the river together side by side, with each helping the other from time to time. Wampum are beads made of clam (quahog) shells used in jewelry or made into strands of a belt. Wampum can be used to tell a story given the design on a belt or can be given as tribute to someone being honored. This call for mutual cooperation served a common interest: There is only one river, and both peoples must protect it to ensure peace, and the continuation of the Natives' fish supply. The two purple rows represent a canoe with Haudenosaunee and a ship carrying Dutch people, each representative of their own people, culture, and way of life. The three white rows of the belt symbolize Sken: nen (peace), Kariwi: io (a good mind), and Kasastensera (strength). These principles keep the two peoples—Natives and immigrants—healthy and in peace (Mitchell, 2006).

The Schaghticoke reservation was initially founded on the western banks of the Houstanic River in eastern New York, as well as western Connecticut in a town now known as Kent, with approximately 400 acres left. Their reservation was established in 1736 by the General Assembly of the Colony of Connecticut. Most tribal members today trace their heritage to their first sachem, Gideon Mauwee. The Schaghticoke people are descendants of Mahican, and the name Schaghticoke means "where the river forks." The Schaghticoke tribe is a state-recognized but not federally recognized tribe. Trudie Lamb-Richmond—recently retired director of public programs for the Mashantucket Pequot Museum and Research Center, cofounder of American Indians for Development, educator, and author of many publications—provided information regarding changes on her reservation and within the tribal community once contact with the Europeans occurred. In the case of the Schaghticoke people, it was the Moravians who overtook their reservation during 1720 to 1740. At the time, Gideon Mauwee was the Schaghticoke Sachem. He had heard about the Moravians while speaking at Mahican. According to Lamb-Richmond, the Moravians were different from the Puritans in that they were less condescending. The Moravians had come to North America to escape persecution in Europe and to promote their religion among the people here. They had no problem living among the Indian people and accepted many of their ways. The Schaghticoke people initially seemed to be able to balance their traditional ways of life with the new people who came to live with them. There was a quote that Richmond-Lamb shared, indicating that balance: "We can't go to your love feasts tonight, we are going to sweat." A sweat is a ceremonial cleansing used to reflect and to heal. A small lodge is made using deer skins wrapped around a frame. Stones are heated in a fire, brought inside the lodge, and water is then placed on the stones, causing a moist, hot environment. Herbs and tobacco are often placed into the fire. Those in attendance will use the time to pray and reflect. This relieves the body and mind of any impurities and keeps life in balance. A lodge keeper typically organizes the sweat in a manner traditional to his tribal heritage.

The offering of gifts, such as cloths, tools, and pots, as well as the joyous singing at the religious services intrigued the Native people. However, this is the point where "everything changed." The tribe had to change to the English way of growing and planting in rows. "The Friendlies" were those tribal members who joined the Moravians and were then required to choose one or the other: the Moravian or the traditional way of life. This is illustrated by changing prayers from the Native language to a new language. Even in the simple matter of prayer, it is believed that when one prays in one's traditional language, it helps to understand the world in a manner unique to one's tribal culture. Therefore, changing prayer to a new language became a very powerful way to change culture.

POPULATION SHIFTS

Severe population declines were experienced by the indigenous people during the early years of first contact with the Europeans for multiple reasons: lack of immunity to disease, germ warfare in the form of smallpox-infested blankets (Calloway, 2013), colonial laws forbidding exogamous marriage between tribal communities (Occom, 2006), and conflict among the tribes as well as with the European settlers. It is estimated that from the time of first contact with the European immigrants in the late 1500s to early 1600s, until the mid-1700s, the population of New England Indians diminished by approximately 90%.

Mohegans lost roughly 93% of their population by 1650, in which year it was reported to have a population of 1,000 citizens. By 1782, the number stood at 135 (Office of Federal Acknowledgment, 1989). Additionally, some tribal leaders were concerned that the political forces of the now dominant force of the settling Europeans opted to move west in the hope of avoiding assimilation and thus loss of culture, traditional ways, and identity (Occom, 2006).

According to notes from Mohegan Medicine Woman Gladys Tantaquidgeon, when she worked as a field agent for the Bureau of Indian Affairs in the 1930s, significant population losses were noted throughout New England. When visiting Gay Head Aquinnah, the estimated population in 1642 was approximately 1,500 (Speck, 1928a.); in 1764, it was 313 people, and by 1929, a mere 200 survivors remained (Barber, 1840).

Other factors that created a loss of people living near the original territory of a tribe were lack of employment or sustainability, causing tribal people to relocate. Many New England Indians participated in the whaling industry. Military service was another factor, beginning with the American Revolution, with 34 Mohegan men fighting alongside the colonists, and active military service continuing to the present day. Alternatively, Indian people were held as indentured servants during the late 1700s to the mid-1800s, with, according to some estimates, as high as 35.5% of all Indians in servitude (Sainsbury, 1978) and 42% of all indentured children in Rhode Island being Indian (Herndon & Sekatau, n.d.).

The Schaghticoke population in Connecticut stood at approximately 500 to 600 people in 1740 shortly after White settlers established the Town of Kent. The number dwindled to less than 100 by the mid-1800s.

The present-day Mashantucket Pequot and Mohegan tribes were once one tribe prior to the early 1600s, when conflict between leadership caused Uncas to separate from the Pequot with his followers, moving to the opposite bank of the Thames River and assuming the old Lenne Lenape clan name, Mohiks (Mohegan) or Wolf People. It is estimated that prior to this split and prior to European contact, the Pequot tribe numbered approximately 13,000. Following two epidemics, one thought to be the bubonic plague during the years 1616 to 1619 and the other smallpox in 1633, the Pequot population decreased to approximately 3,000 individuals (Starna, 1990). Following the Pequot War in 1637, that number further declined to 1,000. By 1935, only 42 Pequot people remained (Hauptman, 1990).

In addition to population loss, as noted earlier, land loss was a common theme throughout New England, with the original territory of Mohegans estimated to be 20,000 acres before European contact, 2,700 acres by the end of the 1700s, and only the parcel of land that the Mohegan Church stands on and traditional burial grounds by 1872 (Fawcett, 1995). In Rhode Island, by 1881, all but 2 acres of the remaining 927 acres belonging to the Narragansett Tribes were authorized for sale by the State of Rhode Island (O'Brien, 2010). The original territory of the Pequot prior to the Mohegan/Pequot split was estimated to be 2,000 square miles at the time of European contact (Starna, 1990), which reduced to 204 acres following various actions by the colony/State of Connecticut (McBride, 1990).

A prevailing strategy of President Jefferson was to restrict the options of the tribal people by reducing the amount of land they were able to hunt and farm on, and, instead, forcing the Eastern Woodlands' Indians to exchange their traditional way of life for a settled, agricultural way of life: paternalistically "better for them" in the long run (Calloway, 2013).

Chief Beverly Cook—a traditional longhouse leader of the Akwesasne Mohawk Tribe—indicates that at the time of contact, the Mohawk territory, known as Mohawk Valley, was estimated to be over 9 million acres, spreading over what is now known as New York, Canada, and Vermont. In 1796, a treaty was entered into with the State of New York, at which time New York asserted its right to land, subsequently confining the Mohawk people to a small parcel of land. Millions of acres of land were lost not only for the Mohawk people but for all members of the Iroquois Six Nations. The Oneida Nation saw their traditional homelands shrink from an estimated 5 to 6 million acres to 0.25 million acres (Calloway, 2013). The Mohawk community is now bisected by the border of the United States and Canada. As a result, the Mohawk community has two of every governmental department serving its citizens. Current population estimates are 8,000 to 9,000 citizens in the United States, and 4,000 in Canada. The present-day tribe resides in what is now considered Mohawk Valley, consisting of 6 square miles of land.

In terms of population shift, Akwesasne villages were more often in the traditional Mohawk Valley, but the people traversed and lived throughout the territory. The Abenaki and refugees from the Oswegatchie Mission came to live with the Mohawk people at St. Regis—a mission established by the French Jesuits to relieve crowding at Kahnawake and to move closer to the Iroquois homelands. This area was prized and continuously used by the Mohawk people because of its good hunting and fishing grounds, in addition to its location near a confluence of several small rivers.

Another major shift in the population occurred during the boarding-school era, in which many young Mohawk people (estimated at 50%–75%), as young as 5 or 6 years old, were sent to boarding schools to become assimilated into the dominant White society. Many remained until age 18. When they returned, the loss of language, traditional culture, and relationships (some to the point of not remembering grandparents) was devastating.

CONFLICTS

In New England, two major conflicts had lasting effects on the indigenous population— the Pequot War and King Philip's War. Conflicts between the indigenous people in New England centered around political and diplomatic disagreements, particularly about the ever-encroaching immigrants and the loss of indigenous rights to use the land in traditional ways (Mandell, 2010). In 1637, the Pequot War was waged against the Pequots by the colonies with the Narragansett and Mohegan tribes fighting alongside the colonists. This led to increasing colonization in southeastern Connecticut and a severe reduction in the numbers of Pequot people. Pequot survivors were dispersed throughout the region—some were sent to live with colonists; some were placed with Mohegan, Narragansett, or Nehantic tribes; some were sent to Bermuda in slavery; and others to the West Indies (McBride, 1990). The war formally ended with the Tripartite Treaty of Hartford (Haynes et al., 1638), but the Pequot tribe was nearly decimated.

King Philip's War was about land use and sovereignty. The way the English settlers used the land and their ever-increasing need for more land was a source of conflict for the Native people. Entire forests were cleared, and traditional hunting and planting areas were fenced in and cut off from the indigenous people. Cattle and pigs were allowed to roam free, consuming the wild food used for sustenance and ruining the clam beds used in the traditional diet. The tribes indigenous to the area were beginning to lack their traditional foods and medicines. The political power was changing in favor of the English. With the decline in the indigenous population, it is estimated that by the early 1640s, there were four Massachusetts settlements totaling approximately 20,000 people. Although his father, Massoit, had previously reached an agreement regarding relations between the settlers and the Wampanoag people, Metacom—named King Philip by the English—banded with other tribes attacking the settlers. Although 25 English towns were destroyed during what is thought to be the deadliest war of this country in proportion to the population, it ended similarly to the Pequot War, with many of the Wampanoag people sold into slavery (O'Brien, 2010). The result of the war was again the decimation of Native peoples, and eventual subjugation to the colonists (Mandell, 2010).

EASTERN WOODLANDS TRIBES

Tribes considered to be Eastern Woodlands tribes can be seen on the accompanying map (Figure 8.1).

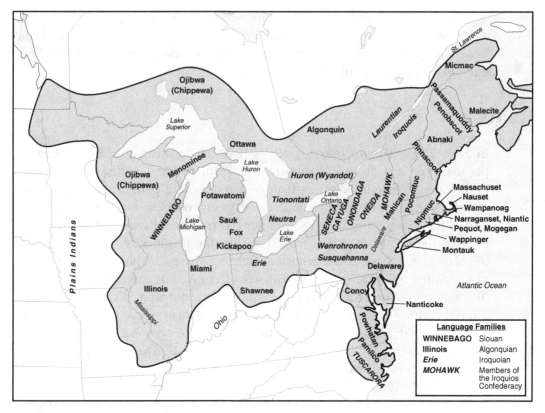

FIGURE 8.1 Eastern Woodlands tribes map.

Source: Reprinted with permission from Encyclopaedia Britannica © 1998 by Encyclopaedia Britannica, Inc.

Using a list of federally recognized tribes and the present-day name of the tribe, the tribes noted in Figure 8.2 can be considered Eastern Woodlands.

MAJOR HEALTH ISSUES IN THE WOODLANDS

A recurring theme for the people I spoke with regarding issues affecting health is pollution and the impact it has had on tribal people. Jill MacDougall, the health director for the Penobscot Nation, discusses the fact that dioxin has contaminated the river, thus affecting the ability to eat traditional foods such as turtles, fish, and eels.

A recent health assessment undertaken in 2010 by Penobscot provided insight into the top five health problems facing its community:

• Diabetes—The Nashville area tribes, which are the tribes east of the Mississippi, have an incidence of diabetes three times the national average, which is a common theme for all tribes in Maine.
• Drug/substance problems

Connecticut
        Mashantucket Pequot
        Mohegan Tribe
Maine
        Aroostok Band of Micmac Indians
        Houlton Band of Maliseet
        Passamaquoddy Tribe
        Indian Township
        Pleasant Point
        Penobscot
Massachusetts
        Mashpee Wampanoag
        Wampanoag Tribe of Gay Head (Aquinnah)
Michigan
        Bay Mills Indian Community
        Grand Traverse Band of Ottowa and Chippewa Indians
        Hannahville Indian Community
        Huron Potawatomi
        Keweenaw Bay Indian Community
        La Vieux Desert Band of Lake Superior Chippewa
        Little River Band of Ottawa Indians
        Little Traverse Bay Band of Ottawa Indians
        Match-e-be-nash-she-wish Band of Pottawatomi Indians
        Pokagon Band of Potawatomi Indians
        Saginaw Chippewa Indian Tribe
        Sault Ste. Marie Tribe of Chippewa
Minnesota
        Bois Forte Band of Chippewa
        Fond du Lac Band of Chippewa
        Grand Portage Chippewa Indians
        Leech Lake Band of Chippewa
        Lower Sioux Indian Community
        Mille Lacs Band of Ojibwe
        Prairie Island Indian Community
        Red Lake Band of Chippewa
        Shakopee Mdewakanton Sioux
        Upper Sioux Community
        White Earth Band of Chippewa
New York
        Cayuga Nation
        Oneida Nation
        Onondaga Nation of New York
        St. Regis Mohawk
        Seneca Nation
        Shinnecock Nation
        Tonawanda Band of Seneca
        Tuscarora Nation
Rhode Island
        Narragansett Tribe
Wisconsin
        Bad River Band of the Lake Superior Tribe of Chippewa
        Forest Country Potawatomi
        Ho-Chunk Nation
        Lac Courte Oreilles Band of Lake Superior Chippewa
        Lac du Flambeau Band of Lake Superior Chippewa
        Menominee Indian Tribe
        Oneida Tribe of Indians of Wisconsin
        Red Cliff Band of Lake Superior Chippewa
        Sokagon Chippewa Community
        Stockbridge Munsee Community

FIGURE 8.2 List of federally recognized tribes and the present-day name of the tribe; the tribes noted here can be considered Eastern Woodlands.

- Alcohol problems
- Obesity—81.6% of the Penobscot community are considered obese compared with the State of Maine's average of 63.7%.
- Cancer

Chief Beverly Cook—a traditional longhouse Akwesasne Mohawk—echoes this problem.

> Environmental issues have had a very real effect on the health and well-being of the Mohawk people. The largest super fund site in the United States was caused by General Motors, which greatly impacted the ability to fish the St. Lawrence River. Fishing as a traditional way of life has all but disappeared. All families used to have "fishing boxes." The inability to eat fish has had a detrimental effect on health, particularly for unborn babies. Fishing has just now begun again, avoiding the longer-living species due to ongoing contamination. (personal communication, December 23, 2013)

So, too, has contamination from the Alcoa and Reynolds companies sickened the cattle normally consuming grasses indigenous to the area that are now contaminated with chlorides (Patterson, n.d.). "In the last 5 years, people have begun growing gardens again with particular interest in heirloom seeds and organic gardening. The lack of a traditional diet has had its effects with the highest rates of diabetes in New York State noted by the Mohawk people" (personal communication, Chief Beverly Cook, December 23, 2013). Heirloom seeds are those that are not produced by man or modified, but are passed down from previous generations of plants.

Gladys Tantaguidgeon, tribal medicine woman and noted herbalist, has lamented the fact that over the ages, pollution has changed the purity and effectiveness of the indigenous plants and herbs traditionally used for healing, indicating that caution needs to be used to ensure that the healing properties are intact when using them for healing purposes. A good example would be the use of tobacco, which is considered to have antiseptic properties but also spiritual properties when used in ceremony. The tobacco used for ceremony was not processed, nor did it contain additives as tobacco today commonly does. As she traveled throughout New England in the 1930s, while working for the Bureau of Indian Affairs, she identified the contaminated water on reservations in Maine (Penobscot and Passamaquoddy) as a pressing health concern.

As Schaghticoke people moved from the reservation to find work and support their families, those who were born in the urban area had a different outlook from those on the reservation. The people living on the reservation still had medicinal plants to use for daily life. Indeed, most people made medicine out of herbs, and kept plants drying in the basement to make into medicinal teas. There was a tendency not to call for a physician unless the illness was very serious.

INDIAN HEALTH SERVICE REGIONAL STATISTICS

The Nashville area Office of the Indian Health Service (IHS) has as an epidemiology program in collaboration with the United South and Eastern Tribes organization, which assists in the understanding of the health status of all tribes within this area in comparison with the general population. The most recent data show that the Nashville area has an age-adjusted diabetes prevalence rate of 22.6%, compared with 11.4% for all of the Indian Health Service, and 6.4% for the United States, all races. Of those diagnosed with diabetes, a higher proportion are women, at 54.6% (USET Diabetes Program, 2013).

Preliminary data on mortality and causes of death for all Nashville area tribes indicate that the average age of death is 59, which is far below that of the United States, all races, at 79. The number of deaths occurring under the age of 45 is noted to be 22% of the tribal citizens in this region, compared with 8% for all United States citizens. The average life expectancy once someone survives past 59 is 80 years, not dissimilar to that in the United States, all races. However, these data could be misleading given the rate of racial misidentification, which is noted at 14%. Misidentification is the incorrect categorization of race, which happens when someone incorrectly identifies the race of an individual or an individual does not correctly or completely fill out the identifier of race when asked. The major causes of death are heart disease, cancer, and diabetes, which account for 75% of all deaths. A comparison of the number of deaths per 1,000 from heart disease and cancer for Nashville area tribes and for the United States, all races, shows that the rates are lower in the former case—0.74 per 1,000 versus 2.81 per 1,000 for heart disease, and 0.49 per 1,000 versus 1.88 per 1,000 for cancer (USET Tribal Epidemiology Center, 2014). Given the low average age of death, it is conceivable, perhaps, that the tribal citizens in this area are dying before they develop heart disease or cancer.

Resources for AI/AN Patients in the Region—Discussion of the I/T/U Health Care System

Each tribe varies in the scope and provision of services available. Generally, medical care from the IHS is available only to federally recognized tribes, not to state-recognized tribes. Federal recognition or "re-recognition" is an extensive process in which tribes that wish to be federally recognized must demonstrate that they have remained a tribe since the time of first contact with the European immigrants with a functioning government and unbroken social and political contact with one another. The IHS is woefully underfunded overall, with the most recent estimate being 56% of need funded (National Indian Health Board, 2014). Additionally, unlike other federal health programs, the IHS is not a mandatory program for federal budget purposes, but is considered discretionary, despite a trust and treaty responsibility on the part of the United States to provide for the health of its first nations. The effect of this budget policy creates a situation in which the funding for IHS actually purchases fewer services each year because the budget does not automatically increase with population growth, medical inflation or new technologies, and is subject to sequestration (see Figure 8.3).

The current administration has increased the budget overall, but the funding is still far below that of the national average health cost per person. The effect of this budget policy is devastating for Indian tribes, with poor health outcomes, lack of access to service, and higher incidence of disease. Additionally, because of restricted resources, rationing of care creates a situation in which tribal citizens enter the system with a higher acuity of illness. Although some tribes have an ability to supplement this funding with privately owned business enterprise revenues, not all are able to do so for lack of access to capital, lack of infrastructure, and remote locations.

The IHS funds several methods of providing health care: direct care, which is operated by Indian Health Service, Urban Indian Health Programs, Tribally Administered Health Programs under Title V Self-Governance Compacts between the Indian Health Service and the individual tribes, and Contract Health Services (CHS; now known as Purchased/Referred care). According to the Indian Health Service (2008), Contract Health Services are utilized in situations in which:

1. No IHS direct care facility exists.
2. The existing IHS direct care element is incapable of providing required emergency and/or specialty care.
3. Utilization in the direct care element exceeds staffing.
4. Supplementation of alternate resources (i.e., Medicare, Medicaid, or private insurance) is required to provide comprehensive health care to eligible AI/ANs.

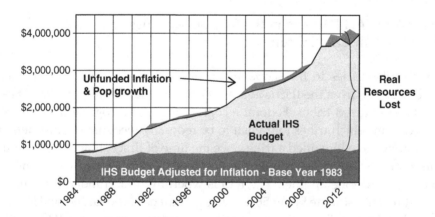

FIGURE 8.3 Diminished purchasing power—a thirty-year look at the IHS Health Services Accounts. Actual Expenditures adjusted for inflation and compared to lost purchasing power when adjusted for inflation and population growth (fiscal years 1984 to 2014).
Source: Roberts (2012).

Contract Health Services—now renamed Purchased/Referred Care—are very important in the context of being able to provide patient care in the most appropriate setting possible, and when there may be no alternative care provider available. Throughout all the service delivery areas for Indian health in the United States, no program offers tertiary care for medically intense needs such as burn care or open-heart surgery. Although 46 facilities offer emergency room and inpatient care, not every tribal citizen has access to those facilities. These facilities typically operate with an average daily patient census of 45 or fewer patients, and only 20 have operating rooms (Oversight Hearing on Contract Health Services, 2009). In areas that have no access to more sophisticated care or specialty providers, CHS is the only mechanism for treatment, but the access is limited by the available funds. Thus, the availability and scope of services not just for Eastern Woodland Indians but for all AI/ANs throughout the United States is extremely varied.

Mohegan currently operates a Title V Self-Governance Compact with the Indian Health Service. There is some provision of direct services on site, but there is a major reliance on purchased or contractual services for those services that are not provided directly. Funding is insufficient for the care of the population, but Mohegan is able to supplement those funds using revenue from its business enterprises. Locally, there are three hospitals within a 20-mile radius from Mohegan with two tertiary facilities within 45 to 50 miles away, indicating that access to care is not as problematic as for tribes in more remote locations.

Unlike Maine tribes in more remote locations, the Penobscot community members have greater access to health care options because of their proximity to Bangor, the location of a major medical center. The Penobscot Nation operates a tribally run clinic. One of the major challenges for Penobscot is a shortage of clinicians.

There are many resources on the American and Canadian side of the Akwesasne Mohawk reservation. Among the Canadian resources are a traditional holistic medicine program, including medicine, use of a diet log, family tree exploration, psychosocial work, and healers involved in behavioral medicine work. People from the United States are regularly referred to this program. On the U.S. side, there is a clinic with a traditional healer in the mental health department and the chemical dependency department. Providers at the clinic include two practice physicians, one part-time internal medicine physician, two nurse practitioners, two pediatricians, and one part-time obstetrician/gynecologist. Another important resource is Contract Health Services for referred care to hospitals and specialty medical providers. There are two hospitals contracting with the tribe for care: one is 12 miles and the other 25 miles away from the reservation. A tertiary-care facility is available, which is approximately 2½ hours' drive from the reservation. For a complete listing of all programs serving the Eastern Woodlands Indian tribes, see Tables 8.1 and 8.2.

Apart from the tribes and tribal programs already listed that have federal recognition, there are state-recognized tribes in these areas that do not have the same federal standing or treaty rights to services. Those tribes in the Eastern region are listed in Table 8.3.

TABLE 8.2 Programs Offered in the Bemidji Area

Federal/Direct Service Programs		
Cass Lake Hospital 425 7th Street NW Cass Lake, MN	Red Lake Hospital Hwy 1 Red Lake, MN 56671	White Earth Health Center 40520 County Highway 34 Ogema, MN 56569

Tribal Health Programs

Bay Mills Ellen Marshall Memorial Center 12124 W. Lakeshore Dr. Brimley, MI 48715	Grand Traverse Band 2300 N. Stallman Road, Ste A Peshwabeeston, MI 49682	Hannahville Indian Community N15109 Hannahville B-1 Road Wilson, MI
Nottaweaseppi Huron Band of Potawatomi 1474 Mno-Bmadzewen Way Fulton, MI 49052	Keweenaw Bay Indian Community Department of Health and Human Services 102 Superior Avenue Baraga, MI 49908	LacVieux Desert Band Health Department P.O. Box 249 Watersmeet, MI 49969
Little River Band of Ottawa Indians Health Department 310 9th Street Manistee, MI	Little Traverse Bay Band of Odawa Health Department 7500 Odawa Circle Harbor Springs, MI 49740	Match-e-be-nash-she-wish Pottawatomi Gun Lake Health Department P.O. Box 281 Dorr, MI 49323
Pokagon Band of Potawatomi Indians Pokagon Band of Potawatomi Health Services 57392 M-51 South Dowagic, MI 49047	Saginaw Chippewa Indians of Michigan Nimkee Memorial Wellness Center 2591 S. Leaton Road Mount Pleasant, MI 48858	Sault Ste. Marie Tribe of Chippewa Sault Ste. Marie HHS 2864 Ashmun Street Sault Ste. Marie, MI 49783
Bois Forte Band of Chippewa Indians 13071 Nett lake Road Net Lake , MN 55771	Fond du Lac Band of Chippewa Min-No-Aya-Win Clinic 927 Trettel Lane Cloquet, MN 55720	Grand Portage Chippewa Indians P.O. Box 428 62 Upper Road Grand Portage, MN 55605
Leech lake Band of Chippewa Indians Leech Lake Band Health Division 6530 US 2 NW Cass Lake, MN 56633	Lower Sioux Community P.O. Box 308 Morton, MN 56270	Mille Lacs Band of Ojibwe 43500 Migizi Drive Onamia, MN 56359
Prairie Island Indian Community 1158 Island Blvd. Welch, MN 55089	Red Lake Band of Chippewa Indians Red Lake Comprehensive Health Service PO Box 249 Red Lake, MN 56671	Shakopee Mdewakanton Sioux 2330 Sioux Trail NW Prior Lake, MN 55372

(continued)

TABLE 8.2 Programs Offered in the Bemidji Area (*continued*)

Tribal Health Programs (*continued*)

Upper Sioux Community P.O. Box 147 Granite Falls, MN 56241	White Earth Band of Chippewa Indians White Earth Band Health Division P.O. Box 418 (Hwy 224) White Earth, MN 56591	
Bad River Band of Lake Superior Chippewa Bad River Health Services P.O. Box 250 Odanah, WI 54861	Forest County Potawatomi Community Health & Wellness Center P.O. Box 396 Crandon, WI 54520	Ho-Chunk Nation Ho-Chunk Nation Health Department P.O. Box 636 Black River Falls, WI 54615
Lac Courte Orielles Tribe of Wisconsin Community Health Center 13380 West Trepania Road Hayward, WI 54843	Lac du Flambeau Band of Chippewa Pete Christensen Center 120 Old Abe Road Lac Du Flambeau, WI 54538	Menominee Tribe Menominee Tribal Clinic P.O. Box 970 Keshena, WI 54135
Oneida Tribe of Wisconsin Oneida Community Health Center P.O. Box 365 Oneida, WI 54155	Red Cliff Band of Chippewa Indian Red Cliff Health Services P.O. Box 529 Bayfield, WI 54814	Sokaogon Chippewa Indian Community 3163 State Hwy. 55 Crandon, WI 54520
St. Croix Chippewa Indians of Wisconsin St. Croix Health Services 4404 State Road 70 Webster, WI 54893	Stockbridge-Munsee Band of Mohican Health and Wellness Center P.O. Box 86, W12802 County Road A Bowler, WI, 54416	

Urban Indian Health Programs

American Indian Health Service Chicago Urban 4081 N. Broadway Chicago, IL 60613	American Indian Health and Family Services of Southeast Michigan (Detroit Urban) PO Box 810 Dearborn, MI 48121	Minneapolis Indian Health Board (Minneapolis Urban) 1315 East 24th Street Minneapolis, MN 55404
Gerald L. Ignace Indian Health Center Milwaukee Urban Milwaukee, WI 532204		

Source: U.S. Department of Health and Human Services (n.d.).

TABLE 8.3 State-Recognized Tribes in the Eastern Region

Connecticut	Eastern Band of Pequot
	Golden Hill Paugussett Tribe
	Schaghticoke Tribe
Massachusetts	Nipmuc Tribe
New York	Unkechaug Tribe
Vermont	Elnu Abenaki Tribe
	Nulhegan Band of the Coosuk Abenaki Nation
	Koasek Abenaki Tribe
	Mississquoi Abenaki Tribe

NURSING IN THE WOODLANDS

In Maine, Penobscot employs two registered nurses—both recruited locally—one employed for 20 years and another for 5 years. One of the nurses is a member of the Passamaquoddy tribe. One nurse, who works 20 hours per week, is specifically dedicated to doing home visits on the reservation for people who are considered homebound, hospital recovery patients, and the elderly. She is responsible for assessment and treatment to ensure safety, good medication management, and overall well-being of those in need of care. This is in keeping with the tribal value of keeping people in the community.

Recruitment of staff is difficult because of shortage of family practitioners, and the tribe has currently hired a staffing firm to assist in the recruitment of family nurse practitioners. It was noted that the other Maine tribes find it even more difficult to recruit health care practitioners as a result of their rural locations, which underscores the need to educate community members in primary care medicine and other specialties with the goal that they will practice in their local tribal communities.

In Connecticut, Mohegan employs a nurse funded by the Special Diabetes Program Initiative, which is funded by IHS to address the prevention and treatment of diabetes using diet and exercise interventions. Advanced practice nurses provide counseling and medication management in a behavioral health program working alongside a Mohegan alcohol and substance abuse counselor. There is a "three-quarter house" available for people recovering from alcohol and drug abuse issues with multiple group offerings for various segments among the population.

The Pequot Nation reports that several people are in nursing school—one is in medical school, and there is currently an intern working in the IHS clinic on site.

Patient Population

As with any discussion of Indian health, important factors that may or may not be considered intangible with regard to population health are the effects of marginalization and federal policy concerning relocation, termination, and assimilation. Assimilation was especially harmful as it was seen as a way the "Indian problem" was to be dealt with: eventual termination of all tribes, with tribal citizens assimilating into the dominant culture, losing their unique culture, identity, health practices, and sovereign governing rights.

Crushing poverty and the inability to provide health care at the same level offered to mainstream America has long-reaching effects and will be felt for decades to come. As previously noted, the incidence of disease among Indians remains much higher than the national average, with a decided lack of resources available to address these health challenges.

Cultural Needs/Issues/Beliefs That Would Be Helpful for a Nurse to Know

Issues affecting the health of the Mohegan population are related to the extreme poverty experienced in the late 1800s and early 1900s. There was a lack of electricity, shared water sources in the form of shallow dug wells, and lack of indoor plumbing. Food was communally shared so that no one would go hungry. Farming and preservation of foods were routine, unlike today's way of life.

Family was, and still is, considered more important than formal care providers. Families are very active, and engaged with the care of their ill family members, with informal care providers being recognized as experts and even called "nurses" earlier in the 20th century. Although they may not have had formal training in the provision of health care, they learned from their mentors and were the people who would be called when someone was ill. A cultural shift that has not necessarily been well accepted is that today, people may be cared for in settings other than the local community by nonfamily members. Culturally, Mohegan people are proud, self-reliant, and humble about accepting care. It is very common to hear someone who is experiencing illness or disability respond to an offer of assistance by saying, "No, I'm fine; please give the care (or service) to someone who really needs it."

There is a belief that illness is the product of bad spirits enticed by failure to live by natural law and failure to participate in traditional ceremonies. Only good spirits bring good medicine (Medicine Trail, personal communication, 2000.). This belief was commonly shared by Delaware Medicine Man Wi-tapanóxwe (Walks-with-Daylight): "In ancient times there was but little sickness among the Indians. The Delaware were greatly blessed because we always kept up pure ceremonies and observed the rules of right living. The Indian was healthy because he ate only clean, pure food and lived close to nature. Then came the new people with their strange ways and food and dreadful diseases" (Hallowell, 1939; Tantaquidgeon, 1972). A reason for ill health would be the departure from traditional ancient foods provided by the Creator (Tantaquidgeon, 1972). Tools used to keep evil spirits away include medicine masks, rattles, eagle feathers, sweet grass, the burning of sage or cedar known as a smudging ceremony, and other various herbs used in healing ceremonies. Additionally, turtle shells were used to administer medicines. This is because the turtle shell represents Mother Earth and, as such, is believed to have powerful healing properties.

When feeling ill or the need to heal, Mohegan people will participate in a sweat lodge, ask for a healing ceremony, or seek herbal remedies. Herbal medicine can be a single herb or simple remedy, or could be compounded remedies containing as many as 10 different substances. When using herbal medicines, the herbalist will offer a prayer to the Creator and to the plants themselves, and will not only choose the plants in a very prescriptive manner but will prepare them in a very traditional manner as well. An herbalist may smoke tobacco as an offering while preparing the herbs.

Shell wampum is considered to have unique healing properties. When approaching a medicine man or herbalist for healing, a string of wampum beads would be offered as a gift (Speck, 1931).

In addition to the actual healing activities, a strong sense of place is very important to the inner and physical well-being of Mohegan people. Mohegan is a community very much connected to the land, which is more important than the building or things the community is surrounded by. "You shall always remain in the land where your Creator is (Medicine Woman Fidelia Fielding)" (Fawcett, 1995). This theme was also shared by Lamb-Richmond stating that the connection to the land becomes spiritual as one gets older.

In a reflection on the particular beliefs of the Penobscot people, Jill McDougall shares some particular cultural sensitivities that would be helpful for nurses caring for Penobscot people. She notes that among the population, in general, there is a high anxiety rate that could affect the time it takes to build a trusting relationship between the patient and the provider. Additionally, it is of great importance to be treated with respect and dignity, not to be "talked down at" or "talked down to" but rather to be treated as an equal partner in the health care team. Cultural sensitivity seminars would be considered very appropriate for those who have never worked within an Indian community.

Although traditional medicines have not been incorporated into the clinic, there is a medicine man living on the Penobscot reservation. Traditional foods are incorporated into the care of Penobscot people to the extent possible, given the difficulties with environmental pollution.

Chief Beverly Cook underscores the importance of exploring with the patient the use of traditional healing. It is important for the care provider to understand that there is diversity among the Mohawk people regarding their willingness to access "Western" medical care and/or their engagement with traditional healing. There is a reluctance to speak about the use of traditional medicine and a fear to disclose too much about it. Mohawk people go to traditional healers regularly and also seek outseers. These traditional healers are very powerful in terms of influencing compliance with the prescribed path to wellness. Cook cited the example of a traditional healer prescribing certain dietary restrictions, such as no meat, sugar, or bread, and the increased likelihood of the person following the diet as prescribed by a traditional healer as opposed to a more mainstream provider. Traditional healers do receive referrals from the clinic, but the Akwesasne people are very likely to self-refer.

Traditional healers are believed to have been given a gift. The community has a tradition of ancient healing medicine societies (such as the bear medicine society, the otter medicine society, emotional healing society, etc.) who use different ceremonies, medicines, rituals, herbs, and songs for different maladies, depending on the particular society to which the person belongs. These societies are not just one medicine man, but a group of people who, once they "have medicine," carry it with them and continually renew their medicine. With this medicine and inclusion in a medicine society, the individual has a great responsibility to honor the gift of healing. When one is healed through medicine people, it is considered a very humbling experience because of the realization that the medicine people are sacrificing their time to administer healing to the individual. This experience is described as emotional, mental, and physical healing. An example given of a healing ceremony is the water drum ceremony, which is used for musculoskeletal healing practices much like ultrasound and touch therapy used to heal broken bones.

Lamb-Richmond echoes much of what Chief Cook discussed about the use of traditional healers. Most important is Native people's beliefs and connections to the natural world. "When medicines are taken from the natural world, Native people believe in their ability to heal" (Trudy Lamb-Richmond, personal communication, January 17, 2014). Her husband was Akwesasne, and they frequently visited with the Mohawk people. She tells of a time she brought her son to a medicine man whom she also describes as a seer. He asked her not to discuss what was wrong with her son. Rather, the medicine man gave him plants and told her son how to prepare them, reminding him that no one else could prepare them for him. Once he was done making the tea, he was instructed to take the roots and bury them properly. When he did so, an eagle flew overhead. She recounts that her son felt better after doing so.

Lamb-Richmond confirms what others noted when discussing the use of traditional medicines. Typically, one gives an offering (such as tobacco) to the Creator before taking a plant. Then while making the medicine, it is important to pray, ask the plant to help you, and give thanks to the plant for helping to heal you. Citing the unique healing qualities of each plant, she discussed the use of sweet flag, which is a very bitter root but known to be good for sore throats, and thus popular among singers and drummers. This root was found underwater, and when digging down into the cold water to harvest this plant, when the person seeking this root found it, his or her hands would warm up. She speaks of the great loss experienced by Native communities as it is becoming less and less common to collect and use traditional plants for healing; feeling "waves of sadness for not doing things as we used to do on the reservation" (personal communication, Trudie Lamb-Richmond, January 17, 2014).

Mashantucket Pequot Tribal Councilor Marjorie Colebut-Jackson reports about the regular use of holistic healing methods, including naturopathic medicine provided by their physician. The use of prayer is common, with an acceptance of spiritual beliefs playing a role in healing (personal communication, Marjorie Colebut-Jackson, January 14, 2014).

Physical Issues

Within Mohegan tradition, individuals with special needs are very much accepted, and are considered to have other gifts to compensate for physical limitations. Wi-taponóxwe commented, "Sometimes the weakest person is chosen by the creator to be powerful in mind. He does that as a matter of pity" (Tantaquidgeon, 1972 p. 6). According to Tribal Nonners Jayne "Kikuk" or "Hilltopper" Fawcett and Loretta "Ponemah" or "She Who Sees Beauty" Roberge, people who had physical disabilities were very adaptive and independent, typically using a sense of humor as a coping mechanism. They shared an example of a woman who had multiple sclerosis still finding a way to chop her own wood.

Mental Issues

In general, Mohegan people held the belief that if one had a paycheck, and a roof overhead, then life was good. There is thankfulness for having basic needs met. When people struggled with mental health issues, the typical response would be: "That's family talk, not something we discuss outside the family." Phrases like "That person is not tied too tight" "or "You don't know beans when the bag is untied" would be used to describe people who, as we would say today, "have issues." There was a general reluctance to engage fully with social workers or behavioral health specialists. Only when someone was unsafe to him- or herself or others would an outside person be consulted or placement be considered. Even when children were living in very poor conditions, the children would not be taken from their homes because, as social workers would note: "There is too much love there." Extended families would support one another during times of difficulty, taking in younger relatives when the adult members of the family were struggling with issues impacting the ability to properly care for the children.

There is an acceptance or willingness to consult a tea-leaf reader, a fortune teller, or someone in the community who has special gifts to aid in the healing process. The reader/fortune teller would intuitively feel the negative energy of the person who was distressed, and try to find something positive to say to shift the mental state of that person.

Health director Jill McDougall, from Penobscot, shared that among the Penobscot people, the issues most commonly seen are high anxiety rates, substance abuse issues, higher sexual and/or domestic abuse rates, historical trauma, avoidance and depression issues, and anger management problems.

As noted earlier, the boarding-school era left the Mohawk people coping with grief, loss of language, loss of relationships, and loss of traditional ways. This has created generations of Akwesasne people who have had to cope with historical trauma and intergenerational trauma, the outward expressions of which were rage, anger, alcohol and substance abuse. Many of the people who attended boarding schools returned to the reservation, and had large families of 12 to 13 children as a result of sexual acting out, as well as the influence of Catholicism. Not having grown up within the confines of a traditional family, and without the affection of an extended family, many of the children who subsequently became parents did not have the modeling necessary to gain the skills to nurture and be part of a family. One hundred percent of the Mohawk people were affected by the boarding-school era, with the effects lasting three or more generations. Additionally, many health problems are experienced because of the social issues that were triggered by this tragic period in time (personal communication, Chief Beverly Cook, December 23, 2013).

Emotional/Spiritual Issues

According to Mohegan informants, earlier religion was nature based, as evidenced by the belief that the Creator and the four winds provide guidance and direction. A conversion to Christianity occurred, but Mohegan is fortunate that tribal elders maintained Mohegan traditions, culture, and language. There is a strong belief that life is a continuum; walking on the life trail from east to west, one eventually becomes a star in the Milky Way when one passes over to the next life.

The physical and spiritual worlds are always considered to be in juxtaposition with one another. Anyone who has a vision is thought to be pure in spirit, and thus blessed by the Creator with that vision (Speck, 1931). The closer one is to death, the closer the spirit world and ancestors will be to guide the person to the next world. As described by her niece and great-niece, when Gladys Tantaquidgeon was in the process of crossing over, she spoke with people in the room, and with people those in the room could not see. Another person had a vision of people walking out of graves. Many traditional Mohegan people find this very comforting. It would be very acceptable for a care provider to explore this with the ill person because it would be deemed as "medicine talking."

Lamb-Richmond speaks of the fact that physical, mental, spiritual, and cultural issues are never considered separate. She quotes Jake Swamp—a traditional chief at Akwesasne—"It is an honor to be human" (Swamp, 1995 p. 1.). Gently reminding others at all times to be thankful for the earth, sky, animals, people, and creator, all of which contribute to well-being. She emphasizes the need to incorporate cultural traditions and beliefs into our healing practices to make those practices most effective.

Life Span Issues With an Emphasis on the Elderly

As with most American Indian and Alaska Native people, Mohegan elders are held in the highest esteem. Besides being consulted by traditional Mohegans for any major decisions that need a prior understanding of Mohegan history, and an appreciation of how a decision should be considered in its context, they are believed to have a responsibility toward the generations past and those yet to come.

Mohegan elders primarily live on traditional homelands in Uncasville, with many elders moving to Uncasville on retirement. A prevailing common theme for Mohegan elders is that they wish to die in place on indigenous lands. Fidelia Fielding, who was the last fluent-speaking Mohegan, noted in her diary, "You shall always remain where your god is" (Prince & Speck, 1903, p. 202), referring to the indigenous homelands. It is very important to them to be surrounded by the good spirits that can be felt in Mohegan by the Mohegan people. As one of our tribal Nonners, Pauline "Red Feather" Brown was recently quoted: "The hill, Mohegan hill, that's home" (personal communication from Pauline Brown to Melissa Tantaquidgeon, date unknown. Her sons, Chairman Kevin Brown and Ambassador/Tribal Councilor Mark Brown, noted that in her last months as she shuttled between the hospital and long-term care facilities, she pined to be home on the hill where she felt most secure.)

Death is considered to be part of the circle of oneness with Mother Earth, which helps the elders avoid a fear of death or growing old. This belief is expressed by Tantaquidgeon-Zobel in her earlier writings:

> A burial ground represents a door to the Spirit Land. It opens only one way, because it is a place from which we would not wish to return. That conviction enables elder Mohegans to avoid a fear of death or growing old. They see life as the joining of a continuum with their ancestors. Death is merely another part of the Sacred Circle of Being—a return to union with the Mohegan homeland. (Fawcett-Sayet, 1995, p. 14)

One of the first initiatives that the Mohegan Tribal Council undertook when revenues from the Mohegan Sun Casino were realized was to develop services for the elder population of the community. Not only was an assisted living facility developed to provide services to people wishing to live in the facility on the reservation, but also a program was developed in consultation with the elders to determine what services would be most important to assist those who wished to live as independently as possible within their own homes. These services include not only physical services but also maintenance, transportation, and socialization opportunities to ensure that the elders have an active role in the tribal community.

The life expectancy of the Penobscot is 64 years (Penobscot Census Book, 2010), which is significantly lower than that of the general U.S. citizen, which is 79 years. Echoing the sentiments of Mohegan elders, most elders wish to age and die in place on the reservation rather than in an institutional setting. In addition to home care services, the Penobscot Nation has a six-bed assisted living facility on the reservation that aids in accomplishing the goal of keeping their elders in the community.

Respect for elders is further validated by Chief Cook. "Elders are treated with the utmost respect" (Chief Beverly Cook, personal communication, December 23, 2013). The Akwesasne prefer to keep parents at home, but this may not always be possible if there is dysfunction in the home, or if there are addiction issues because then the youth are less attentive to grandparents. Two facilities are available on the Canadian portion of the reservation: an inpatient chronic care facility and an "old age home" for those who are more mobile and need less care. The people who work in these facilities love the elderly who reside there because they are from the Mohawk community as well.

One of the ways in which respect is demonstrated for the Mohawk elderly is by immediately seeing an elder when the elder presents at the clinic, regardless of whether an appointment has been made. It is typical of Mohawk elders to loathe "bothering anyone"; thus, it is culturally understood that if an elder is seeking care, the presenting issue must be a matter of great concern to the elder. Similarly, if an elder calls for an appointment, one is given immediately.

When someone is close to death, traditions are a means of "taking you out of yourself and making you part of the circle" (Chief Beverly Cook, personal communication, December 23, 2013). An example of this is the "release ceremony" performed when someone is close to death. Typically, a chief would pray with the person and hold white wampum while praying. With regard to the passing of a tribal member, Lamb-Richmond offers the wisdom that when there is a sacred fire to help that person pass to the next world, the expectation is that it demonstrates the connectedness between those still on this earth and the person who has passed on. It reminds those left behind to respect, acknowledge, and connect to the spirit world, keeping the circle of life intact. Ceremonies surrounding death are extremely important to ensure that the loved one transitions to the next world properly (Kavasch & Baar, 1999). Some tribes believe that the soul and spirit are one and, as such, travel together; others like the Menominee believe that each human possesses two souls: one that lives in the head (intellect) and one that lives in the heart, which after death travels to the spirit world (Kavasch & Baar, 1999).

CONCLUSIONS

The most important implication for a nurse caring for an Eastern Woodlands' Indian is to understand that although there is homogeneity among some practices, there is also much diversity in terms of health beliefs, health practices, and individual engagement in those practices. Some tribal citizens will be very engaged in utilizing all the ceremonial and herbal, plant-based medicines in addition to more modern medicine. Others will only seek out modern medical practices. A nurse caring for an Eastern Woodlands' Indian should spend time exploring the beliefs of the individual and his or her personal connection to the historical ways of healing.

It is especially important to ask the individual whether he or she is, in fact, an Indian person. As mentioned earlier, one cannot simply rely on visual identification but must ask to clarify tribal identification.

Nurses need to understand that healing in the traditional sense involves diet, ceremony, traditional plant-based medicines, spirituality, and a very strong connection to the natural world. Healing is not a linear process but rather a holistic process connecting the individual with all the rich traditions of the people who have gone before him or her. Although some individuals will share exactly what traditional methods of healing they are employing, others may withhold that information based on their cultural norms. The questions a nurse should ask a patient is whether he or she is using methods of traditional healing, whether there is someone from within their tribe who should be contacted to assist in the healing process, and how that individual may be contacted. For instance, a tribal member may wish to have a smudge ceremony (the blessing and purification of the individual using the smoke of burning sage), and it will be important to know how to arrange for this ceremony, who to call, and how to ensure this can happen in what are now typically smoke-free environments. Referrals to traditional practitioners can be considered very routine in some communities.

It is necessary to understand what resources are available to tribal citizens and how those resources are funded. Although all federally recognized tribes are eligible for care from the Indian Health Service, funding is limited, and Indian Health Service is considered the payer of last resort. State-recognized tribes are not eligible for IHS and, therefore, if uninsured, must access other means of funding such as Medicaid. Some mental health and substance abuse treatment centers are regionalized, which means greater travel for the individual to access those services. When dealing with a tribe that has citizens both in the United States and in Canada, there may be services available at one location that are unavailable at another. Familiarizing oneself with the various services available to that tribal citizen is one way to achieve the highest, most appropriate level of care for that person.

Another consideration for nurses is the connection of the individual to a particular place. It is very common for Eastern Woodlands' Indians to express a desire to be returned to their home community. Arranging for home health care to allow for this to happen will be an especially important component of care. Death is typically not something to be feared; rather, it is understood that life is a continuum.

As the nurse completes an assessment of her patient, it is especially important to understand the role of historical trauma and how it impacts the health of the individual in terms of trust for the care provider, rates of depression and anxiety, use of alcohol and drugs for the purpose of self-medication, and the impact of those community members surrounding the person.

Lastly, a big consideration for any nurse caring for the Native American population is the understanding that despite overwhelming changes in circumstances, these tribal Nations have persevered. The impoverished conditions they have faced, the need to change to a very different reality once contact with the Europeans occurred, the difficulties of sustaining the natural ways of life, and the lack of access to and funding for care have negatively impacted the overall health of this population. This is evidenced by the shortened life spans, high incidence of disease, and the fact that many AI/ANs enter into the health care system with a higher intensity of illness. Nurses caring for this population need to be advocates of a better health care system and adequate funding.

ACKNOWLEDGMENTS

With gratitude to all who contributed to this chapter (in alphabetical order): Councilman Hiawatha Brown from Narragansett, Tribal Councilor Marjorie Colebut-Jackson (Mashantucket Pequot), Chief Beverly Cook (Akwesasne Mohawk), Nonner Jayne Fawcett (Mohegan), Trudy Lamb-Richmond (Schaghticoke), Nonner Loretta Roberge (Mohegan), Jill MacDougall (Health Director, Penobscot) and Medicine Woman Melissa Tantaquidgeon Zobel (Mohegan).

CRITICAL-THINKING EXERCISE
♦ Your patient is a tribal elder who is refusing to take medication as prescribed. What questions should you ask to explore this with the elder, and how will you discuss the implications of not taking medications with the elder?

STUDY QUESTIONS
♦ How can you identify a patient as an American Indian/Alaska Native?
♦ Name several different traditional healing practices and how they are used.
♦ Describe what historical trauma is and how it might impact the present health of an American Indian/Alaska Native.

USEFUL WEBSITES
♦ Indian Health Service, www.ihs.gov
♦ National Indian Health Board, www.nihb.org
♦ National Congress of American Indians, www.ncai.org

RECOMMENDED READINGS
Kavasch, B. E., & Baar, K. (1999). *American Indian healing arts: Herbs, rituals and remedies for every season of life*. New York, NY: Bantam Books.
Ransom, J. W. (Ed.). *Words that come before all else: Environmental philosophies of the Haudenosaunee*. (pp. 44–50). Awkewsasne, NY: Haudenosaunee Environmental Task Force.
Tantaquidgeon, G. (1972). *Folk medicine of the Delaware and related Algonkian Indians*. Harrisburg, PA: Pennsylvania Historical and Museum Commission.

REFERENCES

Barber, J. W. (1840). *Outline history of every town in Massachusetts*. Worcester, MA: E. L. & J. W. Barber Pub.

Calloway, C. G. (2013). *Pen and ink witchcraft: Treaties and treaty making in the American Indian history*. New York, NY: Oxford University Press.

Fawcett, M. J. (1995). *The lasting of the Mohegans: Part I*. Uncasville, CT: Pequot Printing.

Fawcett, M.J. (2000). *Medicine trail: The life and lessons of Gladys Tantaquidgeon*. Tuscon, AZ: University of Arizona Press.

Fawcett-Sayet, M. (1995). *Mohegan religion: The land of Mundu, Makiawisug & Moshup*. Unpublished manuscript.

Hallowell, A. I. (1939). Sin, sex and sickness in Saulteaux belief. *British Journal of Medical Psychology, 18*(2), 191–197.

Hauptman, L. M. (1990). The Pequot war and its legacies. In L. M. Hauptman & J. D. Wherry (Eds.), *The Pequots in southern New England: The fall and rise of an American Indian nation* (pp. 69–80). Norman, OK: University of Oklahoma Press.

Haynes, J. Ludlow, R., Hopkins, E., & Miantonomo, S. et al. (1638). *Articles of agreement between the English in Connecticut and the Indian sachems*. doi:http://cslib.cdmhost.com/cdm/ref/collection/p128501coll11/id/3860

Herndon, R. W., & Sekatau, E. W. (2003). Colonizing the children: Indian youngsters in servitude in early Rhode island. In Calloway, C.G. & Salisbury, N. (Eds.), *Reinterpreting New England Indians and the colonial experience* (pp. 137–173) Boston, MA: Colonial Society of Massachusetts.

Indian Health Service. (2008). *Indian health manual (IHM)-chapter 3-contract health services*. Washington, DC: Department of Health and Human Services.

Kavasch, B. E., & Baar, K. (1999). *American Indian healing arts: Herbs, rituals and remedies for every season of life*. New York, NY: Bantam Books.

Mandell, D. R. (2010). *King Philip's war: Colonial expansion, native Resistance and the endof Indian sovereignty*. Baltimore, MD: Johns Hopkins University Press.

McBride, K. A. (1990). The historical archaeology of the Mashantucket Pequots: 1637–1900. In L. M. Hauptman & J. D. Wherry (Eds.), *The Pequots in southern New England: The fall and rise of an American Indian nation* (pp. 96–140). Norman, OK: University of Oklahoma Press.

Mitchell, M. K. (2006). *The Haudenosaunee code of behaviour for traditional medicine healers*. Ottowa, Ontario, Cananda: National Aboriginal Health Organization.

National Indian Health Board. (2014). *National tribal budget recommendations to DHHS-2015*. Washington, DC: Author.

O'Brien, J. M. (1997). *Dispossession by degrees: Indian land and identity in Natick, Massachusetts*. Lincoln, NE: University of Nebraska.

O'Brien, J. M. (2010). Resisting. In R. Warrior & J. Weaver (Eds.), *Firsting and lasting: Writing Indians out of existence in New England* (pp. 145–199). Minneapolis, MN: University of Minnesota Press.

Occom, S. (2006). This Indian world. In J. Brooks (Ed.), *The collected writings of Samson Occom, Mohegan* (pp. 11–12). New York, NY: Oxford University Press.

Office of Federal Acknowledgment. (1989). *Proposed finding document: Summary under the criteria and evidence for proposed finding against federal acknowledgment of the Mohegan tribe of Indians of the state of Connecticut*. Washington, DC: United States Department of the Interior.

Oversight hearing on contract health services: Committee on Indian Affairs, United States House of Representatives (2009). (Testimony of Dr. Yvette Roubideaux, Director of Indian Health Services).

Patterson, N. (n.d.) The fish. In Haudenosuanee Environmental Task Force (Ed.), *Words that come before all else: Environmental philosophies of the Haudenosaunee* (pp. 44–50) Awkwesasne, NY Haudenosaunee Environmental Task Force.

Prince, J.D., & Speck, F. G. (1903, April–June). The modern Pequots and their language. (April–June 1903). *American Anthropologist,* 5(2), 193–212.

Quaquaquid, H., & Ashpo, R. (1789). In Connecticut General Assembly (Ed.), *Petition to the general assembly of Connecticut by the Mohegan Indians.* Hartford, CT: Connecticut Archives. 1666-1820, v.58–59.

Roberts, J. (2012). *Together building on our trust for the health of our people.* Washington, DC: National Indian Health Board.

Sainsbury, J. A. (1978). Indian labor in early New England. *New England Quarterly, 45,* 378–393.

Speck, F. G. (1928a). *Native tribes and dialects of Connecticut* (No. 43). Washington, DC: Bureau of American Ethnology.

Speck, F. G. (1928b). *Territorial subdivisions and boundaries of the Wampanoag and Nauset Indians.* New York, NY: Heye Point.

Speck, F. G. (1931). *A study of the Delaware Indian ceremony.* Harrisburg, PA: Pennsylvania Historical Commission.

Starna, W. A. (1990). The Pequots in the early seventeenth century. In L. M. Hauptman & J. D. Wherry (Eds.), *The Pequots in southern New England: The fall and rise of an American Indian nation* (pp. 33–47). Norman, OK: University of Oklahoma Press.

Swamp, C. J. (1995). *Giving thanks: A native American good morning message.* New York, NY: Lee and Low Books.

Tantaquidgeon, G. (1934). *Personal papers.* Uncasville, CT: Mohegan Archives.

Tantaquidgeon, G. (1972). *Folk medicine of the Delaware and related Algonkian Indians.* Harrisburg, PA: Pennsylvania Historical and Museum Commission.

United South and Eastern Tribes Diabetes Program. (2013). *Targeting diabetes, united south and eastern tribes, Inc.* Nashville, TN: Tribal Epidemiology Center United South and Eastern Tribes.

United South and Eastern Tribes Tribal Epidemiology Center. (2014). *Draft mortality report.* Nashville, TN: United South and Eastern Tribes.

U.S. Department Health and Human Services. (n.d.). Indian Health Service Facilities Locations. Retrieved from http://www.ihs.gov

NINE

Southeastern Woodlands

Lee Anne Nichols

LEARNING OBJECTIVES

+ Explore nursing care for American Indians in the southeast region of the United States.
+ Identify significant historical events and details of Southeastern American Indians as they relate to nursing care.
+ Describe federally recognized and state-recognized tribes.
+ Identify the unique cultural and historical heritage of American Indian tribes in the Southeast.
+ Describe the health disparities of American Indian populations in the Southeast.
+ Identify resources in the Indian Health Program/Tribal Health Program/Urban Health Program (I/T/U) health care system for patients who are members of federally recognized tribes.
+ Identify health care resources and health care systems for patients who are members of state-recognized tribes.

KEY TERMS

+ Civil Rights Act of 1964
+ Confederate states
+ Cultural humility
+ Federal registry of AI tribes
+ Federally recognized tribes
+ Indian removal period
+ Jim Crow laws
+ One-drop rule
+ Racial category
+ Segregation
+ Solid South
+ State-recognized tribes
+ Termination period
+ Trail of Tears

KEY CONCEPTS

+ All-Indian schools and churches
+ Culturally homeless
+ Federal acknowledgment process
+ Federal Indian policies
+ I/T/U health care system
+ Southeastern American Indian tribes
+ Southeastern Indian culture
+ Southeastern tribal history
+ Topical influences on health
+ Tribal membership

The purpose of this chapter is to explore the nursing care for American Indians (AIs) in the southeastern (SE) region of the United States. An 11-state area—Eastern Texas border, Louisiana, southern Missouri, Mississippi, Alabama, Georgia, Florida, North Carolina, South Carolina, Tennessee, Virginia—will serve as the cultural target area for this discussion (Braun, 1988). Many distinctive factors relate to the topographical location, historical events, legal and political issues/events, cultural settings, and health care resources that impact the delivery of nursing care in this area. Populations examined are AIs who are members of federally recognized tribes as well as AIs who are members of state-recognized tribes. Topics include geographical, historical, and political factors of the cultural target area, description of tribal entities in the region, definitions of federally recognized and state-recognized tribes, differences in tribal membership criteria, health disparities, health care resources in the area, I/T/U health care system for members of federally recognized tribes, health care system for members of state-recognized tribes, nursing care provided to tribal members in the region, and demographics and health needs/issues of Southeastern American Indian (SE AI) populations.

AI CHAPTER MODEL

Cultural Humility

Nursing care for SE AIs needs to be delivered within the social and cultural context of each SE tribe. Nurses need to understand their own personal history and culture in order to develop the tradition and incorporation of cultural humility into nursing practice (Meleis, Isenberg, Koerner, Lacey, & Stern, 1995). Cultural humility refers to is an individual lifelong process of self-evaluation and self-critique that allows the individual to be open to other cultural identities. Because of this process, the nurse–client relationship becomes circular and fluid, and is reflective of the value of interconnection that is grounded in AI culture. It is necessary for nurses to examine the social and cultural factors of SE tribes to better comprehend the idea of health from an SE AI's perspective. Understanding this unique cultural perspective will assist nurses in developing a deeper understanding of the health philosophy among SE AIs. Nurses need to understand the social and political environments in which each tribal culture exists. The health of tribal communities is strongly influenced by the historical, political, and social contexts in which SE AI tribes live.

Cultural humility is essential when providing respectful nursing care to the diverse Indian peoples living in the Southeast. Embedded in SE AI culture are values related to circularity, honoring, and numerology. Application of these concepts to nursing care of SE tribes is vital in delivery of care. AIs "think" circularly versus linearly, which is the predominate approach in the SE professional nursing society, and may contribute to lack of understanding in eliminating

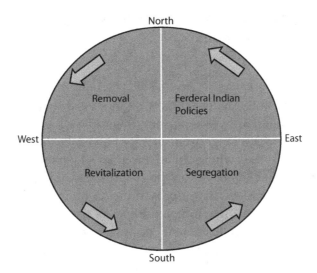

FIGURE 9.1 Circle of revitalization of Southeastern AI/AN.

health disparities among SE tribal members. A circular approach respectful of AI values comprises the format for this discussion. An example is the significant events for SE AIs (although not inclusive) that include removal, federal Indian policies, segregation, and revitalization (Figure 9.1).

The circle represents the interconnections of the removal, federal Indian policies, segregation, and revitalization atmosphere in the tribal SE. Four is a sacred number for SE tribes and represents the four directions on the circle. Removal is located in the west because SE AIs were removed to the West in the early 1800s. Federal Indian policies are located in the north because the federal government responsible for the policies is located in Washington DC, north of the SE AIs. Segregation is found in the east because SE AIs were racially isolated as a group, and geographically sequestered from the tribes removed to the West. Revitalization is in the south because tribal communities live in the SE part of the United States and continue to prosper and thrive in the past, present, and future as Indian nations.

When Cherokees dance at the Stomp Dance they dance counterclockwise to honor their past and ancestors, so the direction of the circle is counterclockwise (Nichols, 2004). Moving counterclockwise interconnects the four significant events that SE AIs experienced (removal, federal Indian policies, segregation, and revitalization), and honors the wisdom and sacrifice of all AIs from "those who have gone before us and those who are yet to come" (Mississippi Band of Choctaw Indians. n.d., para. 9).

Nurses will find merit and significance in the number four, as well. The paradigm of nursing includes four metaparadigm concepts: environment, person, health, and nursing. As nurses care for SE AIs, defining these four concepts from an SE tribal perspective will improve nursing care and decrease health disparities in the SE tribal communities.

HISTORY OF CULTURAL AREA: SOUTHEASTERN TRIBES AND STATE-RECOGNIZED TRIBES

Environment

Fawcett and DeSanto-Madeya (2013) defines *environment* as "human beings' significant others and physical surroundings as well as to the setting in which nursing occurs, which range from private homes, health-care facilities to communities to society as a whole" (p. 6). From an AI perspective, mutual existence with the environment is based on the AI principle of self-determination (Good Tracks, 1973). AIs believe that a person has to be in balance and "walking in step" with the universe (environment) and its natural rhythms (Garrett et al., 2011). The universe or environment encompasses many principles—nature and spiritual world, family, self, and community (Struthers & Lowe, 2003). As nurses assess the environment of SE AIs, both of these definitions are inclusive of the contextual as well as the physical environment that nurses should include in care.

Sacred Lands: SE Geography

Nursing care for AIs is influenced by the geographical differences in the SE region of the United States, which will be the target cultural area for this discussion. Geographical boundaries provide insight into the social and cultural context of AIs in the SE region. Geographical linkages among the SE tribes exist. Within these geographical boundaries are Native people who value circularity and oneness. Several map resources cite different criteria for inclusion required to define the regional boundaries of the Southeast. The U.S. Census Bureau includes 17 states in what is identified as the "south region" of the United States (U.S. Census Bureau, n.d.-a). The population statistics can increase or decrease if the physical boundaries identified by the Census Bureau change. This, in turn, may sway how health care data are collected and how health care policies and programs are implemented.

The Bureau of Indian Affairs (BIA) includes 24 SE states in the section designated as the "eastern region" (U.S. Department of Health and Human Services, Indian Health Service, n.d.). The physical area for the Nashville Area Indian Health Service includes 14 states where 29 federally recognized tribes are located; it also serves individual Indian patients across 24 states in the eastern, southeastern and mid-United States (U.S. Department of Health and Human Services Indian Health Service, n.d). Eleven states are described as the "Confederate States," located in the physical area known as the "Deep South," and this has significance for historical events and the southern cultural milieu of the area (Public Broadcasting Service, Oklahoma Educational Television Authority, n.d.). The "solid south" refers to the southern states' voting patterns prior to the 1960s. This voting trend and "solid blue" map do not happen anymore, as the Deep South votes both Democratic and Republican now.

(Woolley & Peters, n.d.) The geographical region of the "Solid South" has implications for the political ambience of the area. The historical Civil Rights places are located in many SE states such as Alabama, Mississippi, Georgia, and South Carolina. These historical sites are places of significant events related to the Civil Rights movement (National Park Service, U.S. Department of Interior, n.d.-a). The geographical acknowledgment of land sites where historical and political events occurred intertwines and regionally connects the SE states together. Nursing care delivery to SE tribal populations will be affected by these geographical contextual factors in regard to census data for the region, Indian Health Service (IHS; I/T/U) resources available, historical and political events related to civil rights, and southern cultural dynamics.

Sacred Lands: Landscape

Tribes are isolated from each other as well as from other populations. The Band of Poarch Creek Indians in Alabama is approximately 450 miles south of the Eastern Band of Cherokee Indians in North Carolina. Access to health care resources and health care providers is significantly impeded for tribes in times of natural disasters. The southeastern United States includes the flatlands in Texas to the Great Smoky Mountains in Tennessee to the Gulf Shores in Alabama and to the Atlantic Shores of Florida. Some states, for example, North Carolina, South Carolina, and Florida, have Atlantic coastlines, whereas other states like Florida, Alabama, Mississippi, and Louisiana, have Gulf coastlines. Some states have threads of islands offshore, whereas Tennessee is surrounded by land only. The Great Smoky Mountains run along the Tennessee–North Carolina border. The Great Mississippi River either borders or flows through several of the states in the Southeast (i.e., Tennessee, Mississippi, and Louisiana). The vast different physical landscapes of the natural environment are extensive.

Some tribes are located in land areas that leave the tribal peoples vulnerable to threatening weather. Weather pattern changes in some locations have made the region high risk. States located along the borders of the Atlantic Ocean and Gulf of Mexico experience seasonal hurricanes, which can cause loss of lives and destruction to the land, and devastate areas. The most graphic example is Hurricane Katrina, which hit the Gulf States in 2005. The vulnerable New Orleans area was crippled by the hurricane, and thousands of residents became trapped in the city. In the end, almost 2,000 lives were lost in Louisiana, Mississippi, and Alabama to Hurricane Katrina. In response to Hurricane Katrina, efforts were made to assist low-income areas in disaster planning, that is, "planning in the event of an emergency" (Bureau of Minority Health Access, 2009, p. 83). The Chahta Native American tribe in St. Tammany Parish (nonfederally recognized) in Louisiana partnered with The Bureau of Minority Health Access (BMHA) to establish their own emergency preparedness plan in the event of a natural disaster or pandemic flu outbreak (Bureau of Minority Health Access, 2009).

Four Events: Removal, Federal Indian Policies, Segregation, and Revitalization

Removal

A misconception held by the general public is that Indian tribes do not exist east of the Mississippi. The Indian Removal Act of 1830 forcibly relocated Indian tribes, beginning with Choctaws. The Bureau of Indian Affairs Report 1975 provides detailed descriptions of the federal Indian policies from colonial times to the 1970s (U.S. Department of the Interior, Bureau of Indian Affairs, 1975). The earliest federal policy (in 1834) involved forcibly removing and relocating tribes from the eastern and SE regions of the United States to the western areas of the United States, notably the new Indian Territory (Oklahoma). The report mentions how the Five Civilized Tribes—Cherokees, Chickasaws, Choctaws, Creeks, and Seminoles—were involuntarily relocated along with other tribes despite active resistance by their tribal members (U. S. Department of the Interior, Bureau of Indian Affairs, 1975). However, owing to resistance and hiding, significant numbers of Indian people remained in the South after the removal period—Lumbees of North Carolina, the Eastern Band of Cherokees, the Choctaw in Central Mississippi, and the Seminoles in southern Florida. Influences from the removal continue into modern SE AI culture, and still contribute to health disparities and the well-being of these tribes today.

Federal Indian Policies

Two federal Indian policies of significance to SE AI tribes were the reservation policy and the termination policy. After the removal period, the federal government continued to impose policies on AI tribes with the intent to assimilate them into mainstream culture. Around the end of the 18th century, the reservation policy came into existence with the intention of sequestering Indian populations onto lands held "in trust" by the federal government. Indians were pressured into relinquishing traditions and culture (U.S. Department of the Interior, Bureau of Indian Affairs, 1975). After the Civil War, the federal government did not officially recognize any Indian people or tribal entities in the Southeast or "south of the Mississippi" (U.S. Department of the Interior, Bureau of Indian Affairs, 1975). However, in the late 1800s, the Office of Indian Affairs (later renamed BIA) recognized the existence of tribal communities (even if the federal government chose not to) because of the deplorable state of health and extreme poverty of the SE AI people. The federal government assumed responsibility for some of the tribes by placing "land in trust" for them, including the Mississippi Band of Choctaw Indians, Eastern Band of Cherokee Indians, Florida Indian Tribe, Chitimacha Indian Tribe, and Catawba Indian Nation (Cole & Ring, 2012).

The policy on termination of tribes as "wards of the United States" began in the 1950s. The Menominee of Wisconsin was the first tribe whose federal trusteeship was terminated in June of 1954 (U.S. Department of Health, Department of Health, Education, & Welfare, National Institute of Education, 1975). In the Southeast, the Alabama-Coushatta Tribe of Texas and the Catawba Indian Nation of Louisiana had their federal recognition terminated during this time frame. Following the termination period, many tribal entities (including SE tribes) began requesting federal acknowledgment as an Indian tribe. In 1978, in response to the increasing numbers of requests, the Office of Federal Acknowledgment (OFA) was established within the U.S. Department of the Interior, Bureau of Indian Affairs. The OFA oversees the acknowledgment process for Indian groups that wish to petition for federal acknowledgment as Indian tribes and by which they become eligible to receive services provided to members of Indian tribes (U.S. Department of the Interior, Bureau of Indian Affairs, 2013). Since then, over 350 Indian groups have begun the process of petitioning for federal acknowledgment.

Segregation

During the time between 1900 and around the 1970s, historical, societal, and political events and factors focused on the civil rights of African Americans. The social structure of this period related to civil rights events and included both social mood and state laws—racial category and classification, "one-drop rule," Jim Crow laws, segregation, and the Civil Rights Law of 1964. How these laws and social concepts impacted the civil rights of SE Indians is scantily addressed in the literature.

In the pre-Civil Rights South, an American policy existed informally, known as the "one-drop rule" existed informally. This social "rule" defined a person with any ancestry of African heritage as racially Black (Oakley, 2005; Wright, 1994). The "one-drop rule" applied to Indians when they were racially classified as non–African American or African American, therefore allowing the opportunity to segregate Indians. Legally, only two racial categories existed during this period of history, White or Black (Oakley, 2005). This created a biracial society, when in actuality, there were more than two groups (Cole & Ring, 2012). From an Indian perspective, a triracial society really existed, but there was no legal recognition of a racial category for AIs. Tribal people did not identify with either racial category—Black or White. The Indians wanted to distinguish themselves from the African Americans and the Whites in order to retain their recognition by state and federal governments (Cole & Ring, 2012). For example, there were only two racial categories to select from on birth certificates and death certificates. Many Indians felt forced to select White over Black, however, but did not identify with either racial category (Cole & Ring, 2012). This biracial categorization created a mechanism to virtually eliminate the SE Indian populations. After the Civil Rights laws were set in place, many Southern Indians amended their racial category from "White" to "Indian" on their birth certificates (Matte, 2002).

Segregation and the Jim Crow laws forced SE Indians to find ways to preserve their cultural and racial identity (Cole & Ring, 2012). What are known as the Jim Crow laws are policies that mandated segregation in public schools, public places, public transportation (buses), restrooms, restaurants, drinking fountains of Black Americans from Whites. Segregation included the sites of the U.S. military, as well. SE Indians were also segregated in this biracial society. For example, laws prohibited Indian children from attending White-only schools, and Indians did not identify themselves as Black and so did not wish their children to attend Black-only schools either. In response to the segregation laws, an Indian-only system of schools and churches emerged from the influences of Indian groups, White-only school frictions, and state governments. Indian-only churches served as places of religion, schools for Indian children during the week, and public places of social gatherings (Oakley, 2005). Christianity (specifically, Methodist and Baptist) played a powerful role in the social/spiritual retention of their identity as Indian.

To this day, Indian Baptist Churches and Indian Methodist Churches are sprinkled throughout the South. Some state governments, such as North Carolina's, funded Indian-only schools for SE Indian populations (Cole & Ring, 2012). These schools were not affiliated with the BIA. The Office of Indian Affairs (the BIA was known by this name in the 1940s) established Indian school systems for tribes that had land "held in trust" by the U.S. government. (Some historians identified OIA's solutions to education of Indians as another form of segregation.) The Lumbee Tribe of North Carolina developed a well-established Indian-only system of churches and schools in Robeson County. The Poarch Band Tribe sent their Indian children to Indian-only schools (Poach Band, n.d.). In the 1920s, the Reed's Chapel Baptist Church built the Reed's Chapel School for the children of the MOWA Band of Choctaw Indians to attend (Matte, 2012).

The Civil Rights Law of 1964 improved the human and civil rights of SE Indian tribes by increasing the opportunity to identify as AI, revitalized the Indian culture, and paved the way for tribes to move toward self-governance and self-determination.

Revitalization

Leininger and McFarland (2006) refer to *culture* as "learned, shared, and transmitted values, beliefs, norms, and lifeways of a particular culture that guides thinking, decisions, and actions in patterned ways and often intergenerationally" (p. 13). Historical events—removal, termination, segregation—that SE tribes experienced shaped their culture as it exists today. The impact of the federal Indian policies and the segregation laws of the pre-Civil Rights era, which aimed to extinguish SE tribes, are part of history and guide Indian culture today. Some SE tribes emerged into a new Indian society as they tried to reestablish their native identity and gain recognition. Other tribes remain grounded in their tribal identity as a result of their tenacity, and now prosper as a tribal community. Many tribes across the Southeast are revitalizing their culture after the oppression of segregation.

A great source of pride for SE tribes is remaining on traditional lands and resisting removal efforts. Despite the federal policies, the Southeast still has pockets of Indian people living there after the removal period, and the SE tribes share common histories related to the prerelocation and postrelocation. Tribal stories of ancestors resisting relocation efforts are passed orally to new tribal members. The biracial society (Black or White racial categories) that existed before the Civil Rights era strengthened the Indian identity of SE tribes. SE tribes have continued relationships with the tribes relocated to Indian Territory or other U.S. areas. In the 1990s, when historical markers and sites were erected in honor of the "Trail of Tears" march, Western tribes, such as the Muscogee (Creek) Nation, were invited to come and participate.

Cultural commonalities exist across SE tribes, but each tribe has its own unique language, traditions, and culture. The Eastern Band of Cherokees and the Mississippi Band of Choctaw Indians continue to speak in their native language (versus losing their language as an outcome of historical events) as well as do other SE tribes. The Sequoyan Syllabary for the Cherokee Language was created in the 1800s. Indian names in the SE for places and towns were taken to Oklahoma by the tribes relocated to the area. For example, Alabama Indian names like Eufaula, McIntosh, Wetumpka, Chickasha, Tecumseh, and Muskogee can be found in Oklahoma as well. Most, if not all, of the SE tribes are trying to revitalize Native languages by establishing traditional language programs. Native languages are one of the most resilient ways to sustain traditions.

The Mound Builders of the Mississippi culture had a powerful influence on tribes in the Southeast. Members of this culture built platform mounds in the Mississippi area from Ohio to Alabama. One of the larger developed settlements of the Mound Builders is in Moundville, Alabama. Artifacts such as pottery and arrows have been excavated from the mounds (see Figure 9.2). The Mississippi Choctaws preserve the Nanih Waiya Mound as a sacred entity of Choctaw culture.

The SE tribes have other traditions in common, but, again, each tribe is unique. Many tribes sponsor a powwow each year. Traditional clothing in each tribe is similar but each has distinctions. Some of the tribes are attired in a similar traditional dress—the Choctaw women wear a dress and apron, and Florida Seminoles are famous for their elaborate patchwork. Chitimach baskets, Catawaba pottery and baskets, Cherokee baskets and pottery, and Choctaw beading are among the many traditional crafts that continue to be made by members today—(see Figure 9.3). Traditional games, like stickball, are still played, and children and adults are encouraged by the elders to participate. Traditional foods include the hominy that Choctaws prepare, and the Kanuchi that is cooked by Cherokees. Ingredients include dried nuts, dried fruit, fry bread, corn, fish, and small game. Animals depicted in tribal stories are common among the tribes, rabbits (see Figure 9.4), wild hogs, turkeys, eagles, opossums, raccoons, squirrels, and deer. The Cherokee story about Trickster Rabbit

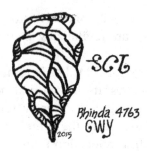

FIGURE 9.2 Arrow with Cherokee word for *arrow*.

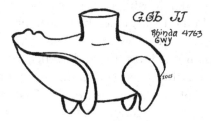

FIGURE 9.3 Frog–shaped pot with Cherokee word for *frog* and *pot*.

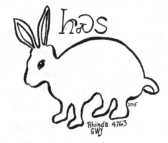

FIGURE 9.4 Rabbit with Cherokee word for *rabbit*.

is shared with children. Stories about the "Little People" are told to children as lessons in discipline. Dancing and music, such as the Stomp Dance, continue to be part of the Indian culture in many tribes. This is both a spiritual and a social dance. Turtle shells are cleaned and used to create shakers for women to wear. One man (men) uses a rattle to accompany his singing, and the other men provide a chorus. Sounds of rattles and turtle shells are considered healing (Portman & Garrett, 2006). Although commonalities of tribes across the SE have been discussed, remember that traditions and culture have special meaning to each tribe. Nurses need to keep this perspective in mind when delivering nursing care for SE AIs.

Nurses should be knowledgeable about the social, historical, and cultural factors of SE tribes to better comprehend the idea of health from a SE AI perspective. Some tribes were able to stay grounded despite their historical impact, whereas other tribes and AI individuals became "culturally homeless" as a result. Many AI people in the SE continue to be disenfranchised, segregated, or isolated and are thus culturally homeless, bereft of an Indian identity. Understanding this unique cultural perspective will assist nurses in assessing the environment of SE AIs when providing health care. This will help nurses to develop a deeper understanding of the health philosophy among SE AIs.

SOUTHEASTERN TRIBES AND STATE-RECOGNIZED TRIBES IN THE CULTURAL AREA

Human Being

American Indians believe that each person is holistically composed of different attributes related to mental, emotional, physical, and spiritual forces, and each characteristic bears the same importance as the others. AI people experience their being in totality, not as separate entities (Struthers et al., 2003). According to Fawcett, "the metaparadigm concept human beings refers to the individual, if individuals are recognized in a culture, as well as to the families, communities, and other groups of aggregates who participate in nursing" (2013, p. 6). There are differences and commonalities between the two perspectives. Nursing care of SE AIs not only focuses on the human aspect but also includes the environment of SE AIs (sacred lands, landscape, removal, federal Indian policies, segregation, revitalization). The SE tribal perspective is holistic, inclusive, and fluid in the relationship between person/client and environment.

Demographics of Tribes in Cultural Area

In April of 2010, the Census Bureau reported the U.S. population as 308.7 million (Norris, Vines, & Hoeffel, 2012). Approximately 2.9 million or 0.9% of the U.S. population self-identified as AI or Alaska Native (AN). Thirty-one percent of American Indian and Alaskan Natives (AI/ANs) live in the southern region of the United States. The number of AI/ANs living in the South increased from 31% to 33%. North Carolina ranked among the top 10 states with the largest population of AI/ANs. The number of federally recognized and state-recognized reservations in 2010 is 334. (Only 2010 Census data for AI/ANs who reported only one race were included in this section.)

Categories of Indian Tribes

Over 60 tribal entities are located across the 11 states in the SE region of the United States. These tribal entities can be divided into three categories.

In the first category, 13 of these Indian tribes are officially recognized by the federal government, and are on the Interior's BIA list of federally recognized Indian tribes in the *Federal Register* (Department of the Interior, Bureau of Indian Affairs, 2012).

The second category includes tribal entities that are officially recognized by state governments but not by the federal government (e.g., the Lumbee Tribe). In addition, some state governments officially recognize AI groups or AI assemblies (i.e., state-recognized groups and special interest organizations in South Carolina) as well (The South Carolina Commission for Minority Affairs, 2015; U.S. Government Accountability Office, 2012). State-recognized Indian tribes include nonfederally recognized tribes, as well. In addition, a federally recognized tribe can be a state-recognized tribe, as in the case of the Band of Poarch Creek Indians in Alabama (Alabama Indian Affairs Commission, n.d.).

The third category includes assemblies of people that self-identify as an AI tribe but are often 501-C nonprofit organizations or special interest organizations (U.S. Government Accountability Office, 2012). These Indian groups are referred to as nonfederally recognized tribes, and are without federal or state recognition.

Definition of an Indian Tribe

The BIA lists the names of federally recognized tribes in the *Federal Register* (Department of the Interior, Bureau of Indian Affairs, 2012). The BIA's definition of a federally recognized tribe is as follows:

> A **federally recognized tribe** is an American Indian or Alaska Native tribal entity that is recognized as having a government-to-government relationship with the United States, with the responsibilities, powers, limitations, and obligations attached to that designation, and is eligible for funding and services from the Bureau of Indian Affairs.
>
> Furthermore, federally recognized tribes are recognized as possessing certain inherent rights of self-government (i.e., tribal sovereignty) and are entitled to receive certain federal benefits, services, and protections because of their special relationship with the United States. (U.S. Department of the Interior, Bureau of Indian Affairs, n.d., para. 5 & 6)

Few federal agencies maintain listings of state-recognized tribes. The National Conference of State Legislators describes state-recognized tribes on their website thusly:

> **Indian tribes or groups that are recognized by the states**. This acknowledges their status within the state but does not guarantee funding from the state or the federal government. State-recognized Indian tribes are not federally recognized; however, federally recognized tribes may also be state-recognized. (National Conference of State Legislators, 2015, para. 1)

Definition of *American Indian* or *Alaska Native*

Racial classification and recognition as an AI/AN is still a subject of debate. (Haozous, Strickland, Palacious, & Solomon, 2014). This issue has particular pertinence for SE tribes because federally recognized tribes are entitled to health services from the federal government, whereas state-recognized tribes are not. Fewer federally recognized tribes exist than state-recognized tribes in the Southeast, and this influences who is acknowledged as AI and who is not federally recognized as Indian. Owing to political changes (i.e., Civil Rights movement, American Indian movement), financial prosperity for many AI tribes, such as through gaming, and increase in tribal populations, the debate about Indianness continues intensely in the SE area of the country. People can self-identify as AI/AN on the U.S. Decennial Census 2010 (see Table 9.1). The 2010 Census, according to the Office of Management and Budget (OMB), refers to an "American Indian or Alaska Native" individual as: "a person having origins in any of the original peoples of North and South America, including Central America, and who maintains tribal affiliation or community attachment" (Norris, Vines, & Hoeffel, 2012, p. 2).

Federally Recognized Tribes

There are 13 federally recognized tribes (Table 9.2) located across the 11 states in the cultural area (Department of the Interior, Bureau of Indian Affairs, 2012; National Conference of State Legislators, 2015). Alabama, Mississippi, North

TABLE 9.1 Percentage of American Indian Population

GEOGRAPHY	POPULATION	PERCENTAGE OF AMERICAN INDIANS (ONE RACE)
United States	316,128,839	1.2
Eastern Texas border	26,448,193	1.0
Louisiana	4,625,470	0.5
Southern Missouri	6, 044,171	0.5
Mississippi	2,991,207	0.6
Alabama	4,833,722	0.7
Georgia	9,992,167	0.5
Florida	19,552,860	0.5
North Carolina	9,848,060	1.6
South Carolina	4,774,839	0.5
Tennessee	6.495,987	0.4
Virginia	8,260,405	0.5

Source: U.S. Census Bureau (n.d.-b).

TABLE 9.2 Federally Recognized Tribes

Eastern Texas border

Alabama-Coushatta Tribe of Texas

Kickapoo Traditional Tribe of Texas

Ysleta del Sur Pueblo

Louisiana

Jena Band of Choctaw Indians

Chitimacha Indian Tribe

Coushatta Tribe of Louisiana

Tunica-Biloxi Indian Tribe

Southern Missouri

None

Mississippi

Mississippi Band of Choctaw Indians

Alabama

Poarch Band of Creek Indians of Alabama

Georgia

None

Florida

Miccosukee Tribe of Indians of Florida

Seminole Tribe of Florida

North Carolina

Eastern Band of Cherokee Indians

South Carolina

Catawba Indian Nation

Tennessee

None

Virginia

None

Carolina, and South Carolina each have only one federally recognized tribe located within their state boundaries. Tribal enrollment ranges from 284 tribal members in the Jena Band of Choctaw Indians to a tribal membership of 15,000 in the Eastern Band of Cherokee Indians. This is based tribal enrollment numbers listed on tribal websites (e.g., Jena Band of Choctaw Indians; Eastern Band of Cherokee Indians; Table 9.3). According to the U.S. Government Accountability Office (2012), the federal recognition of two tribes was terminated and restored; the Alabama-Coushatta Tribe of Texas had their federal recognition terminated on August 18, 1955, and restored on August 18, 1987—the tribe experienced 32-years as a nonfederally recognized tribe; the Catawba Indian Nation had their federal recognition terminated on July 2, 1960, and restored on October 27,

TABLE 9.3 Enrolled Tribal Members of Federally Recognized Tribes in Southeast

TRIBE	TRIBAL MEMBERSHIP BY WEBSITE	AI POPULATION LABOR FORCE REPORT[a]
Alabama-Coushatta Tribe of Texas	1,000	522
Ysleta del Sur Pueblo	1,729	1,169
Jena Band of Choctaw Indians	284	212
Coushatta Tribe of Louisiana	875	887
Chitimacha Indian Tribe	1,300	528
Mississippi Band of Choctaw Indians	10,000	9,199
Poarch Band of Creek Indians of Alabama	3,074	1914
Miccosukee Tribe of Indians of Florida	640	589
Eastern Band of Cherokee Indians	15,000	8,600
Catawba Indian Nation	2,800	1,847
Tunica-Bilox Indian Tribe	Not reported	358
Seminole Tribe of Florida	Not reported	3,680
Kickapoo Traditional Tribe of Texas	Not reported	1,169

[a]U.S. Department of the Interior, Office of the Secretary Office of the Assistant Secretary—Indian Affairs (2014).

1993; the Catawba tribe experienced 33 years as a nonfederally recognized tribe (U.S. Government Accountability Office, 2012).

Since 1978, three tribes have received federal acknowledgment as Indian tribes: the Tunica-Biloxi Indian Tribe effective September 25, 1981, the Poarch Band of Creek Indians effective August 10, 1984, and the Jena Band of Choctaw Indians effective August 29, 1995. The 2010 Census Bureau Federal List of Reservations listed all 13 tribes as having land held in reserve by the federal government (U.S. Census Bureau, n.d.-c). Each of the 13 tribes determines its own tribal membership criteria. The Office of the Interior states, "tribal enrollment criteria are set forth in tribal constitutions, articles of incorporation or ordinances. The criterion varies from tribe to tribe, so uniform membership requirements do not exist" (U.S. Department of the Interior, 2015, para. 2).

State-Recognized Tribes

The National Congress of State Legislators listed 50 state-recognized tribes in the 11-state cultural areas (Alabama Indian Affairs Commission, n.d.; Table 9.4). Virginia and Louisiana have 11 state-recognized tribes. Tennessee and Florida have no state-recognized tribes located in their states. The range for tribes with state recognition extended from three to 11. The percentage of AI/ANs by state on the 2010 Census data ranged from 0.4 in Tennessee to 1.6% in North Carolina (as compared with the 1.2% in the United States; refer back to Table 9.1).

Four state-recognized tribes have state reservations—the MOWA Band of Choctaw Indians in Alabama, the Lower Muskogee Tribe in Georgia, and the Mattaponi Tribe and the Pamunkey Tribe in Virginia (U.S. Government

TABLE 9.4 State-Recognized Tribes

Eastern Texas border

Louisiana

Adai Caddo Tribe

Bayou Lafourche Band of the Biloxi-Chitimacha Confederation of Muskogees

Choctaw-Apache Tribe of Ebarb

Clifton Choctaw Tribal Reservation, Inc.

Four Winds Cherokee

Grand Caillou/Dulac Band of the Biloxi-Chitimacha Confederation of Muskogees

Isle de Jean Charles Band of the Biloxi-Chitimacha Confederation of Muskogees

Louisiana Choctaw Tribe

Pointe-au-Chien Indian Tribe

United Houma Nation

Southern Missouri

None

Mississippi

None

Alabama

Cherokees of Northeast Alabama

Cher-O-Creek Intra Tribal Indians (Cherokees of Southeast Alabama)

Echota Cherokees of Alabama

Ma-Chis Lower Alabama Creek Indian Tribe

MOWA Band of Choctaw Indians

Piqua Shawnee Tribe

Star Clan of Muscogee Creeks of Pike County

United Cherokee Ani-Yun-Wiya Nation

Georgia

Cherokee of Georgia Tribal Council

Georgia Tribe of Eastern Cherokee Indians, Inc.

Lower Muscogee Creek Tribe

Florida

None

North Carolina

Coharie Tribe of North Carolina

Saponi Indian Tribe of North Carolina

Lumbee Tribe of North Carolina

Meherrin Indian Tribe

Occaneechi Band of Saponi Nation of North Carolina

Sappony (High Plains Indians, petitioned as Indians of Person County)

Waccamaw Siouan Tribe of North Carolina

(continued)

TABLE 9.4 State-Recognized Tribes (*continued*)

Eastern Texas border
South Carolina
Beaver Creek Indians
Edisto Natchez Kusso Tribe of South Carolina (petitioned as Four Holes Indian Organization, Edisto Tribal Council)
Pee Dee Indian Tribe of South Carolina
Pee Dee Nation of Upper South Carolina
Santee Indian Organization
Waccamaw Indian People (petitioned as The Chicora Waccamaw Indian People)
Wassamasaw Tribe of Varnertown Indians
Tennessee
None
Virginia
Cheroenhaka (Nottoway)
Chickahominy Indian Tribe
Eastern Chickahominy
Mattaponi Tribe
Monacan Indian Nation
Nansemond
Nottoway of Virginia
Pamunkey Indian Tribe
Patawomeck
Rappahannock Tribe
Upper Mattaponi

Accountability Office, 2012). When a state reservation is located within the state's boundaries, the U.S. Census Bureau (n.d.-d) "works with a governor appointed state liaison to obtain the name and boundary for each state-recognized AI reservation." These data are used to identify state and federal Indian reservations for the Census. State-recognized tribes can be members of the National Congress of American Indians (National Congress of American Indians, n.d.). State-recognized or nonfederally recognized tribes with status as a nonprofit organization are eligible to receive federal funding for certain programs. Between the fiscal years of 2007 and 2010, 26 nonfederally recognized tribes received more than $100 million from federal agencies (U.S. Government Accountability Office, 2012). Tribal membership is determined by each state-recognized tribe and within the governing laws of the state if applicable. Three states have state or Indian commissions that identify state-recognized tribes as well as federally recognized tribes—Alabama, North Carolina, and South Carolina

TABLE 9.5 State Committees and Commissions on Indian Affairs

Eastern Texas border
Texas Commission of Indian Affairs ended operations. http://www.tshaonline.org/handbook/online/articles/mdt38

Louisiana
http://www.gov.state.la.us/index.cfm?md=pagebuilder&tmp=home&navID=85&cpID=564&

Alabama
http://www.aiac.state.al.us/tribes.aspx

Georgia
http://www1.gadnr.org/caic/Documents/parks_policy.html

Florida
http://www.fgcia.com/index.html

North Carolina
http://www.doa.state.nc.us/cia/Default.aspx

South Carolina
http://cma.sc.gov/native-american-affairs/

Tennessee
Tennessee Commission of Indian Affairs ended operations as of June 30, 2010, the expiration of the legal authority for its existence (Tenn. Code Ann. 4-34-101 to 108)
http://www.naiatn.org/

Virginia
http://virginiaindians.pwnet.org/today/index.php

(see Table 9.5). State-recognized tribes and/or nonfederally recognized tribes have found Indian affair commissions useful in negotiating tribal–state issues.

State-recognized tribes can petition for federal recognition through the OFA Federal Acknowledgment Process (FAP) within the U.S. Department of the Interior, Bureau of Indian Affairs. The Interior Department implemented the FAP to handle requests in a uniform manner from various tribal entities requesting federal recognition. The process has been described as cumbersome, costly, and lengthy by nonfederally recognized tribes seeking acknowledgment. Currently, the number of petitions submitted by SE tribes statewise are as follows: Alabama 14, Florida 10, Missouri 11, North Carolina 21, Texas 14, Georgia 6, Louisiana 15, Mississippi 2, South Carolina 13, Tennessee 3, and Virginia 15. Approximately 10 nonfederally recognized tribes from the Southeast have been denied acknowledgment (U.S. Department of the Interior, Bureau of Indian Affairs, 2013). In the case of two Indian tribes in the cultural area, federal acknowledgment was terminated, and then restored by an act of the United States Congress.

Exemplar for Federally Recognized Tribes

The only federally recognized tribe in Alabama is the Band of Poarch Creek Indians (Alabama Indian Affairs Commission, n.d.). The tribe is located near the city of Atmore and in the county of Escambia, Alabama. The Poarch Creek Indians are descendants of the original Creek Nation that existed and lived in Alabama and Georgia (The Poarch Band of Creek Indians, n.d.). The Poarch Creeks were not removed from their tribal lands as many Creek AIs were during the removal period. According to the 2010 U.S. Census Bureau, Escambia County has a population of 37,983. The percentage of persons age 65 or older is 16.2%, as compared with 14.9% for the state of Alabama. The percentage of people who identified as AI/AN (one race) is 3.5% versus 0.7% for the state of Alabama. The percentage of high school graduates or higher is 76.2% in the county versus 83.1% for the state. The median household income (2009–2013) is $30,687 versus $43,253 for the state. The percentage of county residents who live below the poverty level is 25.4% versus 18.6% in the state. The percentage of firms owned by AI/ANs in 2007 was 3.2% in the county versus 0.8% in the state (U.S. Census Bureau, n.d.-b).

The Poarch Creek Indians received federal recognition in 1984, many years after petitioning (The Poarch Band of Creek Indians, n.d.). Currently, the tribe has 460 acres and 1,600 additional acres held in trust. There are approximately over 3,000 enrolled members, about half of whom live near or on the reservation. The Poarch Creek Tribe is the largest employer, including AI and non-AI people, in the area. The tribe has a modern and up-to-date health care facility and health department, and includes a medical clinic, pharmacy with a drive-through window, human services, community health, dental clinic, and diabetic clinic, as well as other services and programs. The tribe is rediscovering their tribal traditions and language, and investing in new ways to preserve tribal culture and history. In 2008, the Alabama Department of Public Health Office of Minority Health compiled a report on the health status of AIs in Alabama (Parmar & Williamson, 2008). This report did not include health data on the Poarch Creek Tribe. The tribes that participated in the survey were state-recognized tribes of Alabama. The Alabama Health Disparities Status Report 2010 did not include health data on AI/ANs because of the small sample size, although racial category and population statistics were described (Alabama Department of Public Health Office of Minority Health, n.d.).

Exemplar for State-Recognized Tribes

The Lumbee Tribe of North Carolina is a state-recognized tribe historically described as present-day descendants of the Cheraw Tribe. A significant number of tribal members live in Robeson, Hoke, Cumberland, and Scotland counties in North Carolina. The tribe has an enrollment of 55,000 tribal members (North Carolina Department of Administration, n.d.). The 2010 Census Bureau reported for select tribal groupings the Lumbee population as 66,922 (U.S. Census Bureau, n.d.-b). North Carolina is one of the states that have more than 100,000 AI/ANs. In 1953, the Lumbee Tribe was recognized by the North Carolina state legislature as a state-recognized tribe. The Lumbee Act of 1956 designated a group of Indians living in North Carolina as Lumbee Indians. The Act also indicated that the Indian group would not be eligible for services that other federally recognized Indian tribes receive (U.S. Government Accountability Office, 2012). Because of the Lumbee Act of 1956, the Lumbee Tribe is not eligible to petition for federal acknowledgment through the OFA. The Lumbee Tribe has been devoted to gaining federal recognition since that time.

The 2010 Census reported the population of Robeson County in North Carolina as 134,168 (U.S. Census Bureau, n.d.-b). The percentage of people who identified as AI/AN (solely) in the county is 39.5% as compared with 1.6% for the state. The percentage of people over 65 years of age is 12.5% as compared with 14.3% for the state. The percentage of high school graduates is 71.1% as compared with 84.9% in the state. Median household income for 2009 to 2012 is $29,806 compared with $46,334 for the state. The poverty level is 31.7% versus 17.5% for the state. The percentage of firms owned by AI/ANs in 2007 was 26.2% versus 1.0% in the state. The tribe does not have a state reservation (U.S. Government Accountability Office, 2012). The tribe offers services for elders, housing, vocational rehabilitation, volunteers, and youth programs. The Lumbee Tribe was one of the largest recipients of the $100 million of federal funds distributed to state-recognized tribes in the years 2007 to 2010 (U.S. Government Accountability Office, 2012).

CURRENT HEALTH PICTURE OF SOUTHEASTERN TRIBES AND STATE-RECOGNIZED TRIBES

Health

For many American Indian people, the concept of health is not only a physical state but a spiritual one as well (Garrett et al., 2011). Fawcett (2013) states that *health* refers to human processes of living and dying. Health for SE AIs involves a spiritual and historical journey to health. The culturally homeless AIs are progressing toward their spiritual health, and reconnecting to the ancestors of the past and to the tribes of today.

Health Data

Health disparities continue to exist for AI/AN populations. Both federal and state agencies document the health disparities, but accuracy of the data and soundness of the methodology are questionable. Haozous et al. (2014) describe how critical it is to collect health data that accurately describe the authentic health needs of the population. Issues with the collection of health data include misclassification of race, small population size, omission from national health reports, and being dropped from analysis for lack of statistical significance (Haozous et al., 2014). An example is the Alabama Health Disparities Status

Report 2010 (Alabama Department of Public Health Office of Minority Health, n.d.), which did not include health data on AI/ANs.

Birth certificate and death certificate misclassification existed with SE states because of segregation laws and racial categories that occurred within a biracial society. This is evident in the OFA process that SE nonfederally recognized tribes go through when petitioning for federal acknowledgment (Bureau of Indian Affairs, 1997). Tribes petitioning may not have population data (i.e., birth certificates, death statistics, and state vital statistics) because of historical events prior to the Civil Rights era, which impacted racial classification. The Census Bureau did not start collecting census data on AIs until after 1900. The health data reported on SE tribes are limited, or not available in regard to tribal-specific health data. Buescher, Gizlice, and Jones-Vessey (2005) advocated that the National Center for Health Statistics (NCHS) rules for coding race in North Carolina be reexamined. The rules imply that a "one drop" criterion categorized someone who is any part of a race (Hawaiian) as belonging to that race (Hawaiian).

Federally Recognized Tribes

Health Indicators

National data on health disparities and health status of SE federally recognized tribes include statistical reports from the Centers for Disease Control and Prevention (CDC), Indian Health Service (IHS), and the U.S. Census Bureau.

The CDC report showed that the death rates for AI/ANs of both genders were nearly 50% greater than those for non-Hispanic Whites during 1999 to 2009. Cancer was identified as the leading cause of death followed by heart disease among AI/ANs. Death rates from lung cancer have not improved. Suicide rates were 50% higher when compared with non-Hispanic Whites. Death rates for AI/AN infants were higher than those for non-Hispanic White infants (CDC, n.d.-a). AI/ANs were more likely to report current smoking and lack of seat belt use than were other racial and ethnic groups (CDC, n.d.-b).

The CDC (n.d.-c) identifies the 10 leading causes of death for AI/ANs in 2013 as cancer, heart disease, unintentional injuries, diabetes, chronic liver disease and cirrhosis, chronic lower respiratory diseases, stroke, suicide nephritis, nephrotic syndrome and nephrosis, and influenza and pneumonia.

The IHS identified diseases of the heart, malignant neoplasm, unintentional injuries, and chronic lower respiratory diseases as leading causes of death in AI/ANs (IHS, n.d.-a). The IHS reports that AI/ANs die more frequently than the U.S. population from chronic liver disease and cirrhosis (368% higher), diabetes mellitus (177% higher), unintentional injuries (138% higher), assault/homicide (82% higher), intentional self-harm/suicide (65% higher), and chronic lower respiratory diseases (59% higher; 2006–2008 rates).

Social Indicators

The median age for AI/ANs is 29 years (U.S. Department of Commerce, Economics and Statistics Administration, U.S. Census Bureau, 2012). The life expectancy of AI/ANs is 4.2 years less than that of all U.S. races (IHS, n.d.-a). The median household income of AI/ANs is $36,252 as compared with $52,176 for the nation as a whole. In 2004, the AI/AN population had a larger proportion of young people and a smaller proportion of older people (U.S. Department of Commerce Economics and Statistics Administration, U.S. Census Bureau, 2004). The AI/AN population of 65 years of age or older is 432,343 (U.S. Census report, 2014). About one out of every four AI/ANs lives below the poverty level (U.S. Department of Commerce Economics and Statistics Administration, U.S. Census Bureau, 2004, p. 3). AI/ANs age 65 or older had a poverty rate of 20% as compared with 7% for the White population (U.S. Department of Commerce Economics and Statistics Administration, U.S Census Bureau, 2004, p. 21). Fifty-eight percent of AI/AN grandparents who lived with their coresident grandchildren were primary caretakers (U.S. Department of Commerce Economics and Statistics Administration, U.S. Census Bureau, 2004). The CDC (n.d.-c) reported that 26.9% of AI/ANs lacked health insurance in 2013. The U.S. Commission on Civil Rights reported that the federal government's rate of spending on health care for Native Americans is 50% less than for prisoners. The IHS has been chronically underfunded consistently for many years (Marlerba, 2013).

Regional Health and Social Indicators

Regional heath data and social indicators for SE AI tribes are limited. AI/AN health data are not included or reported in some states. Individual tribal data are not available to the public owing to the issues related to reporting of the data. The Regional Differences in Indian Health Service 2002–2003 report (IHS, n.d.-b) included social indicators for the Nashville Area Indian Health Service. The user population was a younger population with a lower number of high school graduates, higher number of unemployed males and females over the age of 16, and lower household income as compared with the U.S. population.

There are sources of state health statistics that document health disparities of AIs in the SE, but these are incomplete. There are no uniform tracking systems for the SE AI populations. No data on SE AIs are systematically collected. North Carolina State Center for Health Statistics reports data for AI/ANs in several categories of health disparities. The Louisiana Bureau of Minority Health Access 2009 report, Eliminating Health Disparities "From A Grass-Roots Perspective," (Bureau of Minority Health Access, 2009) provided limited health data or did not include health disparities data on AI/ANs. Alabama compiled a report on the health status of AIs by surveying state-recognized tribes in 2008 (Parmar & Williamson, 2008). However, the "Alabama Health Disparities Status Report 2010" did not include a detailed overview of health data on

AI/ANs (Alabama Department of Public Health Office of Minority Health, n.d.). The spending on health care for SE AIs is not detailed nationally or regionally. Resources for this information were not found in the literature.

New Data Sources for Community Health Concerns

Twenty-six tribes are members of the United South and Eastern Tribes (USET), which include memberships of tribes located from Maine to Texas. In 2010, the USET Tribal Epidemiology Center received funding from the Robert Wood Johnson Foundation to develop an Internet-based system (data portal) for reporting community health data. This data system will provide USET members with community-comparative health population statistics. These data can then be used to profile individual tribal communities and to address public health concerns of each individual tribe's populations (Robert Wood Johnson Foundation, 2013).

Resources for AI Patients in the Region

Health care resources for federally recognized tribes are available through the I/T/U health care system (IHS, n.d.-b). The Nashville Area Indian Health Service is located in Nashville, Tennessee. This area office serves SE tribes, as well as others, and includes the Catawba Indian Nation of South Carolina, the Chitimacha Indian Tribe of Louisiana, the Coushatta Indian Tribe of Louisiana, the Eastern Band of Cherokees of North Carolina, the Jena Band of Choctaw Indians of Louisiana, the Miccousukee Tribe of Florida, the Mississippi Band of Choctaw Indians of Mississippi, the Poarch Band of Creek Indians of Alabama, the Seminole Tribe of Florida, and the Tunica–Biloxi Indians of Louisiana. Each tribe has comprehensive health care systems located on the reservations. No urban clinics are located in the cultural area. The USET is an intertribal nonprofit organization with a membership of 25 tribal entities (www.usetinc .org). This organization is currently assisting tribes with development of tribal-specific health data. State-recognized tribes are not eligible for services through the I/T/U health care system. The MOWA Band of Choctaw Indians (state-recognized) has a health care facility located on its reservation. The Alabama Public Health states that the state-recognized tribes "have identified their usual source of medical care as community-based, private pay, insured, or uninsured" (Alabama Public Health, n.d., para. 2).

NURSING IN THE SOUTHEAST

Nursing

Lowe and Struthers (2001) defined seven dimensions of nursing in Indian communities, which include, in ascending order, caring, traditions, respect, connection, holism, trust, and spirituality. A key responsibility of nursing care is "do no harm" to their AI patients (Nichols, Parker, & Henley, 2008). Nursing in the South was impacted by the Jim Crow laws. One such law written in Alabama was: "Nurses: No person or corporation shall require any white female nurse to nurse in wards or rooms in hospitals, either public or private, in which 'Black' men are placed" (National Park Service, n.d.-b).

Nursing care of SE AIs is a sacred trust that exists between the patient and the nurse. Human dignity is the core value of nursing. The historical factors related to federal Indian polices and segregation of the South will remain in the psyche of SE AI communities for decades, so rebuilding that trust is essential in providing nursing care to the AI populations.

Description of Nursing in the Area

Demographics on AI/AN nurses are limited at the regional level. Most state boards of nursing do not collect racial/ethnic data on their nursing workforce in the South. There are some demographics available at the national level. The IHS faces many workforce challenges in recruitment and retention of health care providers. The vacancy rate for nurses in the IHS is 16% as compared with 5.5% in non-Indian health hospitals. Although there has been an improvement in the nursing shortage, there is expected to be a shortage of nurses by 2020 (American Association of Colleges of Nursing, n.d.-a). Almost 69,000 qualified applicants for admission to nursing schools were turned away from baccalaureate and graduate schools because of the lack of qualified nursing faculty available to teach the programs (American Association of Colleges of Nursing, n.d.-b).

There are approximately 13,040 AI/AN nurses in the United States (Spratley, Johnson, Sochalski, Fritz, & Spencer, 2000, p. 17). In 2009, the National League for Nursing (NLN) reported that 0.3% of full-time nursing faculty were AI. In 2013, the percentage of AI/AN students in generic (entry-level) baccalaureate programs was 0.5 ($N = 965$) AI/AN compared with 71% ($N = 123,442$) for White students (American Association of Colleges of Nursing, 2015). The NLN National Survey on Nursing Programs gave the following report about nursing schools in the South: 44% are vocational practical nursing/licensed practical nursing (VP/LP), 39% associate degree in nursing (ADN), 15% diploma, 35% bachelor of science in nursing (BSN), 35% bachelor of science to registered nurse (BSRN), 31% masters, and 32% doctorate. There are no tribal colleges in the Southeast (www.ed.gov). The number of AI students in nursing programs is inadequate to replace the AI nurses needed, and there are not enough AI nursing faculty to teach the students. In summary, the supply of AI nurses (0.9%) is inadequate to care for the 1.2% population of AIs.

PATIENT POPULATION IN THE SOUTHEAST

Little is known about cultural issues of SE tribes concerning the social and political impact of segregation. American Indians who were afraid to reveal their

Indian heritage are now finding it safe to do so without legal retributions. Many tribes are trying to reconnect their youth with tribal culture. Much needs to be learned about the mental and spiritual needs of disenfranchised AIs in the South. These AIs are culturally homeless because of segregation and the biracial society that existed. AI Baptist and Methodist churches offer safe havens and places for social gatherings and support. Exploration into the mental health of tribal members who are petitioning the federal government for acknowledgment needs to be addressed. According to state statistics, there are significant populations of elders over the age of 65. Many elderly AIs continue to react in society in the manner that was expected during the period of Jim Crow laws; they remain submissive when in public. Many federally recognized tribes and state-recognized tribes offer services for elders. Elders do not respond to nontribal members as health care providers and so will not seek the health care needed.

CONCLUSIONS

Cultural humility is necessary for nurses when caring for SE tribal populations. Nurses have come full circle in learning about SE tribes from a circular perspective and integrating of the four metaparadigm concepts of nursing. Many AIs are culturally homeless in the SE, and many are grounded in their roots. Health disparities still continue, and new approaches that are reflective of the historical past are needed to address them.

CRITICAL–THINKING EXERCISES
◆ Evaluate how to define the four metaparadigm concepts of nursing from an SE AI cultural and health perspective.
◆ Evaluate cultural humility as an individual and how this self-critique would be useful for a nurse in caring for SE AIs.
◆ Discuss the importance of the all-Indian school and churches system that emerged during the pre-Civil Rights era, and the impact this system had on SE AI unity.
◆ Evaluate the triracial system of the pre-Civil rights that existed and the implications for health care disparities and nursing care of AIs.
◆ Describe the factors related to cultural homelessness of some SE AIs and the application of this concept to the nursing care for these tribes.
◆ Explain the problems that exist with health data and the methodology used to collect health data. Explore the relationship these problems have with SE AI tribes.
◆ Apply the historical events to the health disparities that exist in contemporary SE AI tribes.

STUDY QUESTIONS
◆ How do segregation of races and the Civil Rights Movement influence the nursing care for southeastern American Indian tribes?
◆ How is the culture of southeastern tribes different from that of tribes in other regions of the United States? How do these differences impact the delivery of nursing care to SE AIs?

♦ What can nurses do to ensure that southeastern American Indian health data are accurate and reflect the population correctly?
♦ What historical, social, and political forces impacted nursing care delivery for SE AIs? What can nurses do to change health care delivery to meet SE tribal needs?
♦ What are the health disparities of state-recognized tribes?
♦ What resources are available to recruit and retain AI nurses to seek employment in the South?

RECOMMENDED READING

Brown, T., (2014). Disenrollment leaves leaves Natives *"culturally homeless."* Retrieved from http://www.powwows.com/2014/01/27/disenrollment-leaves-natives-culturally-homeless/

United South and Eastern Tribes , Inc. (n.d.). Retrieved from http://www.usetinc.org/

REFERENCES

Alabama Department of Public Health Office of Minority Health. (n.d.). *Alabama Health Disparities Report 2010.* Retrieved from http://www.adph.org/minorityhealth/assets/HealthDisparitiesStatusReport04082011.pdf

Alabama Indian Affairs Commission. (n.d.). *Tribes recognized by the State of Alabama.* Retrieved from http://www.aiac.state.al.us/tribes.aspx

Alabama Public Health. (n.d.). *Alabama American Indians.* Retrieved from http://www.adph.org/minorityhealth/index.asp?ID=3341

American Association of Colleges of Nursing. (n.d.-a). *Nursing shortage fact sheet.* Retrieved from http://www.aacn.nche.edu/media-relations/NrsgShortageFS.pdf

American Association of Colleges of Nursing. (n.d.-b). *Advancing higher education in nursing. Nursing faculty shortage.* Retrieved from http://www.aacn.nche.edu/media-relations/fact-sheets/nursing-faculty-shortage

American Associations of Colleges Nursing. (2015). *Race/ethnicity data on students enrolled in nursing programs. 10-year data on minority students in baccalaureate and graduate programs.* Retrieved from http://www.aacn.nche.edu/research-data/EthnicityTbl.pdf

Braun, M. (1988). Native American culture map: Native American information. In C. Waldman (Ed.), *Encyclopedia of Native American tribes.* Retrieved from http://www.snowwowl.com/mapcontents.html

Buescher, P. A., Gizlice, Z., & Jones-Vessey K. A. (2005). Discrepancies between published data on racial classification and self-reported race: Evidence from the 2002 North Carolina live birth records. *Public Health Reports, 120,* 393–398.

Bureau of Indian Affairs. (1997). *The official guidelines to the Federal Acknowledgment Regulations, 25, CFR 83.* Washington, DC: The Bureau of Indian Affairs, The Branch of Acknowledgement and Research.

Bureau of Minority Health Access. (2009). Eliminating health disparities—"From a grass-roots perspective." Retrieved from http://dhh.louisiana.gov/assets/docs/GovCouncil/MinHealth/HealthDisparitiesReport200809.pdf

Centers for Disease Control and Prevention. (n.d.-a). *American Indian and Alaska Native death rates nearly 50 percent greater than those of non-Hispanic Whites.* Retrieved from http://www.cdc.gov/media/releases/2014/p0422-natamerican-deathrate.html

Centers for Disease Control and Prevention. (n.d.-b). *Facts about racial health risk factors.* Retrieved from http://www.cdc.gov/media/pressrel/r2k0324b.htm

Center for Disease Control and Prevention. (n.d.-c). *American Indian & Alaska Native populations*. Retrieved from http://www.cdc.gov/minorityhealth/populations/REMP/aian.html#10

Cole, S., & Ring, N. (2012). *The folly of Jim Crow: Rethinking the segregated South*. College Station, TX: Texas A&M University Press.

Fawcett, J. and DeSanto-Madey. S. (2013). The structure of contemporary nursing. In J. Fawcett & S. DeSanto Madeya (Eds.) *Contemporary nursing knowledge: Analysis and evaluation of nursing models and theories* (p. 6). Philadelphia, PA: F. A. Davis.

Garrett, M. T., Torres-Rivera, E., Brubaker, M., Portman, T. A. A., Brotherton, D., West-Olatunji, C., Conwill, W., & Grayshield. (2011). *Crying for a vision*: The Native American sweat lodge ceremony as therapeutic intervention. *Journal of Counseling & Development, 89*, 318–325.

Good Tracks, J. G. (1973). Native American noninterference. *Social Casework*, 18(Nov.), 30–34.

Haozous, E. A., Strickland, C. J., Palacious, J. F., and Solomon, T. G. A. (2014). Blood politics, ethnic identity, and racial misclassification among American Indians and Alaska Natives. *Journal of Environmental and Public Health*, 2014, 1–9.

Indian Health Service. (n.d.-a). Indian health disparities. Retrieved from http://www.ihs.gov/newsroom/includes/themes/newihstheme/display_objects/documents/factsheets/Disparities.pdf

Indian Health Service. (n.d.-b). Regional differences in Indian health, 2002–2003 edition, part 2: Population statistics. Retrieved from http://www.ihs.gov/dps/includes/themes/newihstheme/display_objects/documents/RD%2002-03%20Part%202-Population%20Statistics.pdf

Leininger, M., & McFarland, M. (2006). *Culture care diversity and universality: A worldwide theory of nursing* (2nd ed.). New York, NY: Jones & Bartlett.

Lowe, J., & Struthers, R. (2001). A conceptual framework of nursing in Native American culture. *Journal of Nursing Scholarship, 33*(3), 279–283.

Malberba, M. (2013). The effects of sequestration on Indian health. *Hastings Report, 6*, 17–21. DOI: 10.1002/hast.229.

Matte, J. (2002). *They say the wind is red: The Alabama Choctaw—Lost in their own land*. Montgomery, AL: New Books South.

Meleis, A., Isenberg, M., Koerner, J., Lacey, B., & Stern, P. (1995). *Diversity, marginalization, and culturally competent health care issues in knowledge development*. Washington, DC: American Academy of Nursing.

Mississippi Band of Choctaw Indians. (n.d.). *Choctaw traditions*. Retrieved from http://www.choctaw.org/culture/traditions.html

National Conference of State Legislators. (2015, February). *Federal and state tribes*. Retrieved from http://www.ncsl.org/research/state-tribal-institute/list-of-federal-and-state-recognized-tribes.aspx

National Park Service. (n.d-a). *We shall overcome: Historical Civil Rights places in the United States*. Retrieved from http://www.nps.gov/nr/travel/civilrights/sitelist.htm

National Park Service. (n.d.-b). *Jim Crow laws*. Retrieved from http://www.nps.gov/malu/learn/education/jim_crow_laws.htm

Nichols, L. A. (2004). The infant caring process among Cherokee mothers. *Journal of Holistic Nursing, 22*(3), 1–28.

Nichols, L. A., Parker, J. G., & Henley, S. (2008). Exploring global health ethics from an American Indian perspective. In V. Tschudin & A. J. Davis (Eds.), *The globalisation of nursing: Ethical, legal, & political issues*. London, UK: Radcliffe Publishing.

Norris, T., Vines, P. L., & Hoeffel, E. M. (2012). The American Indian and Alaska. *National Vital Statistics Reports, 62*(6), 31.

North Carolina Department of Administration. (n.d.). *Welcome to the Commission of Indian Affairs*. Retrieved from http://www.doa.nc.gov/cia/Default.aspx

Oakley, C. A. (2005, Fall). *Communities of faith: American Indian churches in Eastern North Carolina*. Reprinted with permission from Tar Heel Junior Historian Association, NC Museum of History (Original work published in 2005). Retrieved from http://ncpedia.org/print/723

Parmar, G. & Williamson, D. E. (2008). *Health survey of American Indians of Alabama 2008: Keeping the circle healthy*. Alabama Department of Public Health. Retrieved from http://www.adph.org/minorityhealth/assets/HealthSurveyofAmerIndiansofAL_2008.pdf

The Poarch Band of Creek Indians. (n.d.) *History of the band of Creek Indians*. Retrieved from http://pci-nsn.gov/westminster/tribal_history.htm

Portman, T. A. A., & Garrett, M. T. (2006). Native American healing traditions. *International Journal of Disability, Development and Education, 53*(4), 443–469.

Public Broadcasting Services, Oklahoma Educational Television Authority. (n.d.). *The Confederate States*. Retrieved from http://www.pbs.org/kenburns/civil-war/war/maps/#/detail/the-confederate-states-of-america

Robert Wood Johnson Foundation. (2013, July). *A pilot data portal profiles the health of tribal communities: Helping American Indian officials develop community health profiles as a starting point in addressing health disparities* [Robert Wood Johnson Foundation Program Results Report, Report Grant ID 68433]. Retrieved from http://www.rwjf.org/content/dam/farm/reports/program_results_reports/2013/rwjf407061

The South Carolina Commission for Minority Affairs. (2015). *South Carolina Native American Indian entities*. Retrieved from http://www.state.sc.us/cma/nai_re.html

Spratley, E., Johnson, A., Sochalski, J., Fritz, M., & Spencer, W. (2000). *The registered nurse population: Findings from the National Sample Survey Of Registered Nurses*. U.S. Department of Health and Human Services, Health Resources and Service Administration, Bureau of Health Professions. Retrieved from http://bhpr.hrsa.gov/healthworkforce/rnsurveys/rnsurvey2000.pdf

Struthers, R., & Lowe, J. (2003). Nursing in the Native American culture and historical trauma. *Issues in Mental Health Nursing, 24*, 257–272.

U.S Census Bureau. (n.d.-a). *Geography. Geographic terms and concepts—census divisions and census regions*. Retrieved from https://www.census.gov/geo/reference/gtc/gtc_census_divreg.html

U.S. Census Bureau. (n.d.-b). *State and county quick facts beta United States*. Retrived from http://www.census.gov/quickfacts/table/PST045214/00

U.S. Census Bureau. (n.d.-c). *Geography. 2010 Census—Tribal tract reference maps*. Retrieved from http://www.census.gov/geo/maps-data/maps/2010tribaltract.html

U.S. Census. (n.d.-d). *Geography. Definitions of American Indian and Alaska Native geographic areas. State American Indian Reservations (SAIRs)*. Retrieved from https://www.census.gov/geo/partnerships/aian_tsap.html

U.S. Department of Commerce Economics and Statistics Administration, U.S Census Bureau. (2004). *The American Community—American Indians and Alaska Natives: 2004 American Community Survey Reports*. Retrieved from http://www.census.gov/prod/2007pubs/acs-07.pdf

U.S. Department of Commerce, Economics and Statistics Administration, & U.S. Census Bureau. (2012). *The American Indian and Alaska Native population: 2010 Census briefs*. Retrieved from http://www.census.gov/prod/cen2010/briefs/c2010br-10.pdf

U.S. Department of Health and Human Services, Indian Health Service. (n.d.). *The federal health program for American Indians and Alaska Natives. About us.* Retrieved from https://www.ihs.gov/nashville/index.cfm/aboutus/

U.S. Department of the Interior. (2015). *Tribal enrollment process.* Retrieved from http://www.doi.gov/tribes/enrollment.cfm

U.S. Department of the Interior, Bureau of Indian Affairs. (1975). *Federal Indian policies . . . from the Colonial period through the early 1970's.* Washington, DC: U.S. Government Printing Office. Retrieved from http://files.eric.ed.gov/fulltext/ED107420.pdf

U.S. Department of the Interior, Bureau of Indian Affairs. (2012). Indian entities recognized and eligible to receive services from the Bureau of Indian Affairs. *Federal Register, 77*(155). Retrieved from http://www.bia.gov/cs/groups/public/documents/text/idc-020700.pdf

U.S. Department of the Interior, Bureau of Indian Affairs. (2013). *Office of Federal acknowledgement—Brief overview.* Retrieved from http://www.bia.gov/cs/groups/xofa/documents/text/idc1-024417.pdf

U.S. Department of the Interior, Bureau of Indian Affairs. (2015). *Indian lands in the United States.* Retrieved from http://www.bia.gov/cs/groups/public/documents/text/idc013422.pdf

U.S. Department of the Interior, Bureau of Indian Affairs. (n.d.). *Frequently asked questions: I. Why tribes exist today in the United States.* Retrieved from http://www.bia.gov/FAQs/

U.S. Department of the Interior, Office of the Secretary Office of the Assistant Secretary—Indian Affairs. (2014). *2013 American Indian population and labor force report.* Retrieved from http://www.bia.gov/cs/groups/public/documents/text/idc1-024782.pdf

U.S. Government Accountability Office. (2012, April). *Indian issues federal funding for non-federally recognized tribes.* Report to the Honorable Dan Boren, House of Representatives. Retrieved from http://www.gao.gov/assets/600/590102.pdf

Woolley, J. & Peters, G. (n.d.). *The American Presidential Project. Presidential election data.* [Maps]. Retrived from http://www.presidency.ucsb.edu/elections.php

Wright, L. (1994, July 25). One drop of blood: Annals of politics. *New Yorker*, p. 46.

TEN

American Indian Tribes of the Southwest

Nicolle L. Gonzales

LEARNING OBJECTIVES
- To give an overview of American Indian health in the Southwest
- Historical significance of colonization and its impact on health
- Importance of cultural perspectives on wellness
- A brief overview of health disparities and how they are being addressed
- The importance of diversity in nursing
- Diversity in death, and dying perspectives among tribes

KEY CONCEPTS
- Cultural beliefs
- Cultural safety
- Diversity in nursing
- Environmental justice
- Health disparities
- Historical trauma
- Mental health
- Reproductive health and justice
- Socioeconomic factors

KEY TERMS
- Colonization
- Resiliency
- Spiritual
- Wellness

Each Native American community approaches health and wellness within the context of harmony among the physical body, the spiritual being, the community, and the land in which they live. Historically, Western approaches to promoting wellness within Indian country have not fully grasped this concept, and have only recently begun the process of developing trusting relationships and engaging each Native American community to define "wellness" for itself, rather than defining it for them. As Native American tribes are exercising their sovereignty in reclaiming their land rights, there is also a process underway to reclaim cultural values as the foundation on which communities can begin to heal from centuries of colonization.

This chapter provides an overview of health and wellness of the Southwest region, which includes tribes from New Mexico, Colorado, Utah, and Arizona.

Although indigenous communities in the Southwest do share similarities, each tribal nation is unique in its cultural values, language, and perceptions of its health. Some tribes discussed here have purposely withheld reporting specific vital statistics regarding their communities' health with the intent of protecting tribal community anonymity. To get an overview of the health disparities in the American Indian tribes of the Southwest, the historical context of only a few specific tribes is briefly described from two perspectives: one is the cultural perspective of each tribal community, and the other is the depiction in American history by scholars who have researched and documented the tribe's transformation to the present day by way of observation. Keep in mind that some tribes will not be mentioned in the historical narrative, as some of the events that caused conflicts and population shifts affected multiple tribal communities.

HISTORY OF THE SOUTHWEST AREA

One of the largest American Indian Nations in the United States is the Navajo Nation. The Navajos—or Diné, which they call themselves—live on a reservation that covers 27,000 square miles in northeastern Arizona, northwestern New Mexico, and southeastern Utah (Iverson, 2002). The total number of Navajo members documented in the 2010 census was 173,667. Although the historical origins of this Native American tribe are documented in the context of the Navajo beginning to inhabit the Southwest from the migration of ancestral Athabaskan from the north to the south, archaeological research is still unclear whether this migration was caused by climate changes or other unknown factors. The traditional Diné emergence story as told by oral history describes this time as a difficult journey from the First World to the Fourth World, the transition from one world to the next being caused by chaos and disorder in one world, and a need to keep moving up to the next world in an effort to create order. Each world is represented by color and slowly progresses from a dark to light, depicting the journey from the underworld onto the earth's surface. The present-day "Diné Bikaéyah" or Navajo land lies between the sacred mountains of Blanca Peak, Mount Taylor, San Francisco Peaks, and Hesperus Peak.

Prior to the arrival of Europeans, Navajos were hunters and gatherers. Trade represented an essential dimension of life for the Navajo people, and with the incorporation of horses, trade played a pivotal part in the expansions of Navajo territory.

Prior to the arrival of colonists, the Navajos developed a reputation for not appropriating land in a diplomatic way, but also for not understanding initial ownership of land—meaning that if no one lived on it or near it, but used it only on certain occasions, how could they say they owned it? Although the Navajo had trade relationships with the Pueblo people, the contention over appropriating land continued to be a source of conflict. Relationships with the Comanche and Utes of the region consisted of stealing horses, children, and women.

Although the Navajos have their own beginning in the Southwest, there are 19 federally recognized Pueblos that are located in New Mexico and Arizona. Each Pueblo community has its own story of origin as told by its own traditional oral history, and will be touched on briefly. During the 1300s, some of the Pueblo peoples migrated from the Mesa Verde region to establish villages in what is now New Mexico. The ancient Pueblos used art symbols depicted in rock formations as a means to communicate ceremonial sites and mythology that reflected their spiritual lives. Their emergence story depicts their place of origin, "Shibapu," as a body of water or lake through which they climbed up by way of a ladder from the underworld. Each Pueblo community has its own ceremonial order in which a sacred place called a "kiva" is the center of the community. Each Pueblo community also has its own diverse language and dialect. Prior to the arrival of the Spanish colonizers, the Pueblo people were multilingual.

A pivotal part of each Pueblo community's history is the Pueblo Revolt of 1680, which united all the Pueblo tribal Nations. The Revolt was led by Popé—a Tewa religious leader from San Juan Pueblo—and occurred in retaliation for the Spanish colonizers who perpetrated decades of extortion, violence, and mistreatment of the Pueblo peoples. The unification of all of these tribal nations prevented the Spanish colonial expansion into New Mexico and Arizona. Despite the phenomenal effort to keep the Spanish colonizers out of the New Mexico and Arizona territories, the Spanish returned a few years later to establish rights over the land and the indigenous peoples. It was during this time that the Spanish colonizers made vigorous efforts to replace the cultural rituals of the Pueblo peoples with Catholicism. As part of this expansion, churches were set up in each Pueblo tribal community.

After the Pueblo Revolt of 1680, the Spanish monarchy recognized the Pueblo people as chief resources of Spain, and worked toward ensuring preservation and progress by way of a land grant. In 1684, Governor Domingo Jironza Petriz de Cruzate was given the authority to make Pueblo land grants. Eleven Pueblos were given the title to their grants in 1689. The United States recognized the rights put forth in the Spanish land grants, which were made a part of the Treaty of Guadalupe Hidalgo (Sando, 1976).

The primary food sources of the American Indians of the Southwest territories included hunting wild game like antelope and elk, and additional food sources, such as corn, squash, and beans, were produced through land-based farming. The people of the Hopi, who are located in northeastern Arizona, are well known for their dryfarming, a method that was adopted in response to the drought conditions of the land, and involved planting seeds in dry washes or sand dunes where moisture collected during rainstorms. According to the Hopi emergence story of origin, when they were advancing from the Third World to the Fourth World, corn was given to them. Agricultural cycles marked the timing of ceremonial events, and corn was viewed as "life."

Because of the ongoing land encroachment debate between the Navajo and the Hopi tribe, President Chester A. Arthur established the Hopi reservation in 1882. Like the Navajo, the Hopi understood the land to be of ancestral nature, but this did not stop the Navajo from appropriating Hopi land. Over time, the Navajo took over 1,800,000 acres of the Hopi land as designated by President Arthur. It was not until Congress recognized the problem that they then passed the Navajo–Hopi Settlement Act of 1974, which returned 900,000 acres to the Hopi tribe.

POPULATION SHIFTS

Anthropologists, by means of mummified remains, have studied the epidemiologic characteristics of health within American Indian populations over time, focusing on relationships among environment, culture, and biological conditions (Rhoades, 2000). Native American groups have largely protested the study of their American Indian ancestors in this manner, as they did not have input on excavation and curation of the remains. In 1990, legislation was passed called "Native American Graves Protection and Repatriation Act," which required any federal agency or institution that received federal funding to return unlawfully obtained human and cultural remains taken from Native American territories. This piece of legislation redefined anthropology and allowed for American Indians to exercise their sovereign rights as indigenous peoples for respectful treatment of their deceased ancestors.

Living conditions and food sources greatly influenced Indian health prior to European contact. For example, anthropologists studying ancestral Pueblo children attributed their short stature to a corn-only diet. In contrast, the study of ancestral American Indian remains found the Plains children to be taller, and this difference was attributed to wild plant diets and a wider selection of wild game (Arizona Health Disparities Center, 2013; Martin, Goodman, Armelagos, & Magennis, 1991). Because corn was a primary food source for the tribes of the Southwest, this form of nutrition was low in bioavailable iron; iron-deficiency anemia was common and predisposed them to infectious disease by lowering resistance (Rhoades, 2000).

Historical trends and regional differences in population shifts in Native American tribal communities of the Southwest from precontact are difficult to quantify. Accounts of the Pueblo populations in the 1500s at the time of contact with the Spaniards described them as living in multiple villages of less than 2,000 inhabitants. However, it is important to note that the Franciscan de Benavides, a Spanish priest, reported first figures of population as 60,000 converts. Recent anthropological research acknowledges this as a possible exaggeration of numbers aimed at continuing to receive support from the Crown or private entrepreneurs (Sando, 1976). In the post-Spanish period, the Navajo were estimated to be around 7,000 and living in different small communities of 10 to 40 families sharing defined agricultural and grazing land, according to General Kearny's account in 1846 (Spicer, 1962).

One of the major causes of population shifts in the Southwest territories was the smallpox epidemic of 1630, in which New Mexico's population was reduced by one third. Between 1629 and 1641, the Pueblos' populations declined 68%, and 50% of the Pueblo communities were abandoned. During this period, smaller Pueblo tribes aggregated to larger communities in the Rio Grande region. Besides the smallpox epidemic, Apache raids and food shortages also contributed to these population shifts (Barrett, 2002). After the Spanish colonialists reestablished settlements in 1692, an additional 38% of the population was reduced in the Pueblo communities with a concomitant loss of territories.

Present-day population demographics depicting specific characteristic population shifts for American Indians continue to be problematic for researchers. Variations in reporting and definitional problems make it difficult to measure change. A common thread found throughout was that American Indians were more likely to die from communicable diseases, and regional differences existed in both socioeconomic and health conditions that were explained by regional ecologies and histories of contact with non-Native counterparts (Kunitz, Veazie, & Henderson, 2014).

CONFLICTS

One of the historical events that occurred for the Navajos and Mescalero Apaches was the "Long Walk to Bosque Redondo in 1864," which resulted after the final standoff at Canyon de Chelly—8,500 men, women, and children were forced to march almost 500 miles in harsh wintery conditions (New Mexico Historic Sites, n.d). Three groups made this journey to Bosque Redondo over 3 years. Several hundred Navajo lives were lost on this journey, with some being abducted by slave traders along the way. An additional 500 Mescalero Apaches inhabited Bosque Redondo, but left in the middle of a February night in 1865. While the Navajos occupied Bosque Redondo, the smallpox epidemic struck and 2,321 died within a few months. It was not until 1868 that the Navajos were able to return to their lands. An agreement between the U.S. government and the Navajos was established in the Treaty of 1868, which called for a cessation of war and wrongdoing, delineated reservation lands, and produced a list of provisions that would be upheld by the U.S. government. The actual area covered by the treaty was 3,328,302 acres, and did not include Canyon de Chelly (Iverson, 2002).

Twenty-five hundred Navajos who returned from Bosque Redondo settled in Fort Defiance, while the rest dispersed to the newly created reservation, looking for their prior homelands (Spicer, 1962). Three years after the Treaty of 1868 was signed, 9,500 Navajos appeared for the distribution of sheep and goats, which was committed to by the government as a short-term provision for the tribe to reestablish itself. Three decades following 1900, the Navajo population continued to increase, reaching 40,000 in 1930. Despite the vast number of Navajo people, the actual area of defined reservation land covered by the Treaty of 1868 was 3,328,302 acres and did not include Canyon de Chelly (Iverson, 2002). Over time, additions were made to increase "Navajo Land," which now extends to Utah, Arizona, Colorado, and New Mexico.

In 1874, the commissioner of Indian Affairs called for Navajo children to be educated and for boarding schools to be established. During the 1880s and 1890s, 23 boarding schools were established with the focus on educating Native American children. However, Navajo families were very reluctant to send their children to such places, as it challenged their authority and separated them from their Navajo culture. Diseases also spread quickly through the boarding schools. "Agent C. E. Vandevor reported that of the approximately seventy children attending school in Fort Defiance in 1890, five did not survive the year" (Iverson, 2002, p. 88). Students returning home from boarding schools also reported physical and sexual abuse at the hands of their overseers. This forced assimilation through boarding schools touched the Pueblo communities as well, and nearly destroyed Pueblo culture.

SOUTHWEST TRIBES (Some of the American Indian tribes that inhabit the Southwest are depicted in Figure 10.1)

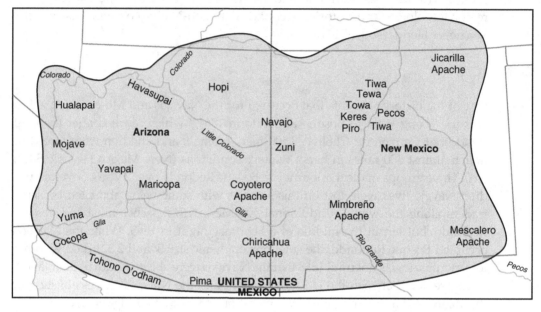

FIGURE 10.1 Map of some of the Southwest tribes.

NEW MEXICO'S PUEBLOS AND RESERVATIONS

The Indians of New Mexico and the locations of pueblos their reservations are indicated in Figure 10.2

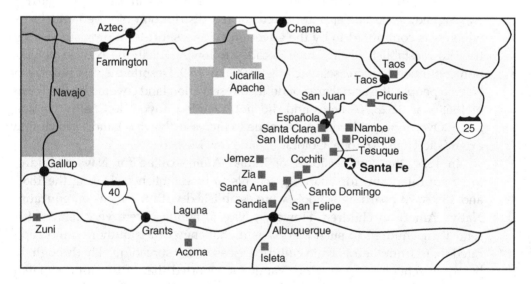

FIGURE 10.2 New Mexico's pueblos and reservations.

Source: New Mexico State Health Assessment (2014–2016).

Table 10.1 presents a list of federally recognized Southwestern tribes by states.

TABLE 10.1 Federally Recognized Tribes of the Southwestern Region

NEW MEXICO	COLORADO	UTAH	ARIZONA
Jicarilla Apache Nation	Southern Ute Indian Tribe and Reservation	**Confederated Tribes of the Goshute Reservation (Nevada and Utah)**	Ak Chin Indian Community of the Maricopa (Ak Chin) Indian Reservation
Mescalero Apache Tribe and Reservation	**Ute Mountain Tribe and Reservation (Colorado, New Mexico, and Utah)**	**Navajo Nation (Arizona, New Mexico, and Utah)**	**Cocopah Tribe of Arizona**
Navajo Nation (Arizona, New Mexico, and Utah)		Northwestern Band of Shoshoni Nation of Utah (Washakie)	**Colorado River Indian Tribes of the Colorado River Indian Reservation (Arizona and California)**
Northern Pueblos		Paiute Indian Tribe of Utah (Cedar City Band of Paiutes, Kanosh Band of Paiutes	**Fort McDowell Yavapai Nation**
Ohkay Owinge (formerly the Pueblo of San Juan)		Koosharem Band of Paiutes, Indian Peaks Band of Paiutes, and Shivwits Band of Paiutes)	**Fort Mojave Indian Tribe (Arizona, California, and Nevada)**
Pueblo of Nambe		Skull Valley Band of Goshute Indians of Utah	Gila River Indian Community of the Gila River Indian Reservation
Pueblo of Picuris		Ute Indian Tribe of the Uintah and Ouray Reservation	Havasupai Tribe of the Havasupai Reservation
Pueblo of Pojoaque		**Ute Mountain Ute Tribe (Colorado, New Mexico, and Utah)**	Hopi Tribe of Arizona
Pueblo of San Ildefonso			Hualapai Indian Tribe of the Hualapai Indian Tribe Reservation
Pueblo of Santa Clara			Kaibab Band of Paiute Indians of the Kaibab Indian Reservation
Pueblo of Tesuque			**Navajo Nation (Arizona, New Mexico, and Utah)**
Pueblo of Taos			Pascua Yaqui Tribe of Arizona
Southern Pueblos			**Quechan Tribe of the Fort Yuma Indian Reservation (Arizona and California)**
Pueblo of Jemez			Salt River Pima–Maricopa Indian Community of the Salt River Reservation
Pueblo of Cochiti			San Carlos Apache Tribe of the San Carlos Reservation
Pueblo of Sandia			San Juan Southern Paiute Tribe of Arizona
Pueblo of San Felipe			Tohono O'odham Nation of Arizona
Pueblo of Santa Ana			Tonto Apache Tribe of Arizona
Pueblo of Santo Domingo			White Mountain Apache Tribe of the Fort Apache Reservation
Pueblo of Zia			**Yavapai-Apache** Nation of the Camp Verde Indian Reservation
Pueblo of Isleta			**Yavapai-Prescott** Tribe of the Yavapai Reservation
Pueblo of Acoma Laguna			
Zuni Reservation and Tribe			
Ute Mountain Reservation and Tribe (Colorado, New Mexico, and Utah)			

165

CURRENT HEALTH PICTURE OF SOUTHWEST TRIBES

Environmental Pollutants

A common thread when discussing health among Native American populations in the Southwest is the historical role that environmental pollutants have played. Between 1945 and 1962, the United States conducted 200 nuclear weapons development tests in this region, which involved uranium mining and processing. Uranium mining and milling was established on the Navajo reservation in the 1940s. Navajo families worked and lived in close proximity to these mines, and were unaware of the harmful impact this had on their health. Uranium mining stopped after 1986, but the legacy of these activities left more than 500 abandoned uranium mines. It also contaminated soil, surface water, groundwater, and rocks in the Four Corners area. Health effects resulting from exposure to these elements have been identified as bone cancer, lung cancer, and impaired kidney function (United States Environmental Protection Agency, 2013).

The U.S. Congress has authorized the Radiation Exposure Compensation Act, which provides partial restitution to those who have developed serious illness after exposure to radiation. In addition, the Indian Health Service has agreed to develop a database to improve cancer case surveillance, review water contamination data, and plans to assess the prevalence of cancer. As part of a 5-year plan to address uranium contamination, the Agency for Toxic Substances & Disease Registry (ATSDR) Prospective Birth Cohort Study was developed to assess the exposure to uranium and other heavy metals as they impact the reproductive birth outcomes in Navajo mothers (United States Environmental Protection Agency, 2013).

Similar pollutants have contaminated soil and water sources in other Native American reservations all over the Southwest. Los Alamos National Laboratories (LANL) is known as the place where the Manhattan project took place to create the first atomic bomb. LANL is located west of several pueblos, and is at the top of several watersheds that feed into the Rio Grande River. Its focus now is thermonuclear weapon design, nuclear reactive research, waste disposal, tritium handling, and radiobiology. The concern with its history and present-day research is how it impacts the environment and the communities surrounding it.

Beata Tsosie-Peña, the environmental justice coordinator at Tewa Women United, and member of San Juan Pueblo, discusses the effects of pollutants on the Native communities of the Rio Grande:

> Even though there have not been health studies to show the impact of Los Alamos National Laboratories, there has been an increase in miscarriages and cancer in the Pueblo communities. The ancestral lands where the men of our community go to hunt and fish were once owned by LANL and recently returned to the tribe. It is plausible that the health effects from multiple and cumulative exposure over time to the chemicals at LANL is what we are seeing in our communities now. (Beata Tsosie-Peña, personal communication, November 25, 2014)

American Indians share a common interest in and understanding of being caretakers of the land, as it holds sacred knowledge and healing medicines. There is also an innate understanding that the land carries the seeds of their history, which it should be protected for future generations. That understanding has led to a resurgence of tribal communities teaching indigenous agricultural practices and of nonprofit organizations like Tewa Women United, which advocates for those most vulnerable by creating a space for dialogue to protect ancestral land.

HEALTH DISPARITIES

It is important to understand the role and meaning of "health disparities" when working with American Indian people, as this is a broad term used to describe the imbalance and inconsistencies in population-specific areas as compared with other populations. These differences have been widely studied in relation to health conditions and behaviors that have been known to cause preventable disease and premature death. The study of these inequalities highlights the characteristics historically linked to discrimination or exclusion that certain populations have systematically experienced over time. Disparities in health status among American Indians, Europeans, and Americans have been recognized for five centuries (Jones, 2006).

Some concepts to consider while reviewing the health status of American Indians are economic and social opportunities and how resources shape living and working conditions. These social factors affect health directly and indirectly, in that education, income, and wealth facilitate making healthier choices (Robert Wood Johnson Foundation, 2008). Although reducing social disparities in medical care is essential, these efforts alone cannot adequately reduce socioeconomic and racial or ethnic disparities in health (Robert Wood Johnson Foundation, 2008).

Scholars have questioned disease susceptibility in American Indian populations over time, but this thought remains:

> Do American Indians have intrinsic susceptibilities to every disease for which disparities have existed? Or, does the history of disparity after disparity suggest that social and economic conditions have played a more powerful role in generating Indian vulnerability to disease? (Jones, 2006, p. 98)

SOCIOECONOMIC CHARACTERISTICS

In keeping with the focus of this chapter, socioeconomic characteristics and major health issues are discussed primarily with reference to New Mexico and Arizona, as that is where the largest populations of American Indians reside. In 2012, a Navajo County Health Assessment was conducted in Arizona, which included American Indians of the Navajo Nation, the Fort Apache Reservation, and the Hopi tribe. It found that in 2011, 33% of all people in Navajo County were living below the national poverty level. Arizona has an 8.4% unemployment rate, whereas those living on the Navajo Nation reservation and off the reservation trust land have a 25.6% unemployment rate. Similar statistics have been recorded for those of the Hopi tribe (21.5%) and the Fort Apache tribe (26.0%). With regard to health care coverage, 20.8% had none, 28.9% did not have a health care provider, and 19.5% could not see a doctor because of cost.

In New Mexico, American Indians make up 10.7% of the population and share similar socioeconomic characteristics of those in Arizona. Specific major health disparities exist for American Indians and have been defined as major and minor disparities, in which the rate of occurrence pertaining to a particular group is higher than that pertaining to the average population in that area (Table 10.2).

TABLE 10.2 American Indian Health Equity: A Report on Health Disparities in New Mexico Report

ILLNESS		DISPARITY RATIO
Major[1] (≥ 2.5) health disparity ratio by NM Department of Health for American Indians		
2010–2012 (rate per 100,000)		
Diabetes deaths	72.1	4.0
Pneumonia and influenza deaths	37.1	2.9
Chlamydia infection	4,679.0	10.6
HIV infections	15.7	3.7
Motor vehicle deaths	37.2	3.1
Homicide	14.7	4.1
Alcohol-related deaths	121.1	3.0
2010–2012 (rate per 1,000)		
Teen births	27.2	6.0
2010–2012 (rate per 100)		
Obesity among adults	39.2	5.7
Minor[2] (1.5–2.4) health disparity ratio by NM Department of Health for American Indians		
2010–2012 (rate per 100)		
Late or no prenatal care	44.4	1.7
Obesity among youth	19.4	2.2
Not had pneumonia vaccination	41.2	1.5
2010–2012 (rate per 100,000)		
Suicide	24.7	1.8
Youth suicide	38.7	2.1

Source: New Mexico Department of Health (2013a).
[1]Defined as a major disparity existing that requires urgent attention.
[2]Defined as a moderate disparity existing that requires intervention.

The 2013 Arizona Health Disparities Report identified the following as the top five leading causes of death for American Indians in the state:

1. Heart disease
2. Cancer
3. Unintentional injury
4. Diabetes
5. Chronic liver disease and cirrhosis

According to the report, the overall prevalence of diabetes during 2008 to 2010 was 14.1%, the highest as compared with that of all other ethnic and racial populations in the state.

The causes of specific health disparities among the American Indian populations of the Southwest are lack of knowledge among individuals regarding disease process or positive personal actions; cultural divisions between the individual and providers; cultural attitudes toward health care among individuals; lack of cultural competency among providers; and lack of availability of and access to health services in the rural, tribal, and inner-city areas. To address these issues, the Tribal Collaboration Act was signed in March of 2009, which required the state to work with the tribes on a government-to-government basis. The overarching goals of this policy are to promote effective collaboration and communication between government agencies and tribes, to promote positive relations between the state and tribes, to promote cultural competence in providing effective services to American Indians/Alaska Natives, and to establish a method for notifying employees of the agency of the provisions of the State–Tribal Collaboration Act and the policy that the agency adopts (New Mexico Department of Health, 2013b). The Arizona Health Department (2013) identified similar strategies for addressing health disparities in the tribal communities, which they outlined in their Health Equity Stakeholders Strategies Report. One of the objectives was to strengthen local, state, and tribal partnerships.

RESOURCES FOR AMERICAN INDIAN PATIENTS IN THE SOUTHWEST REGION

The federal development of health care for American Indians has undergone a gradual evolution since the 1800s. The Snyder Act of 1921, passed by Congress to provide continuing authority for federal Indian programs, identified "relief of distress and conservation of health of Indians" as one of the federal functions (Rhoades, 2000). The Indian Health Care Improvement Act was reauthorized to address health disparities within American Indian populations. It specifically allowed for greater decision making with regard to program operations and priorities set forth by tribes to improve services, and to establish a continuum of care through integrated health care programs for both prevention and treatment of alcohol/substance abuse, social services, and mental health needs of American Indian people (IHS, 2015).

Despite the Indian health policies put in place since the 1800s to improve the health status of American Indians, funding for Indian Health Service is considered "discretionary," and the budget does not reflect the innate need; rather, the lack of funding has created disparities within the health services that American Indians access today.

The Navajo Area Indian Health Service offers services to tribal members of the Navajo Nation, Southern band of San Juan Paiutes, Zuni, and Hopi tribes. Comprehensive health care is provided by way of inpatient, outpatient, and community health programs. There are six hospitals, seven health centers, and 15 health stations. The hospitals range in size from 32 inpatient beds in Crownpoint, New Mexico, to 99 inpatient beds at the Gallup Indian Medical Center. The Navajo Nation sponsors a major portion of the health care delivery system. Its purpose is to ensure that quality and culturally appropriate health care is available and accessible. Additional services in the area are offered in the spheres of nutrition, aging, substance abuse, emergency medical services like ambulance services, and community outreach (Figure 10.3).

The Albuquerque Indian Health Service is located in an urban area and provides health services to 20 Pueblos, two Apache bands, three Navajo chapters, and two Ute tribes. Within this service area are five hospitals, 11 health centers, and 12 field clinics. In addition, it has two specialized care facilities specific to the care of Native youth suffering from substance abuse, as well as a dental clinic.

The Phoenix Area Indian Health Service provides health care to Native Americans in Arizona, Nevada, and Utah. The Phoenix Indian Medical Center is one of the largest health care facilities located near downtown Phoenix. It serves tribal members who live in the urban and rural areas.

Tables 10.3 and 10.4 detail the services offered by these regional Indian Health Service centers.

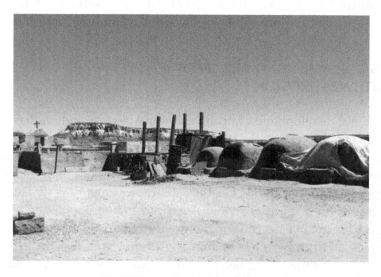

FIGURE 10.3 Zuni Pueblo.
Source: Photo by N. Gonzales (2014).

TABLE 10.3 Southwestern Region Contract Health Services

Contract Health Services for Navajo Area Indian Health

Chinle Comprehensive HC Facility—IHS P.O. Box PH Chinle, AZ 86503	Crownpoint HC Facility—IHS P.O. Box 358 Crownpoint, MN 87313
Fort Defiance SU—IHS P.O. Box 649 Fort Defiance, AZ 86504	Gallup Indian Medical Center—IHS P.O. 1337 Gallup, NM 87301
Keyenta Indian Health Center—IHS P.O. Box 368 Kayenta, AZ 86033	Northern Navajo Medical Center—IHS P.O. Box 160 Shiprock, NM 87420
Tuba City Reg. Health Care Corporation—IHS P.O. Box 600 Tuba City, AZ 86046	Winslow Indian Health Center—Tribal 500 North Indiana Avenue Winslow, AZ 86047
Sage Memorial Hospital-Navajo Health System—Tribal Ganado Mission, P.O. Box 457 Ganado, AZ 86505	Utah Navajo Health System—Tribal East Highway 262 Montezuma Creek, Utah 84534

Contract Health Services for Albuquerque Indian Health Services

Albuquerque Indian Health Center—IHS 801 Vassar Drive NE Albuquerque, NM 87105	Alamo Health Center—Tribal Box 907 Magdalena, NM 87825
Isleta Health Center—Tribal Box 580 Isleta, NM 87022	Isleta Health Center—Tribal Box 580 Isleta, NM 87022
Jemez Health Center—Tribal Box 279 Jemez, NM 87024	Acoma-Canoncito-Laguna SU—IHS Box 310 San Fidel, NM 87049
Jicarilla Apache Nation HC—IHS Box 187 Dulce, NM 87525	Mescalero SU (MSU)—IHS Box 210 Mescalero, NM 88340
Santa Fe SU (SFSU)—IHS 1700 Cerrillos Road Santa Fe, NM 87505	Taos/Picuris—IHS Box 1956 Taos, NM 87571
Ute Mountain Health Center—IHS Box 49 Towac, CO 81334	Ysleta De Sur (YDS)—IHS Box 17579 El Paso, TX 79907

(continued)

TABLE 10.3 Southwestern Region Contract Health Services (*continued*)

Contract Health Services for Albuquerque Indian Health Services (*continued*)

Zuni-Ramah SU (ZRSU)—IHS Box 467 Zuni, NM 87327	Pine Hill Health Box 310 Pine Hill, NM 87327

Contract Health Services for Phoenix Area

Colorado River Service Unit—IHS 12033 Agency Road Parker, AZ 85344	Elko Service Unit— IHS 515 Shoshone Circle Elko, NV 89801
Fort Yuma Service Unit—IHS P.O. Box 1368 Yuma, AZ 85364	Hopi Health Center—IHS P.O. Box 4000 Polacca, AZ 86042
Phoenix Indian Medical Center—IHS 4212 N. 16th Street Phoenix, AZ 85016	San Carlos Service Unit—IHS P.O. Box 208 San Carlos, AZ 85550
Schurz Service Unit—IHS Drawer A Schurz, NV 89427	Uintah and Ouray Service Unit—IHS P.O. Box 160 Fort Duchesne, UT 84026
Whiteriver Service Unit—IHS P.O. Box 860 Whiteriver, AZ 85941	Duck Valley Shoshone Paiute Tribe—Tribal P.O. Box 130 Owyhee, NV 89832
Duckwater Shoshone Tribe of Nevada—Tribal 511 Duckwater Falls Road Duckwater, NV 89314	Fort McDowell Yavapai Nation of Arizona—Tribal P.O. Box 17779 Fountain Hills, AZ 85269
Gila River Indian Community of Arizona—Tribal P.O. Box 38 Sacaton, AZ 85247	Las Vegas Paiute Tribes of Nevada—Tribal 1257 Paiute Circle Las Vegas, NV 89106
Paiute Tribe of Utah—Tribal 440 North Paiute Drive Cedar City, UT 84720	Washoe Tribe of Nevada and California— Tribal 1559 Watasheamu Gardenerville, NV 89460
Yerington Paiute Tribe of Nevada—Tribal 171 Campbell Lane Yerington, NV 89447	Fort Mojave Indian Tribe—Tribal 1607 Plantation Road Mojave Valley, AZ 86440
Ely Shoshone Tribe of Nevada—Tribal 400-B Newe View Ely, NV 89301	

Source: Indian Health Services (2015b).

TABLE 10.4 Southwestern Region Treatment Centers

IHS Youth Regional Treatment Centers

New Sunrise Regional Treatment Center 20 Mockingbird Drive PO Box 219 San Fidel, NM 87049	Navajo Regional Behavioral Health Center PO Box 1830 Shiprock, NM 87420
Desert Visions Youth Wellness Center 198 S. Skill Center Road PO Box 458 Sacaton, Arizona, 85247	

Adult Inpatient Treatment Centers

Rehoboth McKinley Behavioral Health Service 650 Vanden Bosch Parkway Gallup, NM 87301	Nanizhoozhi Center 2205 Boyd Avenue Gallup, NM 87301-7404
New Moon Lodge Treatment Center 579 White Swan Road Ohkay Owingeh, NM 87566	Native American Connections Indian Rehabilitation 636 North 3rd Avenue Phoenix, AZ 85003
Amity Circle Tree Ranch 10500 E. Tanque Verde Road Tucson, AZ 85749	Banner Thunderbird Behavioral Health 555 West Thunderbird Road Glendale, AZ 85306

Pueblo Tribal Health Programs

Eight Northern Indian Pueblos Council, Inc. 327 Eagle Dr. PO Box 969 Ohkay Owingeh, NM 87566	Pueblo of San Felipe Health and Wellness Department PO Box 4339 San Felipe Pueblo, NM 87001	Isleta Health Center Pueblo of Isleta P.O. Box 1270 Isleta, NM 87022

Navajo Nation Health Programs

Navajo Kayenta Public Health Nursing Program PO Box 1390 Window Rock, AZ 86515	Navajo Nation Special Diabetes Project—Central Office P.O. Box 3748 Window Rock, AZ 86515	NNSDP—Window Rock Wellness Center P.O. Box 3748 Window Rock, AZ 86515
NNSDP—Shiprock Service Area P.O. Box 1287 Shiprock, NM 87420	NNSDP—Tuba City Service Area P.O. Box 278 Tuba City, AZ 86045	NNSDP—Fort Defiance Service Area P.O. Box 1610 Fort Defiance, AZ 86504
Navajo Breast and Cervical Cancer Program PO Box 1390 Window Rock, AZ 86515	Navajo Area Agency on Aging PO Box 1390 Window Rock, AZ 86515	Navajo Women, Infants and Children Program PO BOX 1390 Window Rock, AZ 86515

Source: Indian Health Service (2015b).

As an opportunity for tribes to be involved in health, the Community Health Representative program was developed in 1968. This was done to help contain the spread of tuberculosis across several American Indian communities. Today, the Community Health Representative program has grown to more than 1,400 in over 12 service areas. The program contracts with several of the tribes in the area to provide outreach in health in a culturally congruent way.

NURSING IN THE SOUTHWEST

American Indian nurses make up about 1% of the nursing workforce in New Mexico (Ayoola, 2013). The disparity in the diversity of the nursing workforce has been long recognized, and efforts are being made to address this issue. The Navajo Technical University located in Crownpoint, NM, offers an associate nursing degree program and a preprofessional nursing certificate for America Indian students. The University of New Mexico, Arizona State University, and New Mexico State University offer bachelor's degree nursing programs. To increase the number of American Indian nurses, scholarships have been offered by the Indian Health Service and through university-specific funds. As an additional effort to support the American Indian nursing workforce, the Indian Health Service offers clinical placement for students and preference for those interested in working at an IHS site.

Mainstreaming American Indian nurses to work at Indian Health Service sites is secured by payback obligations through their scholarship and loan repayment programs. Despite these efforts to recruit American Indian nurses and retain their services, there remains a shortage. Rural living conditions with limited housing and community resources for families are among the most common reasons why health care professionals do not stay. The urban Indian health care service units provide a more secure living environment, and are generally preferred choices for employment and living.

CULTURAL SAFETY

It is important to understand the influence of racial ideology and that historical trauma is a lived experience for which marginalization has occurred in this population. As a result of dominant influences, American Indians are interacting with complex health care systems, which reflect linear health care models rather than indigenous wellness concepts. Navigating these complex health care systems is problematic and continues to be a challenge for health care professionals and the communities they serve.

The concept of cultural safety is predicated on the understanding that a caregiver's own culture, and the assumptions that follow, impact the manner in which a clinical encounter is played out, and therefore impacts the patients' care (Walker, Cromarty, Linkewich, Semple, & Pierre-Hansen, 2010). The aspects of cultural safety are about minimizing risk to provide a safe healing environment by first acknowledging the cultural differences and then engaging in "self-reflection" in which one's own culture and assumptions are recognized.

This dynamic on the caregiver's part is integral to encouraging individual empowerment and choice. This concept of a culturally safe environment allows for individuals to use the health care system in a manner that supports their healthy lifestyle. Presently, research is being conducted on the recovery and redevelopment of indigenous knowledge systems as a means of achieving self-determination. This in itself is encouraging American Indians to achieve a decolonized methodology to address issues set forth by the communities themselves, rather than for "outsiders" to initiate research that would reflect the needs of the community (Tobin, French, & Hanlon, 2010, p. 50).

CULTURAL BELIEFS

To understand the traditional cultural worldviews from which each American Indian derives his or her identity, it is important to understand the universe from which they operate. The Navajo philosophy about life is that we are all elements of the universe, with life being recognized first as a vibration. Emerging from one world to the next, as described in the Navajo origin story, the four sacred mountains that surround the homelands of the Navajo reservation represent the four cardinal directions and represent the dwelling places of the holy people.

Navajo people consider themselves children of nature and are taught that the earth, sky, sun, moon, rain, water, lightning, and thunder are living kin (Schwarz, 1997). Hence, the Navajo world is holistic, and they recognize that they are part of a larger entity. Through oral history, the Navajo origin stories describe the physical world and the Navajo role in that world. This establishes the meaningful relationship between the community and the cosmos for which Navajos live. A common understanding among Navajos is that the core of social life was given by the holy people, which, if followed, will ensure that harmony is maintained and illness avoided.

Living and thinking in this way represents one of the core values expressed in Navajo culture, namely, that it is important to live and speak in a positive way, as our thoughts have the power to manifest into reality and control events. Living in this way establishes harmony and balance, which if followed, prevents illness. The power of thought in the Navajo culture is taken seriously, and thus it is important not to mention possible outcomes that could be harmful. This philosophy poses a challenge for health care providers working with Navajo people, as much of Western medicine emphasizes physical illnesses and seeks to "cure" by means of biomedical processes.

Despite what Western medicine and research teaches us, American Indians' understanding of the multiple illnesses like diabetes, depression, and obesity are a result of a loss of traditional values and teachings. This was purposely facilitated by acts of assimilation over time by colonizers. Being spiritually weak allows for disease and sickness to take hold. It is for this reason that objects used for prayer and healing are encouraged to be used daily.

It is this very understanding that much of the healing practices and rituals are centered on returning balance and harmony in individuals. However, despite the differences in treatment techniques, similarities exist between Western medical doctors and traditional Navajo practitioners in that they both seek to remove the cause of illness so that the body may heal itself. The difference in each methodology is that the traditional medicine man or woman recognizes the spiritual aspects of illness and seeks to heal and balance these, rather than just seeking ways to heal the physiological illness.

Only recently has traditional medicine been incorporated into Indian Health Service Units on the Navajo reservation. Modern medicine today is just now recognizing the importance of cultural healing practices that have been indigenous to the communities on the reservations. As a nurse working with Navajo patients, understanding the importance of traditional healing practices as an integral aspect of health is vitally important. Additionally, one should understand that a Navajo patient may very well see his or her medicine man first before accessing health care services within a hospital or clinic setting.

Traditional healers are respected and protected in the Native American communities in which they live. Navajo traditional practitioners are believed to have been chosen, or given a gift for healing. Once they recognize this, they undergo an apprenticeship with an elder traditional healer, in which case, learning may span the entire lifetime. During healing ceremonies, the words or songs sung by the practitioners help guide a patient on a healing journey, in which he or she travels among the holy people who have the power to help heal (Joe et al., 2008). In the Navajo culture, there are different types of healers; diagnosticians are consulted to discuss the reasons behind culturally based health problems. Sometimes, a culturally based illness may come in the form of retribution, or as the result of inadvertent contact with something disruptive (Davies, 2001). An example of this might be coming into contact with a deceased body. This could create spiritual disharmony, which is manifesting as an illness.

Traditional healers practice primarily in the privacy of a person's home. Special objects used during ceremonies held to restore balance may be used as forms of protection for individuals to carry while accessing care at hospitals or clinics. It is also important to know that some individuals may not want to share their use of traditional healing practices, fearing that the physicians will disagree with this course of healing. They may also abstain from discussing it to prevent interference with it working properly.

Ceremonial healing practices are not only accessed during times of illness or spiritual unrest; they are also used to ensure good health and harmony. As part of nurturing one's spiritual health, Navajos are taught to begin their day with meditation or prayer. These intentions are set forth for the coming day and are presented in the East direction, for that is where life begins by traditional Navajo trajectory. An offering of corn pollen is also given during this time. For women, pregnancy would be an opportunity to ensure good health and harmony through ceremony, specifically a "Blessingway" ceremony, which emphasizes and accentuates the positive, and reaffirms harmony with the mother and the growing child within.

Despite the very specific healing practices discussed here, it is important to understand that there is diversity among healers within each Native American tribal community. As a result of Western influences, American Indians have adopted different healing approaches as well as beliefs. Within the Pueblo communities of the Rio Grande, the sharing of healing practices between the Spanish traditional healers and Pueblo healers was widely done. Healing plant medicines of the Southwest may have Spanish or Indian names, depending on how their use was taught. Societies of medicine men within the Pueblo communities also carry with them cultural knowledge about seasonal ceremonial dances and songs taught to them by their elders.

Restoring harmony through prayer or receiving blessings for participation in seasonal ceremonial dances are examples of ways in which American Indians of the Southwest maintain their cultural health beliefs. These traditional health beliefs help maintain relationships with all that is in the environment, as well as teaching respect, endurance, care of self, care of family, and care of one's community. The healing properties given by Mother Earth in the form of plant medicines and indigenous healing knowledge passed on through creation stories are a means of survival and resilience. This explains the push for cultural preservation among tribes, for in each aspect of American Indian daily life, they are taught to respect and be in tune with the universe.

PHYSICAL HEALTH ISSUES

Much like sudden illnesses, individuals within the Navajo culture who have disabilities are thought to be in a state of disharmony as a result of breaking a cultural taboo. Another central cultural aspect of Navajo culture is the matriarchal clan system that identifies one's family. It is a serious taboo to marry within a clan from which your partner is identified as being a brother or sister. This would result in disabilities in the individual, or in the children of the couple who married from the same clans. Other examples of "taboos" might be looking at dead animals while pregnant, or attending ceremonies while pregnant that could cause harm to the unborn child. Disabilities might also result from witchcraft, and in such situations, a medicine man or woman is brought in to help the situation.

Additional views on individuals with disabilities are that they are "special" and have a role in one's family to set an example or to teach. Much like a hunter's role is to feed the family or a mother's role is to nurture the children, a "special" person with disabilities has his or her role in the family. Unfortunately, the traditional views on individuals with disabilities do not account for the historical presence of environmental pollutants, alcohol, or illnesses that could have caused these disabilities.

MENTAL HEALTH ISSUES

There are multiple confounding factors that influence American Indians' mental health issues today, one being that American Indians are socially disadvantaged, with varying degrees of cultural discourse as a result of federal policies and colonization. The accumulated stress over time from historical trauma, discrimination, traumatic life events, loss of cultural identity, and loss of ancestral lands has manifested itself in unhealthy lifestyle behaviors. The most significant mental health concerns among Indians/Natives are depression, substance abuse, anxiety, and posttraumatic stress disorder (PTSD; Manson, 2004). Even though Natives recognize that mental health issues within their communities need to be addressed, a stigma is attached to those who do access behavioral health services.

As mentioned earlier, Navajo people are culturally taught that "to live in health is to live in accordance with moral or behavioral codes that strive to maintain harmony between one's self and his/her family, community, environment, and spiritual world" (Avery, 1991, p. 2271). Unfortunately, as a result of boarding schools and forced assimilation that Native children underwent to learn the beliefs, values, customs, and behaviors of the White culture, they have lost touch with the cultural teachings of their elders, which has led to disharmony. It is important to understand the complex belief systems when working with Indians/Natives. Cultural differences exist on many levels, all of which affect an individual's help-seeking behaviors, language and communication styles, symptom patterns and expressions, nontraditional healing practices, and the role and desirability of medical interventions (Comas-Diaz & Griffith, 1988).

The use of traditional healers alongside biomedical services has been widely accepted in the treatment of mental health issues; many Native American-based behavioral health centers use sweat lodges as a form of therapy and spiritual rejuvenation. Even though some of the sweat lodge procedures were primarily adopted from the Plains Indians, sweat lodges are widely accepted in Navajo culture and among some of the tribes in the Southwest.

The federal agency most directly responsible for providing behavioral health services to American Indians is the Indian Health Service. Within IHS, the Mental Health and Social Services Programs branch is responsible for providing culturally appropriate mental health services. However, owing to limited funding, distribution of mental health resources varies from area to area, as resources allocated to IHS are primarily used for acute health care services. What needs to be recognized is that the system of services for treating mental health problems among American Indians is complex, and is often a fractured web of federal, state, local, tribal, and community-based services (Manson, 2004). It is an imperfect system that health care providers and community health care advocates try to navigate for the benefit of their Native clients. It is also another reason that American Indians do not access mental health services; they are unfamiliar with the Western mainstream health care system.

REPRODUCTIVE HEALTH ISSUES

Before Western ideological influences converged with the Native traditional ways of birthing, Indigenous tribes had traditional midwives or family members who attended to births in their own communities. In the Navajo culture, these women were called "baby medicine women" or "umbilical cord cutters." Before the emergence of hospitals, births primarily took place in homes called "hogans." Native women were also thought of as an integral part of the community; they were viewed as sacred life givers, teachers, healers, and warriors. Spiritual role models like Spider Woman, Changing Woman, and Sky Woman shaped much of the traditional teachings surrounding fertility, motherhood, and womanhood. Before the 1950s, plant medicines were used in abundance, and family preparation for birth was a ceremonial process, as each member of the family had a role in the pregnancy and birth. They recognized pregnancy and birth as a sacred time for women and their families.

Things changed drastically for Native women once birth and women's health shifted to hospital-based care centers. Prior to Indian Health Programs' transference to the Public Health service in 1955, diseases of pregnancy and complications of childbirth led to a death rate of 6.2 per 100,000 in the Navajo population, as compared with 1.5 per 100,000 in other ethnic groups in 1953 (Marsh, 1957). Efforts were made to combat the maternal–child health disparities in the Southwest through the placement of nurse-midwives in Shiprock, New Mexico, and Fort Defiance, Arizona. Through this integrated and interdisciplinary approach, there was a significant decrease in the number of premature births and infant mortality. Presently, nurse-midwives attend to over 75% of all births within IHS. According to Knoki-Wilson, "Navajos greatly welcomed CNMs [certified nurse-midwives]" in part because "CNMs often took the lead in partnering with Native healers" (Landwehr & Knoki-Wilson, 2002, p. 25.).

Even though CNMs welcomed the help of Native healers within the health care system they worked in, traditional Navajo women were still hesitant to go to the hospital to birth their babies. The reason for this was that Navajo cultural beliefs surrounding pregnancy advised the mother to avoid contact with death, funerals, or dead animals. If she did not adhere to this, she would have a sick child. Hospitals were known as places where people went to die, and the thought of a Navajo woman going to have her baby in such a place presented a cultural risk to her child. Despite this cultural risk, by 1969, all births on the Navajo reservation took place in the hospital (Waxman, 1990). Unlike other tribes, the Navajo did not see a decrease in births after contact with Spanish settlers or onset of disease. In 1988, over 5,000 Native American women gave birth on or near the Navajo Indian Reservation (Milligan, 1984). By then, a cultural shift had occurred, and 99% of those births occurred in hospitals in accordance with Western biomedicine. As hospital births became more common, it was harder for young women to learn the rituals of childbirth at home. Further compounding the separations of traditional childbearing practices, boarding schools on the reservation deprived young women of the opportunity to learn these practices.

The complex relationship between American Indian women and the Indian Health Service has not always been positive. As part of the government's efforts to assimilate and disempower Native women, in the 1970s, the Indian Health Service oversaw the nonconsensual sterilization of approximately 40% of women of childbearing age (Walters & Simoni, 2002). It is events like this that still resonate strongly for American Indian women, and contribute to the historical trauma they have experienced over the centuries.

Currently, 7.7% of Native American women in New Mexico experience violence during pregnancy, 12.3% experience postpartum depression, and 14.6% have gestational diabetes. According to the New Mexico Pregnancy Risk Assessment Monitoring System (PRAMS) report, 32% of Native American women had inadequate prenatal care, which is higher than that for all other ethnic mothers in 2010. Barriers to prenatal care over the last decade have consistently been lack of transportation, lack of cultural understanding of the need for prenatal care, health care system difficulties with getting an appointment, and the lack of financial means to pay for services.

There is currently a shift in Native American women's health in that tribal communities are slowly beginning to reclaim their cultural birth rites as indigenous people and there is much focus on recovering traditional birth knowledge by increasing the number of Native American midwives and choosing to have an out-of-hospital birth. Native American women, who are aware of their ancestral history, view this as an expression of sovereignty over their bodies, and are asserting their preference for indigenous birth rites as life givers (Figure 10.4).

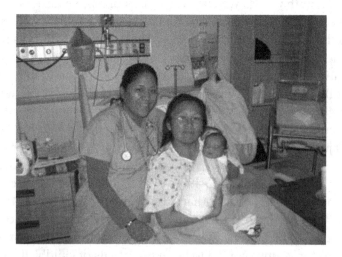

FIGURE 10.4 Navajo midwife, Chinle, AZ.
Source: Gonzales (2011).

EMOTIONAL/SPIRITUAL ISSUES

Navajos and many of the American Indians of the Southwest do not view their spirituality as "religion" that requires attending church on Sunday, but as "life ways," which are a set of teachings and cultural practices defined by the holy people or spiritual deities to live a healthy life. Dawn prayers with corn pollen or white cornmeal, participation in seasonal ceremonial dances, adhering to cultural taboos and avoiding dead animals when pregnant, entering a kiva or a hogan from the East are all examples of this. Spiritual harm can manifest as physical illness, thus requiring traditional healing intervention to correct the imbalance and return individuals to their place in the spiritual universe. Each inner spiritual being has relationships with the earth, with other spirits (living and dead), and with powers both animate and inanimate (Perrone, Stockel, & Krueger, 1989).

Corn is viewed as having healing powers to enhance and to rebalance our thinking. For this reason, corn pollen and white cornmeal are used as part of healing practices (Morgan, 2006). One's mind should always hold positive thoughts, as this leads to a healthy emotional state. Our inner "spiritual being" requires care and attention, in much the same way as our bodies require food and water. It is through our creation stories, spiritual teachings, and relationship to the earth that we have a sense of "self."

In the Pueblo culture, no word translates as "religion." Spiritual life permeates every aspect of daily life. "To maintain a relationship between the people and the spiritual world, various societies exist, with particular responsibilities for weather, fertility, curing, hunting and pleasure or entertainment" (Sando, 1976, p. 22). Individuals who belong to certain spiritual societies within the Pueblos hold an important place in the community. Despite contact with the Spaniards, Pueblo communities still practice their spiritual rituals just as their ancestors did when they lived in pit houses. One way the Spaniards did influence Pueblo communities of the Southwest was by bringing in the Catholic belief system. Owing to the Spaniards' attempt to force their religion on the Pueblo people, the latter were forced to take their beliefs underground. The Pueblos interfaced their own cultural practices with the Catholic religion in an effort to maintain their own beliefs. Despite the existence of these two mutually distinct socioceremonial systems, the Pueblos primarily recognize their ancestral ceremonial and spiritual belief system in their daily lives.

LIFE-SPAN ISSUES WITH AN EMPHASIS ON THE ELDERLY

Elders, much like family in American Indian communities, are respected and held in high regard. Elders are viewed as teachers, holders of ancestral knowledge, and are a central part of families, as they are often sought out for their wisdom. In the Navajo culture, which is primarily matriarchal, elders are viewed as leaders in all aspects of spiritual living and in matters of ceremony.

On the Navajo reservation, elders generally live in hogans and take part in community ceremonies like the "Enemy Way Ceremony," or what some people call a squaw dance. Much of Navajo traditional homelands are remote, and many elders still live there and tend sheep at various camps. These places are called "sheep camps." Historically, the Navajo people moved from various camp sites; today, some of the elders still live in this manner; they have winter homes and summer homes.

As employment opportunities are limited, Navajo men and women may drive hours to work off the Navajo reservation. This leaves much of the responsibility of raising children to their elders. Although some outsiders might view this as neglect on the parents' part, elders teach their grandchildren the Navajo language and about the traditional ways of living that are being lost today. Grandmothers, who are known for their weaving skills, are able to pass on their knowledge to their granddaughters this way. As elders are sought to teach cultural traditions, they are also cared for by family and extended family.

Within the Pueblo culture, many of the elders speak their ancestral language, and are part of special spiritual societies. They are often sought out as "Indian godparents" for naming ceremonies, and to open discussions of importance with prayer. When going to an elder home to ask for their guidance or participation in a naming ceremony, cornmeal is offered out of respect for their sharing of wisdom.

Tribal communities of the Southwest have different views on death, but a common understanding is that all "living" elements have a life cycle. Much like the creation story in the Navajo culture, the preparing of one's spirit takes 4 days. The Pueblo culture also adheres to this belief. There are very distinct differences between the Navajo and the Pueblo on how they view death and dying.

In the Pueblo societies, families of loved ones who have died are advised not to be alone for 4 days, as the spirit is still around and could take them too. Much like the Catholic belief system, a wake is held in the family's home so that the family can say their goodbyes. Depending on which spiritual society the person belonged to, the burial time and place are determined by the spiritual group. Feasting on the fourth day is a common practice, in which community members will come to be with the family.

The Navajo believe that it is a cultural taboo to be around death. Doing so puts one's spirit at risk for disharmony, and makes the individual vulnerable to illness, which is why they limit contact with those who have died. After a family member has died and has been properly prepared for burial, the family will ask a medicine man to perform a ceremony to correct any imbalances that might have occurred in the process. Out of respect for the loved one and the knowledge that spiritual harm could be present, the family cannot have ceremonies like the "Blessingway" or coming-of-age ceremony for young women for at least 4 to 10 days after someone has passed on.

As a result of assimilation, historical trauma, and non-Natives' efforts to appropriate sacred knowledge of tribal Nations, American Indians have become more private in their sharing of ceremonies and wisdom of this nature. Out of respect for the different worldviews on "life" and "death" in American Indian communities, developing trusting relationships is necessary for the caregiver in a biomedical health care system. Death and dying are delicate subjects for all cultures, and being sensitive to the family's cultural ways is vital.

CONCLUSIONS

Despite the daily reminders of loss that American Indian people face, such as loss of ancestral land bases, traditional family systems, language, and healing practices, using cultural foundational belief systems that promote positive thinking can strengthen resilient qualities. Resilience is seen as a force or a drive that leads individuals to achieve self-actualization, altruism, wisdom, and harmony. The energy or source of resilience is believed to come from the collective unconscious spirit, and from the social, ecological, and spiritual environment (Richardson, 2002). Resilient qualities have been identified as spirituality and ceremonial participation, cultural identity, tribal values, children's education, language and stories, political relationships and factors, and communal interdependency (Belcourt-Dittloff, 2006). It is hoped that as American Indians continue to interface with Western biomedical health care systems, health care professionals will support their resiliency behavior.

Tribal nations are actively pursuing ways to reclaim Native cultural values by encouraging language immersion programs and using indigenous wellness frameworks to define their vision of "healthy beginnings," which are all acts of resiliency. Nurses can help foster this process of recovery in tribal communities and with American Indian patients by advocating a culturally safe environment in the hospital setting where life and death converge. Furthermore, it is important to take the time to develop trusting relationships to truly understand the worldview from which Native people navigate. The depth and complexity of American Indian health is more than what you see in the statistical numbers. Rather, it is a ripple of trauma that has been endured over time by systematic acts of acculturation and domination.

CRITICAL-THINKING EXERCISE

♦ You have just moved to Chinle, Arizona, to work at the Chinle Comprehensive Health Care facility. You just recently finished nursing school, and have lived in an urban area for the past 3 years. This IHS facility is the only hospital providing obstetrical service for miles, with 700 deliveries occurring each year.

It is your first 12-hour shift as a nurse and you encounter Jessica, a 21-year-old, gravida 1 para 0 (G1P0), who is 38 weeks pregnant and thinks she is in labor. She has had limited prenatal care throughout her pregnancy. She reports that the reason for this is that she has had limited transportation and lives 1 hour away. Her grandmother, who is Navajo, brought her to the hospital today. Her grandmother only speaks Navajo, but Jessica speaks English. After evaluation, the midwife on call advises Jessica to go home, as she is not in labor. When educating Jessica on when to return for care, you find few written materials for her to take home regarding term-labor precautions. After this experience, you are asked to develop educational material for pregnant mothers that includes term labor, breastfeeding, postpartum changes, and sexual health. When you are discussing the plan of care for labor and delivery with her family, what would you incorporate into this plan? Who would you include when developing educational material? What challenges might you expect to encounter?

Answer:

Data: Research books and articles on Native American perspectives on pregnancy and health; talk to elders, traditional healers, and midwives. Research community health websites for information on sexual health, pregnancy outcomes, barriers to prenatal care, and community resources for new mothers and teens.

Whom to involve when developing written material? Does the tribe have a breastfeeding task force; home visiting network; parenting support groups; sexual health outreach organizations; social services; Women, Infants, and Children programs?

Challenges: Limited culture-specific information.

DISCUSSION QUESTIONS

◆ Review and discuss the impact of historical trauma that AI/ANs of the Southwest experienced since contact with Spanish colonizers.

Answer: Look to the Long Walk, boarding schools, and population shifts for the Southwest region. Impacts of these events have shaped health, resources, AI/AN identity, and relationship with the U.S. government.

◆ Describe some ways you can apply resiliency and cultural safety concepts into the care you will provide as a nurse working in the Southwest with AI/AN patients.

Answer: Use wellness methodologies to approach education and care, with an emphasis on cultural preservation. Encourage the use of ceremonial items in the hospital setting, offering the use of traditional healers if available at your location. Engage patients to express their expectations of care. Encourage the intake of traditional foods indigenous to the community.

◆ Discuss the differences in beliefs surrounding death and dying between the Navajo and Pueblo tribes of the Southwest.

Answer: The Navajo believe that being around death and preparing for death is taboo. It is to be avoided to prevent spiritual imbalances. The Pueblo culture views death as the beginning of a journey, an event surrounded by family. Planning for death is not discussed, but is a ceremonial process undertaken by the family.

USEFUL WEBSITES

Albuquerque Area Indian Health Board, http://www.aaihb.org
Albuquerque Area Indian Health Services website, https://www.ihs.gov/albuquerque
Eight Northern Indian Pueblo Council, Inc., http://www.enipc.org
Los Alamos Historical Document Retrieval & Assessment Project, http://www.lahdra.org
Navajo Uranium Report 2013, http://www.epa.gov/region9/superfund/navajo-nation/pdf/NavajoUraniumReport2013.pdf
New Mexico Department of Health, http://nmhealth.org
Tewa Women United, http://www.tewawomenunited.org/

RECOMMENDED READINGS

Adair, J. (1988). *The people's health: Anthropology and medicine in a Navajo community.* Albuquerque, NM: University of New Mexico Press.

Dutton, B. P. (1983). *American Indians of the southwest.* Albuquerque, NM: University of New Mexico Press.

Echo-Hawk, W. R. (2013). *In the light of justice: The rise of human rights in native America and the UN declaration on the rights of indigenous peoples.* Golden, CO: Fulcrum Publishing.

Lovell-Harvard, D. M., & Anderson, K. (2014). *Mothers of the nations: Indigenous mothering as global resistance, reclaiming and recovery.* Bradford, ON: Demeter Press.

Maracle, L. (1996). *I am woman: A native perspective on sociology and feminism.* British Columbia, Canada: Press Gang Publishers.

Porter, R. O. (1999). *Sovereignty, colonialism, and the future of the indigenous nations: A reader.* Durham, NC: Carolina Academic Press.

Shoemaker, N. (1999). *American Indian population recovery in the twentieth century.* Albuquerque, NM: University of New Mexico Press.

Shwarz, M. T. (2008). *I choose life: Contemporary medical and religious practices in the Navajo world.* Norman, OK: University of Oklahoma Press.

Waters, F. (1963). *Book of the Hopi: The first revelation of the Hopi's historical and religious worldview of life.* New York, NY: Penguin Group.

REFERENCES

Arizona Health Disparities Center. (2013) *Arizona health equity stakeholders strategies.* Phoenix, AZ: Arizona Department of Health.

Avery, C. (1991). Native American medicine: Traditional healing. *Journal of the American Medical Association, 265*(17), 2271, 2273.

Ayoola, A. (2013). *Why diversity in the nursing workforce matters.* Princeton, NJ: Robert Wood Johnson Foundation.

Barrett, E. M. (2002). The geography of the Rio Grande Pueblos in the seventeenth century. *Ethnohistory, 49*(1), 123–169.

Belcourt-Dittloff, A. E. (2006). *Resiliency and risk in Native American communities: A culturally informed investigation* (Doctoral dissertation). University of Montana, Missoula, MT.

Comas-Diaz, L., & Griffith, E. (1988). *Clinical guidelines in cross-cultural mental health.* New York, NY: Wiley.

Davies, W. (2001). *Healing ways: Navajo health care in the twentieth century.* Albuquerque, NM: University of New Mexico Press.

Fort Sumner Historic Site/Bosque Redondo Memorial. (n.d.). Retrieved November, 20, 2014, from http://www.nmstatemonuments.org/bosque-redondo

Gonzales, N. L. (2011). Navajo midwife. Indian Health Services, Chinle Service Unit. Gonzales private collection.

Gonzales, N. L. (2014). Zuni Pueblo Ovens. Zuni Pueblo, NM. Gonzales private collection.

Indian Health Service. (2015a). Indian Health Care Improvement Act. Retrieved from https://www.ihs.gov/ihcia/

Indian Health Service. (2015b). Locations. Retrieved from https://www.ihs.gov/locations/

Iverson, P. (2002). *Diné: A history of the Navajos.* Albuquerque, NM: University of New Mexico Press.

Jones, D. S. (2006). The persistence of American Indian health disparities. *American Journal of Public Health, 96*(12), 2122.

Joe et al. (2008). *A case study: Office of native medicine.* Tucson, AZ: University of Arizona Press.

Jones, D. S. (2006). The persistence of American Indian health disparities. *American Journal of Public Health, 96*(12), 2122–2134.

Kunitz, S. J., Veazie, M., & Henderson, J. A. (2014). Historical trends and regional differences in all-cause and amenable mortality among American Indians and Alaska natives since 1950. *American Journal of Public Health, 104*(3), 268–277.

Landwehr, G. A., & Knocki-Wilson, U. (2002). *Nurse-midwifery within the Indian health service: 1965–1980* (Master's thesis). Yale University, New Haven, CT.

Manson, S. M. (2004). *Cultural diversity series: Meeting the mental health needs of American Indians and Alaska natives.* Washington, DC: National Technical Assistance Center for State Mental Health Planning.

Martin, D. L., Goodman, A. H., Armelagos, G. J., Magennis, A. L. (1991). *Black Mesa Anasazi health: Reconstructing life from patterns of death and disease.* Carbondale, IL: Southern Illinois University Press.

Marsh, J. L. (1957). *Health services for Indian mothers and children. Children, 4:* 203-207.

Milligan, C. B. (1984). Nursing care and beliefs of expectant Navajo women (part 1). *American Indian Quarterly,* 8(2), 83–101.

Morgan, F. (2006). *Living a long healthy life: According to Navajo teachings.* Chinle, AZ: Office of Native Medicine.

New Mexico Department of Health. (2013a). *American Indian health equity: Report on health disparities in New Mexico.* Santa Fe, NM: Author.

New Mexico Department of Health. (2013b). *State-Tribal Collaboration Act July 31, 2013 Agency Report.* Santa Fe, NM: Author.

New Mexico historic sites, (n.d.). Fort Sumner Historic Site/Bosque Redondo Memorial Retrieved November, 20, 2014, from http://www.nmstatemonuments.org/bosque-redondo

Perrone, B., Stockel, H. H., & Krueger, V. (1989). *Medicine women, curanderas, and women doctors.* Norman, OK: University of Oklahoma Press.

Rhoades, E. R. (2000). *American Indian health: Innovations in health care, promotion, and policy.* Baltimore, MD: Johns Hopkins University Press.

Richardson, G. E. (2002). The meta theory of resilience and resiliency. *Journal of Clinical Psychology, 58*(3), 307–321.

Robert Wood Johnson Foundation. (2008). *Overcoming obstacles to health: Report from the Robert Wood Johnson Foundation to commission to build a healthier America.* Princeton, NJ: Author.

Sando, S. J. (1976). *The Pueblo Indians.* San Francisco, CA: The Indian Historian Press.

Schwarz, M. T. (1997). *Molded in the image of changing woman: Navajo views on the human body and personhood.* Tucson, AZ: University of Arizona Press.

Spicer, E. H. (1962). *Cycles of conquest: The impact of Spain, Mexico, and the United States on the Indians of the southwest 1533–1960.* Tucson, AZ: University of Arizona Press.

Tobin, P., French, M., & Hanlon, N. (2010). Appropriate engagement and nutrition education on reserve: Lessons learned from the Takla Lake First Nation in Northern BC. *Journal of Aboriginal Health, 6,* 49–57.

United States Environmental Protection Agency. (2013). *Federal actions to address impacts of uranium contamination in the Navajo Nation: Five-Year Plan Summary Report.* Retrieved November 29, 2014 from http://www.epa.gov/region9/superfund/navajo-nation/pdf/NavajoUraniumReport2013.pdf

Walker, R., Cromarty, H., Linkewich, B., Semple, D., & Pierre-Hansen, N. S. (2010). Achieving cultural integration in health services: Designs of comprehensive hospital model for traditional healing, medicines, foods and support. *Journal of Aboriginal Health, 6,* 58–69.

Walters, K. L., & Simoni, J. M. (2002). Reconceptualizing Native Women's Health: An indigenist stress-coping model. *American Journal of Public Health, 92*(4): 520–524.

Waxman, A. (1990). Navajo Childbirth in Transition. *Medical Anthropology,* 12, 118.

ELEVEN

Great Basin

Lillian Tom-Orme

LEARNING OBJECTIVES

♦ To describe the geography, history, and cultural ways of major tribal nations of the Great Basin
♦ To explain at least two factors that affect the access and quality of health care for the Great Basin tribal nations
♦ To discuss the nursing needs in the context of social determinants of health and health disparities and geography

KEY TERMS

♦ American Indians/Alaska Natives
♦ Colonies
♦ Great Basin
♦ Indigenous people
♦ Native Americans
♦ Nevada
♦ Reservation

KEY CONCEPTS

♦ Health disparities
♦ Social determinants of health
♦ Tribal sovereignty

This chapter provides a brief historical background of four main tribal groups that reside within the Great Basin of the western United States. Each tribal group has a number of bands, but they will be discussed in general. Although each band is unique and would prefer to be treated individually, it is not possible to appropriately characterize their uniqueness in this chapter. An overview of their tribal history is covered to provide some context for the reader. Finally, a description of their health, and specifics of nursing in this population, will be discussed.

As depicted in Figure 11.1, the Great Basin covers a large area in parts of eastern California, southeast Oregon, Utah, southern Idaho, western Wyoming, and all of Nevada. This is the home of four primarily Numic-speaking tribes, including the Shoshone, Paiutes, Goshutes, and Utes (Figure 11.2). The region is characterized by what is called basin and range, mountains that lie north

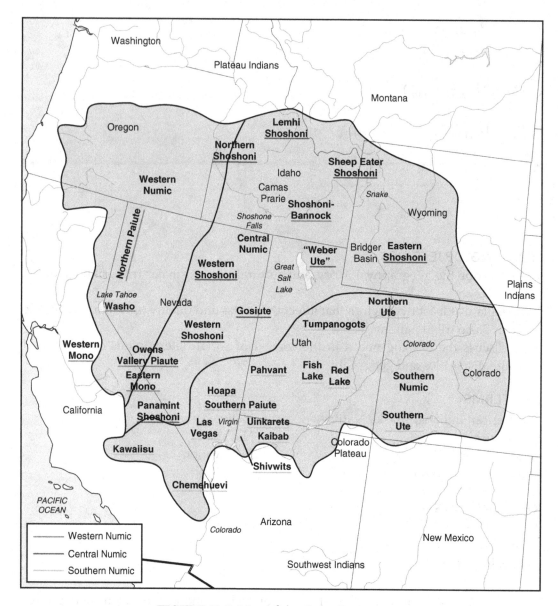

FIGURE 11.1 Map of the Great Basin area.

and south with valleys or a desert basin in-between them, between the Rocky Mountains and the Sierra Mountain.

THE GOSHUTES

Goshute History

The Goshutes (*Gosuite*) make up two small tribes with lands in the states of Nevada and Utah. Deep Creek Reservation—home to the Confederated Tribes

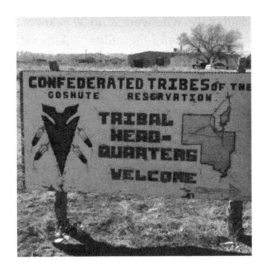

FIGURE 11.2 Welcome sign in Ibapah, Utah.
Courtesy of Lillian Tom-Orme.

of the Goshute Indians—straddles the state boundaries of Utah and Nevada, northeast of Ely, Nevada, and about 60 miles south of Wendover, Nevada. Ibapah is the central community on this reservation.

The other reservation is located in Skull Valley, located near Tooele, Utah, about 90 miles from Salt Lake City—this is home to the Skull Valley Band of Goshute Indians of Utah. Both areas are primarily desert Country, but with nearby mountains, and are sparsely populated.

As with all American Indian tribes, the Goshutes suffered at the hands of Europeans. Spanish slave traders and European fur traders came into Goshute lands in the early 1800s, and later, miners crossed through on the way to California (Defa, 2003). In the latter 1800s, Mormon ranchers and farmers encroached on the land, took more fertile land and water, both treasured commodities, as most of this region is desert land. Goshutes had lived in this region for thousands of years as hunter–gatherers. Staples were pine nuts, seeds, roots, insects, and large game, including deer, elk, and sheep. With the establishment of ranches, they could no longer live off the land because of the decrease in available territory. Mormons established missions in the region to convert the Goshutes to Mormonism. As a result of close Mormon association, their homeland shrank to about a 1,000-acre farm on present-day Deep Creek (Defa, 2003).

In 1912, 80 acres in Skull Valley were established as a reservation, and later in 1919, the land was increased to almost 18,000 acres for use by the Goshutes. The Deep Creek Reservation was established in 1914 with close to 35,000 acres for their exclusive use. Today, Deep Creek has over 100,000 acres. With the reservations came government mandates, including boarding schools for children, vocational education for adults, and further restrictions on land use.

One important historical event was the Goshute uprising in 1918, which came about when Goshutes refused to comply with the Selective Service Act of

1917 that required all males who were 21 to 30 years of age to comply with conscription and possible service in the military. Although the Goshutes had not yet been given citizenship, their federal agent insisted they register. Tensions eventually decreased, and 163 men registered (Defa, 2003).

Ultimately, the Goshutes were pushed into adopting a sedentary way of life as farmers, and to adopt a foreign form of government that the Whites used. Deep Creek Goshutes adopted their own constitution and bylaws in November 1940. The Skull Valley Reservation was formed in 1917 to 1918 by executive order of the federal government. The two groups chose to remain as two separate tribes—Deep Creek and Skull Valley—rather than consolidate as one tribe (Defa, 2003).

Today, the Skull Valley Reservation is uniquely located, surrounded by environmental toxins: nearby are the Dugway Proving Grounds, which store nerve agents and weapons-testing grounds; the Tooele Army Depot has nerve gas incinerators and serves as a weapons-testing facility; Intermountain Power plant is a coal-powered generating facility; and MagCorp is a magnesium production plant generating chlorine gas. Knowing this, the tribe asked to house high-level radioactive waste for boosting their economy, but the U.S. government and the state of Utah nixed the plan as it would put millions in jeopardy if an accident or leak should happen (Jeffries, 2007). Over time, reservation life played havoc on them as they struggled to maintain some of their traditional lifestyle while keeping up with modern demands. Unemployment and alcoholism became challenges for them. Because Deep Creek Goshutes live in three different counties and two different states, there are many demands on them to answer to jurisdictional issues. There are about 120 tribal members, and the tribal headquarters are located in Salt Lake City.

Health Care for the Goshutes

State and county boundaries create situations in which people have to decide where and how far to travel for health care. If on the Utah side, they travel to Wendover or Salt Lake City. If on the Nevada side, they travel to Ely, Wendover, or Elko, Nevada. According to a community health representative (CHR) who provides transportation for dialysis patients, it is an all-day job for her to transport patients for dialysis to Salt Lake City or Bountiful, Utah. She drives people to other doctor's appointments, which is a daylong job for her, but she enjoys being able to help people, as many have no other means to obtain care (C. Steele, personal communication, 2014).

For the Deep Creek population, there is a clinic in Ibapah; most travel to Elko, Nevada, and some are referred to Salt Lake City for specialty care. Skull Valley people recently opened a clinic in Salt Lake City called Sacred Circle. There is no clinic in Skull Valley; however, many tribal members have been enrolled for care through the Patient Protection and Affordable Care Act (Rosenbaum, 2011) and enjoy better access to health care services. This also eliminates the need for tribal members to travel to Ft. Duchesne, Utah, 120 miles away, for Indian Health Service care (L. Bear, personal communication, January 26, 2015). Many of the Skull Valley people live in Salt Lake City, whereas only a small number, about 30 people, live on the reservation.

The Deep Creek Goshutes have an array of health-related services managed by a health director. Close coordination with the Southern Bands Clinic in Elko, Nevada, and several state programs in Utah are a daily occurrence (C. Steele, personal communication, September 4, 2015). Unfortunately, people are exposed to and consume high-fat, high-calorie snacks and beverages. Diabetes is a major health problem. Sadly, these desert people were once extremely knowledgeable about 81 species of plants and took seeds from over 40 of them (Smith, 2011).

Goshute children are sent on a 120-mile round trip to Wendover, Nevada, or some attend public school in Tooele, Utah, whereas others attend boarding school out of state and still others move out of the community (C. Steele, personal communication, September 4, 2015). Preservation of indigenous language and culture is a concern for most tribes, as expressed to the Native American Legislative Committee at the 2010 Utah Legislative session (Jefferies, 2010; Native American Legislative Liaison Committee, 2010). Skull Valley Goshutes are proud of one student's current enrollment in a nursing program, and one just completed some type of phlebotomy program and is working in a hospital (L. Bear, personal communication, January 26, 2015).

THE PAIUTES

History of the Paiute Tribe of Utah

There are a number of Paiute tribes throughout Utah, Nevada, and parts of Idaho, eastern California, and western Wyoming. The early Paiutes—referred to as the Southern Paiutes—traveled throughout southern Nevada, Utah, and northern Arizona as hunter–gatherers. This land has mountains and valleys with springs, where they formed camps at different times of the year. Clothing was made from rabbit skins or deerskin for winter wear, whereas summer wear was usually cliff-rose bark or breech cloth. Nuts, seeds, plants, and small animals were gathered from valleys, whereas pine nuts and larger animals were harvested from higher elevations. People moved in small family groups, forming a band, as the desert environment could only support this type of arrangement.

As with other American Indian cultures, the Paiutes enjoy social dancing and singing. They made flutes out of elderberry or juniper wood; drums, gourds, and rattles were also made and used for ceremonies and dances. They made bows, arrows, arrowheads, buckskin clothing and moccasins; they wove cradleboards, baskets, and used rabbit skin for clothing and blankets. They continue to make these items today (Paiute Indian Tribe of Utah, 2015a).

The Paiute Indian Tribe of Utah (PITU) was federally recognized on April 3, 1980; they celebrate this important occasion every year in their Restoration Gathering and Powwow. The PITU consists of five bands: Cedar, Indian Peaks, Kanosh, Koosharem, and Shivwits. They have a population of close to 1,000. Their reservation is composed of 11 different tracts of land through-out four counties of southwestern Utah.

The PITU had separate reservations prior to the introduction of Public Law 762 by Utah Senator Watkins on January 9, 1954, which terminated their federal recognition. To regain recognition was a difficult process that took over 25 years (beginning in 1970 under President Nixon), and was realized with the help of Indian lawyers (Paiute Indian Tribe of Utah, 2015b).

In recent times, the PITU made health care more accessible to their popu-lation by opening physician assistant–staffed health centers in four locations: Cedar City Paiute Medical Clinic, Kanosh Paiute Medical Clinic, Koosharem Paiute Medical Clinic, and Shivwits Paiute Medical Clinic. The health program offered at these clinics provides a number of wellness programs, including weight loss, nutrition, fun runs, health fairs, and other physical activities that they promote through their newsletters (Paiute Indian Tribe of Utah, 2015c). Southern Utah University, located in Cedar City, has an Intergovernmental Internship Cooperative (IIC) that aims to develop and "expand relationships with the regional Paiute Tribes to offer Paiute youth education and career devel-opment opportunities" (Southern Utah University, 2011, p. 1). The IIC appears to be a promising program for the Paiute youth in this region. Southern Utah University has a nursing program; I am not aware whether nursing has been included in the internship program.

The Southern Paiutes

Another grouping of Southern Paiutes includes the Kaibab Paiute in north cen-tral Arizona, Las Vegas Tribal colony in Nevada, Moapa Paiutes in Nevada, and the San Juan Southern Paiute in northern Arizona. All of these bands and tribes are related in some way; many formed family groupings in their earlier history as a foraging mainstay. The San Juan Paiutes have intermarried with Navajo over the years. And, in fact, "Paiute lands north of the Arizona border and south of the San Juan River in Utah were proclaimed in 1907 as the Paiute Strip Reservation, which was placed under the jurisdiction of the Western Navajo Agency. Unfortunately for the Paiutes, in 1922, the Paiute Strip was integrated into Navajo lands" (Allen, 2013, p. 1).

Since they were recognized as a tribe in 1990, the San Juan Southern Paiute tribe, with 300 members, has been busy contacting those who have moved out of the area for tribal enrollment. Those still living on the reservation live near Paiute Mountain (known as Navajo Mountain or Naatsis'áán to the Navajo), Tuba City, Cow Springs, Hidden Springs, and White Mesa. Several have farms at the bottom of Paiute Canyon. According to two elders, older Paiutes took in Navajos who were escaping the Kit Carson roundup in the mid-1800s to move Navajo to Bosque Redondo for imprisonment (Paiute elder, personal communication, 2014). Now, the Paiutes are negotiating with the Navajo for their portion of the land back. Their health care is included within the Tuba

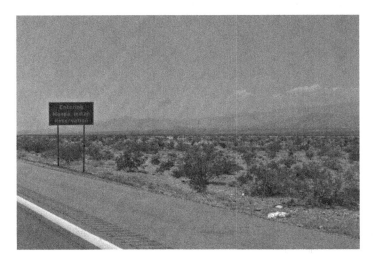

FIGURE 11.3 Entering Moapa Indian reservation.
Source: P199 Wikimedia Commons.

City Comprehensive Health Care facility, a PL 638 program that also serves the Navajo and Hopi Tribal members.

The Moapa River Indian Reservation is located northeast of Las Vegas, in Nevada, with a land base of 71,954 acres of primarily desert terrain. They have a population of close to 300. *Moapa* is a Paiute word for *muddy*, named after the river that flows into Lake Mead. The Moapa Paiutes farmed that area prior to and shortly after the reservation's establishment. Unfortunately, they lost much of the irrigable land and were given mostly desert land.

Toiyabe Indian Health Project, Inc.

Tribes in California are not organized as service units; rather, they are called projects. Thus, the Toiyabe Indian Health Project, Inc. incorporates Benton Paiute Reservation, Big Pine Reservation, Bishop Reservation, Bridgeport Indian Colony, Fort Independence Reservation, Lone Pine Reservation, and the Timbisha Shoshone tribe. These are small tribes located in eastern California, from Death Valley to areas south of the Reno area. In this catchment area, there are three community health centers located in Bishop, Lone Pine, and Coleville, CA. The Bishop center has a dialysis center; a family services program that includes mental health, substance abuse treatment, prevention and outreach services; optometry; public health, including public health nursing, nutrition education and counseling, diabetes education and prevention, injury prevention, community health representatives, and a Centers for Disease Control and Prevention (CDC)-funded community wellness program. An outdoor exercise center was opened; a newsletter is printed to inform the communities of available services; and referrals and contract health services are coordinated with local providers. Most clinical staff is non-Indian.

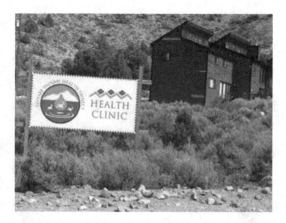

FIGURE 11.4 Toiyabe Indian Health Project in Coleville, California.
Courtesy of Lillian Tom-Orme.

THE SHOSHONES

History of the Northwestern Band of Shoshone

According to the 2010 U.S. Census, the Shoshone population consists of 13,767 individuals. Fort Hall, Idaho, is home to approximately 6,000 members of Shoshone and Bannock tribes. Many Shoshone bands that have been placed on various reservations are all related in some way to other bands, through clan relations and extended family. The Shoshones of Fort Hall are from three different bands that once hunted and gathered food throughout northern Utah, southern Idaho, northern Nevada, and western Wyoming (University of Utah American West Center, 2008).

The Shoshones are part of the Uto–Aztecan linguistic stock and speak the Numic dialect. They called themselves "the Valley people." They hunted buffalo, elk, deer, moose, and antelope in the higher elevations. Animal hides were used for clothing and shelter; meat was sundried and used in the winter months. When they migrated to northern Nevada, they collected pine nuts, which they also stored for winter. Their winter home was in southern Idaho, where they fished, and which also sustained them during the cold season. The horse was introduced to them from their Plains neighbors, enabling the Shoshones to expand their migration patterns.

By the 1840s, emigrants, fur traders, and Mormons began to migrate west, and began encroaching on their lands. The bands protected their lands as best they could, but many incidents occurred in which Shoshone were killed unprovoked.

On January 29, 1863, 200 army volunteers led by Colonel Patrick Edward Connor from Camp Douglas (later Fort Douglas) in Salt Lake City attacked a group of 450 Shoshone men, women, and children, who were camped on the Bear River. The killing spree lasted 4 hours in the early hours of that morning, and 350 Shoshones were slaughtered. This was one of the most violent events in Utah's history; the Shoshone commemorate the anniversary of the Bear River Massacre every year.

Following this tragedy, settlers poured into Shoshone land unabated to claim their homesteads. Some Shoshone who were now homeless were moved to the Fort Hall reservation; a small group refused to move. They claimed some land under the Homestead Act, and they lived in northern Utah until 1987 when the federal government recognized them as an independent tribe. They are now the Northwestern Band of Shoshone Indians.

Health Care for the Northwestern Band of Shoshone

An Indian Health Service health center in Ft. Hall serves the ambulatory health needs of both the Shoshone–Bannocks and the Northwestern Band. The facility serves over 13,380 American Indian and Alaska Natives (AI/ANs), and they record approximately 37,294 ambulatory patient visits per year (Indian Health Service, 2015a). The facility is staffed by a full complement of physicians, nurses, dentists, and others. The tribe operates the Tribal Contract Health Service, Diabetes, and Community Health Nursing Programs. Referrals are made to specialists and local private hospitals.

History of the Eastern Shoshone

The Eastern Shoshone are the descendants of the famous Chief Washakie. They were settled in Wyoming on the Wind River Reservation under the Fort Bridger Treaty of 1868. In 1877, the northern Arapahos were settled on the same reservation.

Health Care for the Wind River Shoshone

There are two Indian Health Service clinics in Wyoming for both tribes in Fort Washakie (Shoshone) and in Arapaho (for the Arapaho). The clinic user population is approximately 11,000 AI/AN people. The clinics are staffed by physicians, nurse practitioners, psychologists, dentists, dietitians, public health nurses, and optometrists (Indian Health Service, 2015b). Specialty services are arranged within the clinics, and referrals for inpatient care are made to two hospitals in nearby Lander, Wyoming, or Riverton, Wyoming.

Diabetes is the fourth leading cause of death among AI/ANs on reservations in Montana and Wyoming. On the Wind River Reservation, diabetes affects the lives of about 12% of adults, or 917 persons (Alliance to Reduce Disparities in Diabetes, 2011). Overweight and obesity are major health problems, and 71% of the residents have a body mass index (BMI) greater than 30.0. Wind River has teamed up with others to address diabetes and its complications by offering diabetes self-management classes, workshops for the providers, cultural workshops, and nutrition and physical activity programs. Wind River is part of the Indian Health Service Billings Area, and participates in the Montana–Wyoming Tribal Council and the Rocky Mountain Tribal Epidemiology Center (Rocky Mountain Tribal Epidemiology Center, 2015).

The Duckwater Shoshone

The Duckwater live in Railroad Valley in high desert Country in northern Nevada. Farming and ranching are the main industries there, along with government jobs. Students can attend public school or the private Shoshone elementary school on the reservation. Students attend the community college in Elko, Nevada, and some go to the University of Utah in Salt Lake City, about 4 hours away.

Te-Moak Tribe of Western Shoshone

The Te-Moak tribe consists of four small bands in northeastern Nevada with a total population of 1,143, located on reservation lands in Elko, South Fork, Battle Mountain, and Wells, Nevada. Owing to their isolation, their first contact with Europeans was in the period between 1827 and 1846, when fur traders came into their territory. Later, emigrants on the way to California disturbed their peaceful ways of existence as hunter–gatherers. Gold and copper were found in the mountains and brought an influx of White settlers, which gave way to skirmishes; thus, the name Battle Mountain (Figure 11.5). The area is located near the Humboldt River and other small rivers and springs, important to earlier groupings of Shoshone and Paiute who made it their territory. In the early 20th century, the government attempted to move all Shoshone to the Duck Valley Reservation along the Nevada–Idaho border, but most refused (Te-Moak Tribe of Western Shoshone Indians of Nevada, 2015).

Health Care for the Te-Moak Bands of Shoshone

The Elko Service Unit of the Indian Health Service, located in Elko, Nevada, serves 7,200 members of the Te-Moak Bands of Shoshone, which include Duckwater, Ely, and four colonies—Battle Mountain, Elko, South Fork, and Wells—as well as the Goshutes. A number of Shoshone bands are organized as colonies, which are small reservations within an established city (Indian Health Service, 2015c).

The Southern Bands Health Center in Elko offers ambulatory health care and has a staff of two physicians, two physician assistants, one dentist, and a psychologist. Nurses staff a 24-hour hotline. The community health program includes public health nursing, mental health, and environmental health. In addition, Ely, located south of Elko, operates a small clinic.

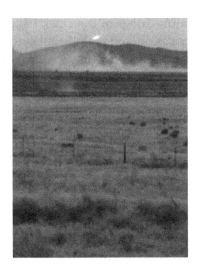

FIGURE 11.5 Dust devils near Battle Mountain, Nevada.
Courtesy of Lillian Tom-Orme.

Owyhee Shoshone–Paiute Tribes of Duck Valley

The land used for centuries by several bands of Shoshone and Paiutes in south-west Oregon and northern Nevada was crossed by the Oregon and California Trails in the mid-1800s. Dealing with White encroachment led to tensions with the settlers and resulted in the establishment of Fort Boise in Idaho, the signing of the Bruneau Treaty in 1866, and the Bannock War in 1868. The Shoshone reservation was established in 1877, and expanded in 1886 for the Paiutes. The Paiutes joined the Bannocks in the Bannock War, were later moved to prison camps in Yakima, Washington, but later moved back to Duck Valley, at which time the reservation was expanded. In the early days, people lived in earthen willow and sagebrush huts using plants from their environment to construct dwellings. They were hunters and gatherers that used the Duck Valley region as their homeland, and wisely used resources for their basic needs. In 1884, the federal government attempted to move both tribes to Ft. Hall, Idaho, and to open up Duck Valley to settlers, but the tribes successfully resisted this mandate.

Today, farming and ranching are primary industries, occupations that were encouraged by the government upon the establishment of the reservation. The Reorganization Act of 1934 allowed them to draft a tribal constitution and bylaws. Tourism, including fishing and hunting, are managed by the tribe.

Health Care for the Shoshone and Paiutes of Duck Valley

The Owyhee Community Health Facility in Owyhee, Nevada, provides health care to the Shoshone–Paiute tribes of the Duck Valley Reservation in northern

Nevada (Shoshone-Paiute Tribes of the Duck Valley Indian Reservation, 2015). Some of the other services offered include behavioral health counseling, health education, managed care, substance abuse counseling, and diabetes education.

In 1937, a hospital was built on the reservation, but it was closed in 1976. Today, the Owyhee Community Health facility serves the Shoshone and Paiute tribes. Tribal membership is approximately 2,000, with 1,700 living as active residents on the reservation. A tribally operated hospital is shared with the non-Indians in the area. Health-related programs include social services, community health, and behavioral health.

The Indian Health Service administrative Schurz Service Unit covers about three quarters of western and southern Nevada while the Elko Service Unit covers the northwestern section of the state. Duck Valley, Elko, Ely, and Duckwater are within the Elko Service Unit. All others are in the Schurz Service Unit. The Schurz Service Unit, located in Schurz, Nevada, serves Shoshone, Paiutes, and Washoe Tribes and Bands, a service population of about 12,000 on 13 reservations and colonies (Indian Health Service, 2015d).

Fort McDermitt Paiute and Shoshone Tribe

The Fort McDermitt Paiute and Shoshone Tribe reservation, established in 1936, straddles the borders of northern Nevada and southern Oregon. It was once a military reservation to protect westward migration—the stagecoach route—the valley in which Fort McDermitt is located in prehistoric Lake Lahontan (Poff, n.d.).

Today, the people are involved in farming, ranching, and mining. Say When Casino provides some income for the tribe. As indicated by tribal Chairman Tildon Smart, tribal members have engaged in working in a variety of settings, including mining, firefighting, ranching, and local government work (National Museum of the American Indian, 2014).

Much progress is being made, but there are challenges too, as described by former Chairman Billy Bell in his testimony to the Indian Law and Order Commission in 2012. Mr. Bell describes the high rates of domestic violence, alcohol and drug abuse, and the lack of proper resources, including a shelter for victims of abuse, police facilities, and detention centers on the reservation, adequate court personnel and even availability of a prosecutor, judge, and police officers (Bell, 2012).

THE UTES

Ute History

The Ute population of Utah and Colorado numbered 11,491 in the 2010 Census. This discussion will be limited to the Northern Utes, and excludes the southern and Ute Mountain Utes of Colorado. The Northern Utes, numbering about

4,200, reside in the Uintah Basin of northeastern Utah and comprise three Ute bands: the Uncompahgre, Uintah, and White River. The reservation is called the Uintah-Ouray (U&O) Reservation.

The over 4,200 Northern Utes' tribal members are divided between those living on the reservation and those living elsewhere. They have approximately 1.3 million acres of trust land, on which they operate a cattle business and mine for oil and natural gas. In addition, they have several tribal enterprises, including small businesses, a tribal feedlot, and water systems (www.utetribe.com/).

The U&O Service Unit of the Indian Health Service serves the Paiutes, NW Band of Shoshone, and Goshutes of Utah, but is located much too far from any of the other tribes. Only the Northern Utes have direct access to the clinic, but are at least a 5-hour drive away. Health care services include general medical clinics, surgical follow-up, prenatal and pediatric care, dental and optometry services. Specialty clinics are offered by visiting consultants. The center is staffed by physicians, a physician's assistant, dentists, an optometrist, nurses, and pharmacists. Referrals and emergency care are offered at the Duchesne County Hospital in Roosevelt, Utah (Indian Health Service, 2015e). Community health is coordinated through the tribal community health programs. The tribe operates a federally funded Special Diabetes Program, has a family services program, an alcohol treatment program, and an air quality monitoring program.

NURSING IN THE GREAT BASIN

The best description of nursing in the Great Basin comes from Naomi Mason, a Shoshone nurse, who was educated in San Francisco and later at Idaho State University. She describes her experience as a public health nurse during the tuberculosis era, having to track infectious disease contacts, and later dealing with diabetes and alcoholism, and observing in more recent times the lack of child care knowledge and skills in young mothers. Her nephew, Dr. Steve Crum, attempted to locate her so she could speak with me, but we were unable to find her in time for this publication (Mason, 2014).

For the most part, nurses working in the Great Basin region are involved in rural nursing, with small communities located in isolated regions of Nevada, Idaho, Utah, Arizona, and California. Tribal lands near the cities of Las Vegas and Reno have access to amenities available there. Most Great Basin American Indians live in small towns, as depicted in the map and figures included in this chapter. Referrals are made to hospitals and specialty care in Salt Lake City, Reno, Las Vegas, Phoenix, and other places.

Nurses are required to be flexible and have various skills to apply for positions in hospital nursing, clinic nursing, as well as public health nursing. Because communities are small and people tend to move on and off reservations, nurses need to be adaptable to changing family dynamics. Good knowledge of health promotion and disease prevention as well as skills in these areas are beneficial as accidents and chronic diseases are the main causes of mortality. Conditions attributed to lifestyle behaviors, including tobacco use, lack of physical activity, poor nutrition, and social determinants of health issues are areas of concern and require health education and policy development.

Perhaps the greatest need is education of the local Native students in the health professions so that they can provide culturally safe and sensitive health care to the indigenous people of the Great Basin. Challenges facing the Great Basin tribes are that there are no local tribal colleges or casinos providing local economic support enjoyed by other tribes in the Country. Families and local communities also need to encourage good educational programs that develop and encourage Native students to pursue college and professional education. Today, there are few American Indian nurses or other health professionals in Nevada.

Naomi Mason (2014) attributed her outside interests to her mother, who read a lot and inspired Naomi's own curiosity about "the world outside of Owyhee, outside the United States. I think that's what she did for us" (p. 16). Although Mason left the reservation to complete her high school and college education, she later returned to finish her nursing career among her people, the Shoshone of Elko and Owyhee.

In a nursing workforce report in 2014, of eight American Indian nurses responding to the survey, seven were employed in urban areas, and the eighth nurse's employment location was undetermined (Griswold, Etchegoyhen, & Packham, 2014). Overall, 65% of rural and frontier nurses are educated at the associate-degree level and tend to work in hospital settings. Nurses in urban areas are educated at the baccalaureate (30%–36%) or associated-degree levels (27%–32%), and a few have master's or doctoral degrees. Nurses from the Great Basin tribes are needed to provide health care to eliminate health disparities as they are the ones who understand the languages spoken and the cultures practiced by the local communities.

CONCLUSIONS

All the tribes listed in Figure 11.1 were at one time hunters and gatherers of the Great Basin region, which is characterized by mountain ranges and valleys. Small bands migrated between these topographies for food and shelter, depending on the season and availability of resources. Many were related by clan, band, or family, but when settled on reservations, they were scattered across Nevada, parts of California, Idaho, Oregon, and Wyoming. Today, they are federally recognized as unique tribes, and have a nation-to-nation relationship with the U.S. government, making them eligible for a number of resources, including health care.

Except for a couple of reservations, all are included under the Phoenix Area Indian Health Service and service units, including Schurz, Uintah-Ouray, and Owyhee. Ft. Hall and Wind River fall under the administration out of Billings and Northwest Portland Areas. Those in California are subsumed under the California Area Indian Health Service.

As documented in a field hearing before the Commission on Indian Affairs, called "Healthcare without an IHS Hospital: Overtaxing the Contract Health Services," Nevada tribes and health directors lamented the severe shortage of contract health service funding, and the bureaucracy that seemingly disapproves most referrals unless they are "life or limb" situations. They sought the establishment of an Area Office in Nevada and a hospital to serve the needs of the 27 tribes that live in remote locations. Among the challenges identified were that contract health funds run out within 5 months of the new fiscal year (by May or June) and only life or limb cases are then approved for referral to a non-IHS provider; in addition, many providers no longer accept referrals because of lack of payment by the tribe or IHS program. The nearest IHS hospital is in Phoenix, Arizona, nearly 1,000 miles away for some tribes; Nevada tribes are unable to access these services.

Espey and colleagues (2014) noted that in the Southwest, which would include Phoenix Area tribes, death rates among AI/ANs, regardless of cause, exceeded those among Whites (1,251.4 vs. 926.2). For AI/AN males, accidents, heart disease, cancer, chronic liver disease, and diabetes were the top reasons for mortality between 1999 and 2009. For AI/AN females, the top five reasons for death were cancer, heart disease, accidents, diabetes, and chronic liver disease. Heart disease, cancer, and diabetes-related mortality could be attributed to changes in lifestyle and lack of health care access. Accidents are related to motor vehicle crashes, poisoning, and falls. Chronic liver disease is related to cirrhosis, alcoholism, and hepatitis. Many of these conditions could be prevented or their complications delayed. Among younger AI/ANs, under 25 years of age, suicide rates are nearly 50% higher as compared with those among non-Hispanic Whites of the same age group.

These conditions provide many opportunities for nurses and other health care providers to perform health–promotion and disease–prevention activities. However, there are few AI/ANs entering the health profession. None of the tribes in the Great Basin area have their own tribal college, and many do not have easy access to a community college. Most nurses who are staffing the health facilities are non-AI/AN.

There is a critical need for local schools to introduce health professions to AI/AN students, and to encourage them to take courses that will help them reach those potentials. Some tribes have newsletters, which also serve as a potential medium to introduce health professions.

STUDY QUESTIONS
♦ What are some possible reasons for the lack of indigenous nurses from the Great Basin area?
♦ Name and discuss some differences and similarities among the Great Basin tribes.
♦ Discuss the relevance of social determinants of health in the context of the health status of Great Basin tribes.

USEFUL WEBSITES

♦ Tribal Groups and Tribes of the Great Basin, http://www.bia.gov/cs/groups/webteam/documents/document/idc1-029026.pdf

TRIBES OF THE GREAT BASIN

♦ The Goshutes
  Skull Valley Band of Goshute Indians of Utah
  Confederated Tribes of the Goshute Reservation, Nevada and Utah
♦ The Paiutes
  Big Pine Paiute Tribe of the Owens Valley, California
  Bishop Paiute Tribe, California
  Bridgeport Paiute Indian Colony, California
  Burns Paiute Tribe, Oregon
  San Juan Southern Paiute Tribe of Arizona
  Moapa Band of Paiute Indians of the Moapa River Indian Reservation, Nevada
  Paiute Indian Tribe of Utah (made up of Cedar City Band of Paiutes, Kanosh Band of
    Paiutes, Koosharem Band of Paiutes, Indian Peaks Band of Paiutes, and Shivwits
    Band of Paiutes)
  Paiute–Shoshone Tribe of the Fallon, Nevada
  Fort Independence Indian Community of Paiute Indians of the Fort Independence
    Reservation, California
  Fort McDermitt Paiute and Shoshone Tribes of the Fort McDermitt Indian
    Reservation, Nevada and Oregon
  Kaibab Band of Paiute Indians of the Kaibab Indian Reservation, Arizona
  Las Vegas Tribe of Paiute Indians of the Las Vegas Indian Colony, Nevada
  Lone Pine Paiute–Shoshone Tribe, California
  Lovelock Paiute Tribe of the Lovelock Indian Colony, Nevada
  Summit Lake Paiute Tribe of Nevada
  Utu Utu Gwaitu Paiute Tribe of the Benton Paiute Reservation, California
  Walker River Paiute Tribe of the Walker River Reservation, Nevada
♦ The Shoshones
  Reno-Sparks Indian Colony, Nevada
  Death Valley Timbi-sha Shoshone Tribe, California
  Duckwater Shoshone Tribe of the Duckwater Reservation, Nevada
  Ely Shoshone Tribe of Nevada
  Northwestern Band of Shoshoni Nation, Utah
  Shoshone Tribe of the Wind River Reservation, Wyoming
  Shoshone–Bannock Tribes of the Fort Hall Reservation, Idaho
  Shoshone–Paiute Tribes of the Duck Valley Reservation, Nevada
  Te-Moak Tribe of Western Shoshone Indians of Nevada (Four constituent bands:
    Battle Mountain Band; Elko Band; South Fork Band; and Wells Band)
  Winnemucca Indian Colony of Nevada
  Yerington Paiute Tribe of the Yerington Colony & Campbell Ranch, Nevada
  Yomba Shoshone Tribe of the Yomba Reservation, Nevada

♦ The Utes

Southern Ute Indian Tribe of the Southern Ute Reservation, Colorado

Ute Indian Tribe of the Uintah & Ouray Reservation, Utah

Ute Mountain Tribe of the Ute Mountain Reservation, Colorado, New Mexico & Utah

REFERENCES

Allen, K. (2013, October 13). Paiutes seek land, acknowledgement from Diné neighbors. *The Navajo Times* (p. 1). Retrieved form http://www.navajotimes.com/news/2013/1013/103113paiutes.php#.Vh1l02Em5aQ.

Alliance to Reduce Disparities in Diabetes. (2011). *Reducing diabetes disparities in American Indian communities (Wind River reservation).* Retrieved from http://ardd.sph.umich.edu/eastern_shoshone_tribe.html.

Bell, B. (2012). *Testimony of the Honorable Billy A. Bell, Tribal Chairman of the Fort McDermitt Paiute and Shoshone Tribe and President of the Inter-Tribal Council of Nevada before the Indian Law and Order Commission Hearing.* Retreived from http://www.aisc.ucla.edu/iloc/resources/documents/ILOC%20FH_Scottsdale, AZ_011312_Testimony_Bell.pdf

Defa, D. R. (2003). The Goshute Indians of Utah. In F. S. Cuch (Ed.), *A history of Utah's American Indians.* Salt Lake City, UT: Utah State Division of Indian Affairs, Utah State Division of History.

Espey, D. K., Jim, M. A., Cobb, N., Bartholomew, M., Becker, T., Haverkamp, D., & Plescia, M. (2014, June). Leading causes of death and all-cause mortality in American Indians and Alaska Natives. *American Journal of Public Health, 104*(Suppl. 3), S303–S311. doi:10.2105/AJPH.2013.301798

Griswold, T., Etchegoyhen, L., & Packham, J. (2014, May). *Registered nurse workforce in Nevada: Findings from the 2013 National workforce survey of registered nurses.* University of Nevada School of Medicine Health Policy Report. Reno, NV: University of Nevada School of Medicine.

Indian Health Service. (2015a). *Portland area.* Retrieved from https://www.ihs.gov/portland/index.cfm/healthcarefacilities/forthall/

Indian Health Service. (2015b). *Billings Area.* Retrieved from https://www.ihs.gov/billings/?module=bao%5Fsu%5Fwindriver.

Indian Health Service. (2015c). *Phoenix area.* Retrieved from https://www.ihs.gov/phoenix/index.cfm/healthcarefacilities/elko/

Indian Health Service. (2015d). *Phoenix area health care facilities.* Retrieved from https://www.ihs.gov/phoenix/index.cfm/healthcarefacilities/

Indian Health Service. (2015e). *Uintah-Ouray service unit.* Retrieved from https://www.ihs.gov/phoenix/index.cfm/healthcarefacilities/uintahouray/

Jefferies, S. M. (2007). *Environmental justice and the Skull Valley Goshute Indians' proposal to store nuclear waste.* Retrieved from http://epubs.utah.edu/index.php/jlrel/article/viewFile/58/51

J. Land, Resources, and Environmental Law. Vol27 (2): 409–429.

Mason, N. (2014). *Great Basin Indian Archive, GBIA 034* (Oral history interview by Norm Cavanaugh, April 23, 2014). Elko, NV: Great Basin College. Retrieved from http://www.gbcnv.edu/gbia/manuscripts/oral_histories/GBIA034_NaomiMason_04232014.pdf

Mason, N. (2014). Oral history by Norm Cavanaugh. Great Basin Indian Archives, Great Basin College, NV. Retrieved from http://www.gbcnv.edu/gbia/manuscripts/oral_histories/GBIA034. aaccess_NaomiMason_04232014.pdf

Native American Legislative Liaison Committee. (2010). September 1, 2010. *Minutes of the Utah Native American Legislative Liaison Committee.* Retrieved from http://www.le.utah .gov/Interim/2010/pdf/00001744.pdf

National Museum of the American Indian. (2014). *Meet Tildon Smart, chairman of the Fort McDermitt Paiute Shoshone tribe of Nevada and Oregon.* Retrieved from http://blog .nmai.si.edu/main/2014/03/meet-native-america-tildon-smart.html.

Paiute Indian Tribe of Utah. (2015a). *Paiute culture.* Retrieved from http://www .utahpaiutes.org/about/culture/paiute-dancing.aspx.

Paiute Indian Tribe of Utah. (2015b). *Paiute history.* Retrieved from http://www .utahpaiutes.org/about/history/

Paiute Indian Tribe of Utah. (2015c). *Journey to wellness newsletter, 5*(5): 1–12. Retrieved from http://www.utahpaiutes.org/about/departments/tribalmemberservices/health/ forms/Health%20Department%20Newsletter.pdf.

Poff, B. (n.d.). *The Paiute and Shoshone of Fort McDermitt, Nevada: A short history.* Retrieved from http://oregonexplorer.info/data_files/OE_location/lakes/documents/fort- mcdermitt.history.pdf.

Rocky Mountain Tribal Epidemiology Center. (2015). *About us.* Retrieved from http://www.rmtec.org/about/

Rosenbaum, S. (2011). The patient protection and the affordable care act: Implications for public health. *Public Health Reports, 126*(1):130–135.

Shoshone-Paiute Tribes of the Duck Valley Indian Reservation. (2015). *Owyhee Community Health Facility.* Retrieved from http://www.shopaitribes.org/ochf/ochf.html.

Smith. E. 2011. Goshute subsistence. American Indian health and diet project. http:// www.aihd.ku.edu/foods/Goshute.html. accesses 10/12/15.

Southern Utah University. (2011, September). *Intergovernmental Internship Cooperative newsletter, 1, 1.* Retrieved from http://www.utahpaiutes.org/about/newsandevents/docs/ IIC%20September%202011%20Newsletter.pdf.

Te-Moak Tribe of Western Shoshone Indians of Nevada. (2015). *History and culture.* Retrieved from http://www.temoaktribe.com/history.shtml.

University of Utah American West Center. (2008). *We shall remain: Utah Indian curriculum project: A brief history of Utah's Northwestern Shoshones.* Retrieved from http:// utahindians.org/Curriculum/pdf/TribalHistories/shoshonehistory.pdf.

USer 199, Moapa Indian Reservation, Nevada, United States. April 30, 2013. Wikimedia Commons/Accessed May 18, 2015. https://upload.wikimedia.org/wikipedia/ commons/a/a2/Moapa_IR.JPG.

TWELVE

California Indians

Bette Jacobs

LEARNING OBJECTIVES

♦ To describe the distinct history of American Indians in California
♦ To understand the diversity of American Indians who reside in California and the origins of California residency (such as a historic tribe with dissolved and reconstituted identity, as part of directed migration in federal Indian policy, or as part of modern social mobility that attracts Indians as well as others to centers of vibrancy)
♦ To explain the advantages and disadvantages of Indian self-determination in a large, diverse state
♦ To know the health indicators for California Indians and discern the meaning of relevant disparities and disparity groupings
♦ To appreciate the measurement challenges associated with ethnic identity, tribal affiliation, and ethnic health indicators for American Indians generally and American Indians in California in particular
♦ To describe tribal lands and the ways health services are delivered for American Indians in California
♦ To identify the dynamic and futuristic profile of American Indian health in the context of a state that experienced ambiguity associated with changing federal relationships, migration, and assimilation and apply these futuristic conditions to overall health practice for American Indians
♦ To explain the relevance of demography, policy, and culture for nurses practicing with American Indians
♦ To promote American Indians to become health care leaders
♦ To describe opportunities, choices, and risks that can chart a new path for improved health for American Indians

KEY CONCEPTS

♦ Adaptation
♦ Assimilation
♦ Burden of disease
♦ Colonization

♦ Cultural revitalization
♦ Culturally competent nursing
♦ Dynamic culture
♦ Federal relations

♦ Harmony
♦ Health behavior
♦ Health service access
♦ Health service effectiveness

♦ Health service financing
♦ Health service utilization
♦ Relocation

KEY TERMS
♦ Alaska Natives (AN)
♦ American Indians (AI)
♦ Civil rights movement
♦ Federal recognition of tribes
♦ Gaming
♦ Indian Health Service (IHS)
♦ Indians

♦ MediCal (the California Medicaid program)
♦ Missions
♦ Occupation
♦ Tribal government
♦ Tribal health service

Among all the American states, California has the largest number of American Indians. California Indians are distinctive for a variety of reasons. The first is that California has the largest state population, so it follows that it would rank with high numbers for many ethnic groups. The second is the magnificent and messy history that is part of Indians belonging in California. The third is the history of civil rights and the parallel American Indian story that flourished along with California political activism. California is also the state with the largest number of nurses and, likely, the largest number of American Indian nurses. These facts draw attention to the importance of California to American Indians and to nursing in America.

The unique existence of American Indians in California and their continuing struggles and steps forward paint a picture that defines areas for improvement in health care for this population. The American Indian health experience presages issues that the rest of the country and the world will face in responding to people who have an ancient claim to stake and little legal or social understanding of their place that is in alignment with any proprietary claims. Concern for group health status is a paramount responsibility in planning, designing, and delivering health care services.

The distinctiveness of American Indians in California represents a remarkably dynamic and resilient culture within a large state at the forefront of ethnic diversity and ethnic admixture. The worldwide phenomenon of migration, both forced and voluntary, has accelerated and characterizes a new vibrancy that the Western world is experiencing. This has long been the California experience. California has the largest number of American Indians among the 50 U.S. states, and the most within-group diversity of American Indian tribes among all the states. Nevertheless, American Indians/Alaska Natives (AI/ANs) are a very small proportion (0.4%) of the California population, compared with their proportion (2%) in the overall U.S. population. California AI/ANs are an aging population. Although the highest proportion (92.3%) of the Latino community is under age 65, AI/ANs have the smallest proportion of people under age 65 (71.6%), exceeding even the commonly noted aging of Whites in California (76.3% under age 65).

The health status of Indians in California is similar to that of indigenous populations in the rest of the United States and the world in terms of disparity and health risks. Yet, in addition to higher rates of elders, there are other key health behavioral attributes that should inform culturally appropriate health services. American Indians/Alaska Natives in California, for example, are more likely than any other group (including Whites) to have a usual source of health care, and, at the same time, are the most likely of any other group to delay getting prescription drugs or medical services (UCLA Center for Health Policy Research, n.d.). This juxtaposition points to a profound disconnect for positive health behaviors, and posits a particular challenge in shaping health services.

HISTORY

The colonization of the United States is at the heart of any story about American Indians. In the eastern United States and pushing westward across the Great Plains and Mountain States, European colonization informed federal policy and the eventual definition of American Indian identity and course of history. In addition, in the northeastern United States, Indians figured prominently in a proxy war between England and France. The ultimate conquest and subjugation of Native peoples throughout the 19th century resulted in the reservation and treaty model that reverberates today.

The backdrop for California Indians is different. In California, the age of European exploration was a period from 1542 to 1769; then came the Spanish colonial period from 1769 to 1821, until Mexico became independent from Spain. California was mostly a Mexican territory until 1848, when it was annexed by the United States. The U.S. Congress approved California as a state, with an authorized state constitution and state government, in 1850. The only way to understand American Indian health in California is to know its unique history.

Many California Indians experienced the Spanish invasion and aggregation into settlements organized around missions. Missions established from San Diego to San Francisco between 1796 and 1823 were called the Las Californias Province of the Viceroyalty of New Spain. The indigenous people of this area became known as Mission Indians. Unlike the dominance of English settlements in the northeast, Spain sent soldiers and priests rather than families to establish their territory in the New World. Indians relocated to missions by enticement or force, and labored in subsistence agriculture. The intent of missions was to convert souls to the Church; this was the purpose of sending priests to live in the Western hemisphere.

The nature of these early encounters defined the following decades of relationships between the Whites and Indians. Mortality rates were high in the 18th and 19th centuries, particularly from infectious disease, and particularly for Indians who were naïve to new infectious agents and subjected to life on the margins. Measles was a cyclic infectious disease new to Indians, and, consequently, caused high rates of mortality.

Some Mission Indians attempted revolt at various times and were killed. A malaria epidemic in 1832 to 1833 devastated many people who lived or traveled in California during that time, profoundly affecting a declining American Indian population. Separate from Mission Indians were inland central tribes and California tribes north of San Francisco.

Russia founded the Russian American Company (RAC) in 1799 as a business formalizing their busy, profitable fur trading work in Alaska and along the Pacific Coast. Parts of what is now known as Alaska were called New Russia, and the general reference of New Russia extended down the Pacific Coast. Russian Orthodox priests sometimes followed settlements established by the fur trade. As sea otters and seal supplies were depleted in the far north and Alaska Native/Alaska Indian relations with Russians in this area deteriorated, Russia pushed more definitively farther down the Pacific Coast. Fort Ross, California, was built by Russians in 1812 as a trade center near the abundant sea otter grounds and as an agricultural center to supply its occupation in Pacific Rim lands. It was the southernmost Russian settlement in North America.

Interestingly, Fort Ross was the site of the first windmills and shipbuilding on the West Coast. Fort Ross is located in Sonoma County, just north of San Francisco. Today, the old settlement is part of the Fort Ross State Historic Park. As Russian competition in the fur trade with the British Hudson Bay Company and the Spanish in the early 19th century heightened, and demands on Russia in the Crimean War intensified, Russia sold Fort Ross to the United States in 1842. The sale of Fort Ross by Russia to the United States occurred 8 years before California statehood and 25 years before Russia sold Alaska to the United States.

Indians were residents of these land areas. Indians were not named as property in land transfers even though they occupied land in the areas where the legal transactions took place, and it was typical of the era to speak about people in terms of property. The West Coast region of North America was sparsely populated. Life was subject to circumstance and the environment. Infectious disease was the predominant threat to human life everywhere at this time, and epidemics could be devastating. The malaria epidemic threatened northern California and Fort Ross in 1833. The smallpox epidemic of 1837 wiped out most Indians in the Sonoma and Napa California areas. These episodic events combined with the surge of migration consequent to the 1849 Gold Rush weakened the presence of the many, small diverse tribes in the region.

California Indian tribes and languages outnumbered the different tribes and languages in the areas we now recognize as American states. Naturally, some of these tribes overlap along the borders of Nevada, Oregon, Arizona, and Mexico. Scholars have identified more than 100 distinct language dialects among the indigenous people who lived in the area we now know as California. Although we use the term *tribes*, the social and political structures of the original California Indians were more like interrelated villages than tribes.

As with all northern hemisphere Indians, there was no written language. Culture and knowledge were anchored and transmitted in lifestyle, spoken language, and storytelling. California Indians were accustomed to varied languages and likely learned quickly to speak the languages of newcomers.

The famous geography and climate of California includes some rugged, difficult terrain or seasonal times. There were active volcanoes still shaping the environment. In general, however, California Indians lived in an environment of abundance, plenty, and beauty. Among the notable enduring arts that California Indians were known for was basket weaving. Though there was massive fragmentation of the indigenous people in California and many stories have been forgotten, one creation story, *The Earth Dragon* (which follows), was preserved from Northern Coast Indians by Gifford and Block (1930). It poignantly points to the history, interaction, and harmony with nature characterizing a California Indian experience. Creation stories contain explanations and empiricism associated with repeated observations over time, reflect values, and teach ways of survival.

Although history does not give us a dominant cultural face of California Indians, the remarkable facts connecting them to this place is striking because, without such a deep anchor and identity, circumstances suggest that the peoples would easily and quickly have faded into oblivion. Note that this story depicts the dramatic young mountains, the rocky coastline of the great Pacific Ocean, and weather patterns typical of northern California; note also the relatively detailed human anatomy apparently advanced in its understanding for the era. There is poetry inherent in the conceptualization of creation.

The Earth Dragon

Before the world was formed, there was another world with sky made of sandstone rock. Two gods, thunder and Nagaicho, saw that old sky being shaken by thunder. "The rock is old," they said. "We'll fix it by stretching it above, far to the east." They stretched the sandstone, walking on the sky to do it, and under each of the sky's four corners, they set a great rock to hold it up. Then they added the different things that would make the world pleasant for people to live in. In the south, they created flowers. In the east, they put clouds so that people would not get headaches from the sun's glare. To form the clouds, they built a fire, then opened a large hole in the sky so that the clouds could come through. In the west, they made another opening for the fog to drift in from the ocean.

Now the two gods were ready to create people. They made a man out of earth and put grass inside him to form his stomach. They used another bundle of grass for his heart, round pieces of clay for the liver and kidneys, and a reed for the windpipe. They pulverized red stone and mixed it with water to form his blood. After putting together man's parts, they took one of the man's legs, split it, and turned it into a woman. Then they made a sun to travel by day and a moon to travel by night.

However, the creations of the gods did not endure, for every day and every night it rained. All of the people slept. Floodwaters came, and great stretches of land disappeared. The waters of the oceans flowed together; animals of all kinds drowned. Then the waters completely joined, and there were no more fields, mountains, or rocks, only water. There were no trees or grass, no fish or land, animals or birds. Human beings and animals had all been washed away.

The wind no longer blew through the portals of the world, nor was there snow, frost, or rain. There was no thunder or lightning, because there were no trees to be struck. There were neither clouds nor fog, nor did the sun shine. It was very dark.

Then the earth dragon, with its great, long horns, got up and walked down from the north. It traveled underground, and the god Nagaicho rode on its head. As it walked along through the ocean depths, the water outside rose to the level of its shoulders. When it came to shallower places it turned its head upward, and because of this, there is a ridge near the coast in the north on which the waves break. Far away to the south, it continued looking up and made a great mountain range.

In the south, the dragon lay down, and Nagaicho placed its head as it should be and spread gray-colored clay between its eyes and on each horn. He covered the clay with a layer of reeds, then spread another layer of clay. On it, he put some small stones, and then set blue grass, brush, and trees in the clay.

"I have finished," he said. "Let there be mountain peaks on the earth's head. Let the waves of the sea break against them."

The mountains appeared, and brush sprang up on them. The small stones he had placed on the earth's head became large, and the head itself was buried from sight.

Now people appeared, people who had animal names. (Later when Indians came to live on the earth, these "first people" were changed into their animal namesakes.) Seal, Sea Lion, and Grizzly Bear built a dance house. One woman by the name of Whale was fat, and that is why there are so many stout Indian women today.

The god Nagaicho caused different seafoods to grow in the water so that the people would have things to eat. He created seaweed, abalones, mussels, and many other things. Then he made salt from ocean foam. He caused the water of the ocean to rise up in waves and said that the ocean would always behave that way. He arranged for old whales to float ashore so people would have them to eat.

He made redwoods and other trees grow on the tail of the great dragon, which lay to the north. He carved out creeks by dragging his foot through the earth so that people would have good fresh water to drink. He created many oak trees to provide acorns to eat. He traveled all over the earth making it a comfortable place for men.

After he had finished, he and his dog went walking to see how the new things looked. When they arrived back at their starting point in the north, he said to his dog: "We're close to home. Now we'll stay here." Therefore, he left the world where people live, and now he inhabits the north (Gifford & Block,1930).

This creation story is clearly situated in northern California. Its English translation uses simple language to describe phenomena that transcend millennia. The observations over time are prospective in voice, recognizing metaphysical but not magical forces in nature. This creation story, as is common to many Indian stories, reveals how culture can be grounded in a natural empiricism. Small groups living in California over centuries had the indigenous experience. They were dependent on land, nature, and its variations. Encounters with interior tribes for trade and the gradual introduction of explorers were a different experience than settlers with families and military coming en masse as happened in the East. The introduction of White people to California Indians occurred incrementally.

Consequently, California Indians did not have the same types of wars and treaty agreements with the U.S. government as did many other Indian groups. When California became a state in 1850, certain provisions were made to stipulate things such as the fact that Indians could not testify against a White man, and that a White man could petition a court to indenture an Indian child. As was the case for all American Indians, California Indians were not eligible to vote as U.S. citizens until 1927.

Immediately after statehood, the aboriginal land title was explicated in court systems. In 1851, the U.S. Congress enacted the Lands Claim Act to formalize land ownership consequent to the purchase of California from Mexico as part of a state within the United States of America. This Act exempted land in occupation or possession by any Indian tribe. The act also authorized the U.S. president to create five military reservations in California for tribal purposes. The federal government gave sovereign land status to the Hupa Indian Reservation in far northwest California in 1864. In 1876, President Grant established nine Indian reservations in California by executive order, which at that time included the Morongo Mission Indian Reservation in Riverside County. Over time, courts revisited the legal status for California Indians. There has not been a consistent approach used. In one such judgment (1901), it was determined that Indians were not to be included as landowners in the purchase agreement, stating the view that Mexico had perceived that Indians had abandoned their lands.

A group of tribes brought a land claim to the California court that was eventually argued before the state by Earl Warren in 1941 and resulted in a settlement for Indians of $5 million. After World War II, the federal Indian Claims Commission Act (n.d.) resulted in a $29 million award for California Indians' compensation in exchange for their land claims. The federal Indian Reorganization Act (IRA) of 1934 intended to secure rights for AI/ANs. Indians were to have a degree of self-determination with federal aid for a time in order to achieve self-sufficiency. This was the era of institutional diminishment and intentional assimilation. The federal assimilation programs profoundly affected the demographics of Indians in California.

In the late 1940s and early 1950s, the federal government enacted plans to foster assimilation through relocation. This relocation was different from the 19th-century Indian Removal Act, which stains American history as a violent and legally ambiguous assault on the Indian people and a violation of rights, agreed to by treaty. The relocation methods of the mid-20th century came in the form of employment programs and financial relocation packages for Indian people and, in some cases, termination of federal recognition of tribes in the march toward assimilation and self-sufficiency. In the initial response to these policies, more than 100,000 Indians left their reservations between 1917 and 1945 to find employment. Likely, also, because two world wars occurred around this time, social forces fostered Indian people to move to be near family stationed at military bases. American Indians, even before being entitled to vote, have been strong and highly proportionate participants in the U.S. armed forces. Then, as now, data were not kept about families who moved residency back and forth from city to reservation in rhythm with work and family obligations. Therefore, we can trace a surge of AI/AN migration into California while lacking precise numbers.

It is estimated that in 1900 there were 16,000 California Indians. That number languished with termination policies and land compensations that "bought out" Indian ownership and Indian identity. Assimilation was the dominant helping paradigm to address the plight of the American Indian. In the mid-20th century, period policies of relocation and termination formalized, and California had two major destination cities established to employ Indians who left reservations throughout the United States. San Francisco and Los Angeles (and eventually Oakland) were recipient cities, and became sites for urban Indians and urban Indian centers.

This century posed a dramatic demographic turnaround of a different type. California tribes did not grow through birth rates. Federal relocation programs had a profound effect on the number of Indians in California. Other forces drew Indians from across the United States to California. Therefore, among all the states, California now has the largest number, though not the highest proportion, of AI/ANs. In the 2010 Census, nearly 800,000 California residents identified themselves as American Indian or Alaska Native.

The mid-20th-century migration of AI/ANs to California evoked greater sympathy and political strength for resident California Indians. The political activism of the 1960s erupted in a sentinel event in the modern history of the American Indian: The occupation of Alcatraz in 1969. A convergence of historic streams was ignited when the island of Alcatraz in the San Francisco Bay was decommissioned as a federal prison. By the mid-1960s, there was a concentration of American Indians in the San Francisco Bay area. Many of the Indian youth had been part of the relocation program and had grown up in California. American Indian student groups from Berkeley and San Francisco State University led the action planning and occupation of Alcatraz.

In the 1960s, youth were inculcated with civic activism associated with minority rights and change. A cadre of elder Indians had done their generational part advocating long term for rights, self-determination, and recognition and were present on the island or in the Bay Area to see the Indians of All Tribes join this action. More American Indians had received advanced education, including education in professions, such as law, and, as has always been the case, there were certain sympathetic Whites present who championed equality and advancement. The idea was to test the notion that decommissioned federal lands (Alcatraz was a federal prison decommissioned in 1964) would revert to Indian land. It is also the case that occupation creates a position of strength. From the position of a court challenge and the physical claim of occupation, American Indians climbed into boats and headed to Alcatraz.

American Indians from across the country came to join forces and lived on the island for 18 months. Alcatraz is now a national park with a plaque documenting the brief history of its occupation by AI/ANs. The event preceded the controversial activism of AIM (American Indian Movement, n.d.) and set the stage for American Indians to be part of the national conversation on civil rights. California tribes and Rancherias have gained federal recognition and energy to reclaim or even "reinvent" place, language, heritage, and culture. Recognition and place have led to a renaissance for the descendants of California Indians. Tribal gaming has fueled growth within California Indian communities, and outsiders have evinced keen interest in learning the story of California Indians. It has enhanced certain capacities for self-determination and preferred coalitions.

California is a youthful, vigorous state where population has exploded and diversity is "the norm." There is no real ethnic majority in the state of California. The many different cultures that occupy the state are also at the forefront of people with mixed race. Immigration into California has been its defining feature throughout the 20th and early 21st centuries. To examine California Indians is to examine a future that many communities and service systems will experience.

HEALTH PICTURE OF CALIFORNIA INDIANS

American Indians in California are a diverse group, and have been so since before the age of exploration and encounter. Diversity of Indian groups accelerated early in mid-20th century California. Migration for military, jobs, and relocation programs illuminated a simmering political activism that marks a California experience and shone a light on American Indians. The phenomenon of population growth from multiple sources creates a large corporate data set (about 800,000 self-identified Indians in the state of California) for health information about California. However, unlike states with dominant tribes, subgroup data by tribal affiliation in California is broken into extremely small denominators because there is so much diversity among American Indians in California. Even though California has the largest number of American Indians among all the states, group data by age or condition must be interpreted with a lens of within-group diversity. Group data by tribal affiliation also gives a picture with very small denominators and a vast array of confounding variables, reflecting the diverse history and experience. Nevertheless, the data are substantial to provide guidance, insight, and direction for informed decision making.

A distinct feature of the health picture of California Indians is the elder nature of this ethnic group, and the accompanying health concerns and health disparities that make for a complex cocktail of health challenges. The California Health Interview Survey reveals a major contrast in aging: only 71.6% of AI/ANs are under age 65, whereas 92% of Latinos are younger than age 65. This gap is stunning. The evidence is even more marked as it significantly exceeds public concern for an aging White population (where 76.3% are under age 65). Chronic conditions and limitations associated with normal aging is a key focus for health planning. The group that might be considered the emerging elderly (that is 55–64 years old) is poised to exacerbate mortality rates and the burden of illness for California Indians in the future. In an article about the health of AI/AN elders in California (Satter, Wallace, Garcia, & Smith, 2010), the authors point to the "crest of a chronic disease epidemic." The largest health disparity between AI/ANs and non-Natives is in this 55-to 64-year-old subgroup, particularly in relation to diabetes (a rate of 26%) and asthma (18%). Further specific risks show the need for coordinated attention in the emerging elderly cohort. Cancer screening rates are seriously low (29% vs. 12% of AI/AN women in this age group have never had a test for cervical cancer, and 29% vs. 16% of AI/ANs have not had colon cancer screening). AI/ANs over age 65 have more accidental falls than any other racial or ethnic group in California (22% vs. 14% for all other races).

Health of the elderly is not simply a sum of health behaviors from the past but ongoing health behaviors that accumulate and complicate disease and injury. Many untoward health behaviors for California Indians are associated with low socioeconomic status and, indeed, Indians typically live below 200% of the federal poverty level. Almost one in five California Indians in the 55 to 64 age group uses tobacco, the highest of any group. To contextualize this further for this cohort, the landmark surgeon general's report on tobacco was released in 1964 when the people in this emerging elderly Indian cohort were young children. They have grown up knowing the risk associated with tobacco use, the social and financial sanctions to discourage it, and experienced universal and local antitobacco messaging. The choice to use tobacco is shaped by many factors. The disparity in this case underscores how distant and nonresponsive California Indians have been, and continue to be, from those types of mass wellness initiatives.

Diabetes and its cascading consequences feature prominently in health disparity data for California Indians as it does for American Indians everywhere. Satter et al. (2010) refers to diabetes as a fellow traveler along with health conditions such as hypertension, heart disease, and stroke. Diabetes is a major contributor to amputations, blindness, and surgical complications. Living with diabetes requires vigilance. Efforts to be vigilant can be compromised by circumstances of low socioeconomic status, circumstances that range from lack of resources to a diminished sense of hope and optimism about the future.

High rates of obesity predispose one to type 2 diabetes and interfere with effective management of the disease. Ethnic groups with a social history of marginalization are plagued by diabetes and its rampant physical damage. For California Indians, the pattern points to a perilous path: the emerging elderly (ages 55–64) have higher rates of obesity than those who are over age 65 with no gender differences (Satter et al., 2010). These contrasting age cohort data may be modulated by the high proportion of California Indians over age 65 as extreme aging leads to greater frailty and weight loss. Nevertheless, some alarm is warranted as the accumulation of physical demands from obesity adds to the overall decline of body function, organs, and joints, and ultimately to physical suffering.

Health services are available to California Indians in many forms. Health care access has been a long-time proxy for understanding health disparities and mechanisms to solve health problems. It is highly warranted and a social obligation not to be shirked. However, access to health services is only part of the picture of health status, and just one element in designing and delivering health care services. By itself, access to health care is not a determinant of health. One of the most remarkable and informative data from the California Health Interview Survey is that AI/ANs are more likely than any other ethnic group in the state, including Whites, to have a usual source of health care. Nevertheless, AI/ANs are also more likely than any other group in the state to delay getting prescription drugs or medical services (UCLA Center for Health Policy, n.d.). The juxtaposition of these two formidable facts is consistent with troubling data on persistent tobacco use, low rates of cancer screening, and rates of preventable disease/complications in the context of access to care. A correlate that is not measured but can be deduced is a degree of suffering from symptoms or disease progression. Of all the duties for health providers, the duty to avoid, diminish, or eliminate suffering is paramount. For nurses, care for suffering is nearly synonymous with the name of the profession. Culturally competent care is a dimension to be examined in ensuring that the American Indians receive the care they need and want.

Culturally competent care for AIs has been promoted for the past 45 years as a powerful mediating variable to improve health and well-being. It is a central element of curricula and continuing education. The capacity to deliver culturally competent care is an ongoing challenge as knowledge and sensitivity are component parts of cultural competence for caregivers. Cultural competence is also relevant at a system level. The interface of people in the health care delivery environment is critical to utilization of health services, compliance with recommendations, and participation in healthy behaviors. Although health care providers have increasingly received training in culturally competent care, the health care delivery environment is far from being patient centered, and therefore begs the question as to whether or not such a system can be culturally competent. The data on availability of and access to health care for California Indians and the data on poor follow-up suggest that the goodness of fit with the system and Indian patients is a major issue.

A patient-focused health care system would necessarily involve cultural competence and understanding of social and community attributes in determining health outcomes. The translation of increasingly sophisticated science and technology into personalized care has been the premier goal of health equity. The past decade has brought new tools and a new language into this arena. There is promise for extending better health care for all with scientific advances. With every advance comes a prospect of side effects. Personalized medicine is an approach that brings high levels of technology and data sophistication to the field of prevention, prediction, and treatment. It is sometimes called "precision medicine." Personalized medicine as a general term suggests greater empathy, patient involvement, and reciprocity in health care services. Although it can and should include those things, the predominant tool in personalized medicine is the application of genomic science. It is not part of a generalized effort for empathy, involvement, and reciprocity. The particular mapping of individual DNA provides more data about individuals, families, and communities. There is dramatic promise in scientific circles about capabilities associated with genetic mapping. In some conditions, such as the field of pharmacogenomics for companion drugs based on genotyping of certain cancers, application of the science yields better clinical decision making and better health outcomes. This is true, for example, for American Indian women with breast cancer. The overall capacities for personalized medicine, however, remain mostly a process with great promise as science is refined.

Personalized medicine using genomic science brings new issues of concern. Genetic testing is a sensitive matter for many people; minorities, more than others, tend to be reluctant to embrace its application wholesale. For American Indians, genomic science has its modern horror story (Jacobs et al., 2010). The Havasupai case is an example of one thing that can go wrong. Tribal elders and tribal leaders are pressured by sophisticated professionals to embrace participation in trials obscured with dense scientific terms. One of the roles that nurses can play is to sort hype and results as well as participation and control (Figure 12.1).

Now, some tribes have resolutions not to participate in genetic studies. Tribal resolutions, however, cannot overrule individual consent to participate. It is also not true that consent is required for various kinds of genetic testing. The history of American Indians and "helpers" has been reviewed here with a wide lens. It is not a history of trust. A history heightens understanding that good intentions on the surface—in person and on paper—can run away with malignant effects on our people. The power of technology, the force of enthusiasm aligned with preliminary results, and even mandates that certain actions be done can be changed with a stroke of the pen when policies, regulations, or laws are changed. The military has long collected genetic samples, which are stored.

National Institutes of Health (NIH)-funded studies, which promise to use genetic samples for only one purpose (cf. Havasupai), actually have access to samples when other rules are made. In January 2015, President Obama, in concert with NIH, mandated the formulation of a national genetic data bank.

	HUGO COUNCIL (1996)	UNESCO (1997)	HGDP (1997)	AIATSIS (2000)	HIS (2001)	AMA (2001)	WHO (2002)	NHMRC (2003)	UNESCO (2003)	NIGMS (2004)	UNESCO (2005)	CIHR (2007)
Community Consultation												
In protocol development			y	y		y	y	y		y	y	y
Before collection of samples	y		y	y	y	y	y	y	y	y		y
Embodies respect for cultural differences	y	y	y	y	y		y	y	y	y	y	y
Formal community approval required			y		y	y	y	y		y		y
Sample collection and informed consent												
Done in a culturally sensitive manner		y	y	y	y		y	y	y	y	y	y
Discussion of a collective harm (e.g. group discr) as part of inform consent process		y	y	y	y		y	y	y	y	y	y
Use and storage of biological materials												
Potential uses defined prior to sample collection				y	y	y	y	y	y	y		y
Provision for withdrawal of samples (IW or CW)		IW, CW	IW, CW			IW	CW	IW, CW	IW	IW, CW	IW	IW, CW
Discussion of secondary uses with contributors (DI or DC)			y	DI			DC		DI	DI,DC		DI,DC
Secondary uses require community approval					y	y	y	y	y	y		y
Prioritization of research uses												
Should benefit contributing population	y	y	y	y	y		y	y	y		y	y
Clear position on commercial applications	y	y	y	y			y				y	y
Post-research obligations												
Ongoing research updates to participating communities	y		y	y		y	y	y	y	y	y	y
Community review of study findings before release			y	y	y		y	y	y	y		y
Need to develop local capacities		y	y						y		y	y

FIGURE 12.1 Guidelines for genomic research with indigenous populations.

Source: Jacobs et al. (2010).

y signifies that the subprinciple is included in the indicated guideline(s).

What is the threat and why is it important? Disease, experimental interventions, and "helping" genetics as a tool for racial ethnic identification are not accepted generally at this time.

POTENTIAL TO CHANGE TRIBAL AFFILIATION

Another issue related to racial ethnic identity that is generally not addressed directly in data analyses is the issue of racial misclassification. This is a matter that is troubling for all ethnic groups because of common sources, and especially for American Indians because of long-standing identity issues around federal relations and blood quantum. Racial identifiers are an issue for all international indigenous people.

Health services for California Indians range across a wide spectrum: private insurance, Medicare, Medicaid, Medicare/Medicaid (note: Medicaid is called MediCal in California), Indian Health Service (IHS), tribal health services, California Indian Health Services, local nonprofits incorporated for Indians living in an area, and specially established programs within large study or demonstration groups (such as the UCLA American Indian Health Center and Native American Research Centers for Health (NARCH) grants in San Diego—explained in the next section).

The vast variety of health service sources moves accessibility closer but can be confusing, even to people in the Indian health care field. It is assumed and communicated that if one does not belong to the local tribe, no health services are available (Satter et al., 2010). This is sometimes true and sometimes not, depending on policy, procedures, and persistence. Because most California Indians are not descendants of California tribes but come from tribes outside of California, this utilization obstacle is one factor in the choice of service, particularly services intended to be culture specific for American Indians. National health reform may improve access for California Indians caught in actual or perceived barriers, although the implementation of the Patient Protection and Affordable Care Act (ACA), although aggressive, has been volatile.

Examples of Health Services in California

Nurses who are seeking out specific tribal experiences in California will find a variety of services to work with. Examples of places with health services are the Hupa Reservation in northern California, and the Morongo Indian Reservation in Riverside County (high desert near Palm Springs; Figure 12.2). Native American Research Centers for Health are funded and administered in collaboration with the Indian Health Service and the National Institutes of Health–National Institute of General Medical Sciences. NARCHes are made up of a cooperative agreement between a tribal body and an academic institution (IHS, 2015). They carry out research projects and mentor students and

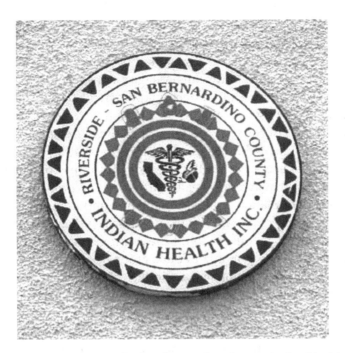

FIGURE 12.2 Riverside–San Bernardino County Indian Health.

other health professionals in the research arena. Nurses interested in nursing research would find this a unique venue. There is one such NARCH of southern California tribes in cooperation with the University of California at San Diego. And in urban areas, there is the California Consortium for Urban Indian Health (2015). They state that their mission is "to facilitate shared development resources for our members and to raise public awareness in order to support a health and wellness network that meets the needs of American Indians living in urban communities."

CONCLUSIONS

A large number of American Indians live in California. In this state, there is no dominant American Indian tribe. The indigenous people of California were relatively small groups dispersed across a vast and highly varied landscape. The early encounter of outsiders and unique history further shapes the story of California Indians. Massive immigration into the state, particularly in the 20th Century, included resettlement of American Indian tribes from across the country to the state. This migration and concentration contributed to California's serving as a focal point for the civil rights of American Indians.

The diversity of tribes and heritage make health care for American Indians in California a topic of special interest. Analyses should be conducted through the context in which they live. Although American Indians are higher in absolute numbers in California than they are in most states, California has 40 million residents, making it the most populous state in the country; therefore, even with a large number of Indians living there, the proportion of American Indians in California is relatively small. It should be noted, however, there is no clear majority of people with European heritage among Californians, and this places California at the forefront of a demographic trend that the rest of the country seems to be following.

Health needs of American Indians (including Alaska Natives) in California have been documented in statewide and regional efforts. There are many different portals of access to health care. Indeed, surveys of American Indians in California show that access to health care is less of a problem for AIs in the state than for other population groups. Of signature importance are data demonstrating that this group of AIs are less likely to use health care services even though they are available, less likely to fill prescriptions, and less likely to engage in preventive behaviors than other ethnic groups. Most significantly, the "emerging elderly" (55–65 years of age) are in the cohort who have been part of mass public health messaging campaigns throughout their lives and still are among the most at risk in their health behaviors. These outcomes are disturbing in terms of two focal interventions: access to health care and health promotion messages. These findings underscore the critical nature of culturally competent care and the need to design culturally competent health care systems that will make access to health care and health promotion effective tools to improve health. Nurses can play a key role in shaping these changes. The findings also suggest that nursing research should probe beyond access to health services and rigorously examine those elements of care that lead to positive health outcomes.

Ethnic/racial classification is a key component of vital health measures: morbidity, mortality, and burden of disease. Misclassification is an ongoing concern in health data and may be a particular problem for California Indians who are not living on or near their tribal lands. Asking the patient or the family to self-identify this information is important during intake, as well as listening and asking respectful questions about traditions that affect health. The need to create culturally competent health systems in a large, complex state offers major challenges and opportunities. There are many tribal-specific, regional, and national health initiatives involving American Indians that take place in California. The most influential research and programs are interdisciplinary and increasingly sophisticated. Emerging science and technologies, such as genomics, present benefits (and possibly new barriers) to the improvement of the health of American Indians in California. Nurses can play an essential role in bridging the critical gaps in health care delivery, health planning, and science. The need to educate more American Indian and Alaska Native nurses at highly skilled levels is imperative. Equity in health care is a common good. California Indians live in a place where change is abundant. By enhancing what we know about culturally competent care, we can bring the best practices to people who need it most, while honoring and preserving the culture and traditions kept alive by resilient American Indians.

STUDY QUESTIONS

♦ How did the indigenous people of California found between San Diego and San Francisco become known as Mission Indians?

♦ What part did the California Gold Rush play in the health of America Indians and Alaska Natives in California?

♦ How did the social and political structures of the original California Indians differ from those in other parts of the nation?

♦ How can understanding the unique California history of indigenous people affect the health provider–patient relationship and, therefore, outcomes? Give an example.

RECOMMENDED READINGS

American Indian Movement. (n.d.). Retrieved from http://www.indians.org/articles/american-indian-movement.html

California Health Interview Survey. (n.d.) Los Angeles, CA: UCLA Center for Health Policy Research. Retrieved from http://healthpolicy.ucla.edu/chis/Pages/default.aspx

Reports of the Surgeon General. (1964). *Surgeon General's Advisory Committee on smoking and health* (Public Health Service Publication No. 1103). Washington DC: Office of the Surgeon General, U.S. Department of Health and Human Services. Retrieved from http://www.surgeongeneral.gov/library/reports/

REFERENCES

California Consortium for Urban Indian Health. (2015). Retrieved from http://ccuih.org/

Gifford, E. W., & Block, G. H. (1930). American Indian myths and legends. In *California Indian nights* (pp. 107–109). Lincoln, NE: University of Nebraska Press.

Indian Claims Commission Act. (n.d.). *National Indian Law Library*. Retrieved from http://www.narf.org/nill/resources/icc.html

Indian Health Service. (2015). *IHS research program—Native American research centers for health (NARCH)*. Retrieved June 25, 2015, from https://www.ihs.gov/Research/index.cfm?module=narch

Indian Reorganization Act, or Howard-Wheeler Act, 48 Stat. 984. (1934, June 18). Retrieved from https://www.iltf.org/resources/land-tenure-history/historical-allotment-legislation/indian-reorganization-act

Jacobs, B., Roffenbender, J., Collmann, J., Cherry, K., Bitsói, L. L., Bassett, K., & Evans, C. H., Jr. (2010). Bridging the divide between genomic science and indigenous peoples. *Journal of Law, Medicine & Ethics, 38*(3), 684–696.

Satter, D. E., Wallace, S. P., Garcia, A. N., & Smith, L. N. (2010). Health of American Indian and Alaska Native elders in California. Retrieved from http://health policy.ucla.edu/publications/Documents/PDF/Health%20of%20American%20 Indian%20and%20Alaska%20Native%20Elders%20in%20California.pdf.

UCLA Center for Health Policy Research. (n.d.). *2011–2012 race and ethnicity health profiles*. Los Angeles, CA: Author.

THIRTEEN

Pacific Northwest/Plateau

C. June Strickland

LEARNING OBJECTIVES

+ Trace the history of American Indians/Alaska Natives in the Pacific Northwest (PNW), discuss the two major cultural groups (Coastal Salish and Plateau people), and outline the strengths of the people
+ Discuss the demographic and geographical data, including the mix of rural tribal reservations, as well as urban AI/AN populations
+ List the top causes of mortality for AI/ANs in the PNW based on epidemiology data, and discuss the priority programs being undertaken to address the major health concerns
+ Describe the structure of health services delivery in the PNW region for American Indian/Alaska Natives, including the major organizations
+ Discuss the role of nursing in addressing the health needs of American Indian/Alaska Natives
+ Integrate information gained in this chapter to address questions posed at the conclusion of this chapter
+ Be acquainted with key resources and websites for additional information on PNW American Indian/Alaska Native health

KEY CONCEPTS:

+ History of Pacific Northwest American Indians
+ Pacific Northwest American Indian data
+ Structures of health services for Pacific Northwest Indians

KEY TERMS

+ Pacific Northwest (PNW)
+ The American Indian Health Commission (AIHC)

The Pacific Northwest region of the United States is a land of snowcapped mountains, coastal rain forests, and high desert plateaus. It is the home of two major American Indian/Alaska Native (AI/AN) groups, the Coastal Salish and the Plateau people. Washington, Oregon, and Idaho are the states that comprise the PNW. In this chapter, the goal is to provide information about the AI/ANs in the PNW, the structure of health services available to them, and their major health concerns. We also consider the role of nursing and nursing services in the region. In all, it is suggested that AI/ANs experience major health disparities in the PNW region. Although the tribal communities are strong and have taken a major leadership role in their health care management, and although many programs have been developed to address health-related concerns, many health disparities persist. Data misclassification makes planning a challenge, and problems with access to services continue to exist for the many people who reside in rural remote communities. The terrain can pose travel challenges, and tribes struggle to recruit and retain health providers. Although the structure of health care and the multiple organizations involved in AI/AN health care in the region provide a major resource to ensure collaboration, the need for creating an infrastructure that links state government priorities to tribes is well recognized. Urban Indian health is a priority concern as well. Although the tribes have made great strides in cultural resurgence, in gaining control of health care, implementing prevention programs, and these efforts are having an impact on health, much additional work is needed. In this chapter, we ask for critical thinking and pose questions that nurses might ask about the contributions nursing can make to address this important area of health disparity. In all, it is suggested that the creation of a sustainable infrastructure that links academic institutions, particularly schools of nursing, with tribes, urban facilities, and regional AI/AN organizations is a vital step in addressing AI/AN health disparities in the PNW.

HISTORY OF AMERICAN INDIANS/ALASKA NATIVES IN THE PACIFIC NORTHWEST REGION OF THE UNITED STATES

The AI/ANs of the PNW, who have been residing in the region for 8,000 to 10,000 years, are thought to have come into the region from Siberia across the Bering Strait, and migrated south into the land that is now the United States (von Aderkas, 2005). The land provided an abundance of food for fishing, hunting, berry picking, root digging, and resources in cedar and plants for clothing and shelter (Ruby & Brown, 1988). Clothing and homes of coastal AI/ANs were made of cedar, as were fishing nets and rope; the Plateau People made homes of mats and clothes of buckskin (Ruby & Brown, 1988). Coastal AI/ANs crafted totem poles and engaged in carving small items and canoes; weaving of cedar–bark baskets was practiced across the region (Ruby & Brown, 1988; von Aderkas, 2005). The Sahaptian and Salishan languages were spoken across the Plateau, and a number of dialects were spoken among the AI/ANs of the coast such as Wakashan and Yahonan (Ruby & Brown, 1988). Jefferson (2001) noted that the Lushootseed language was the primary language of the coastal Indians in the Puget Sound area.

Cultural values were fostered through child-rearing practices reported by early researchers (Haeberlin & Gunter, 1952; Hawthorn, 1965; Lewis, 1970); they noted that the child was taught his or her place in the larger social order. Giving, not hoarding, was a strong value well demonstrated in the potlatch;

values, such as tribal and group orientation, rugged individualism, concern for the land, and honesty and respect for the spoken language, were fostered in parenting (Haeberlin & Gunter, 1952; Hawthorn, 1965; Lewis, 1970). Child-rearing was considered permissive by the early anthropologists writing about the PNW AI/ANs. They noted that the child was greatly valued and expected to be independent at an early age; teaching was done by role model (Haeberlin & Gunter, 1952; Hawthorn, 1965; Lewis, 1970). Spiritual strength was enhanced through traditional practices such as the spirit quest, prayer, dancing, and practice of the religions set forth by prophets such as Smohalla (Ruby & Brown, 1988).

Trade between the coastal and plateau peoples occurred via the Columbia River, which provided fishing and water transportation for the Plateau People; shells, furs, and fish formed part of the traded goods (Ruby & Brown, 1988). Contact with the outside European world began with the arrival of the Spaniards along the Pacific Coast in the 1790s (Ruby & Brown, 1988; von Aderkas, 2005). The Hudson Bay Company brought French fur traders, and Christian and Catholic missionaries brought additional Europeans into the region between 1790 and 1850 (Ruby & Brown, 1988; von Aderkas, 2005).

The 1850s were a time of unrest, war, and struggle with the U.S. government as efforts were made to create reservations and outbreaks of smallpox decimated the AI/AN populations. An ash explosion of Mount St. Helens resulted in prophetic visions seen by Smohalla, a member of the Shahaptian Wanapum tribe, part of the Plateau People, which resulted in the emergence of the Longhouse religion, the Wa'Shat Longhouse (Ruby & Brown, 1988; von Aderkas, 2005), in response to the impact of the cultural influence of non-Indians moving into the region. Chief Leschi (Nisqually) led the Indian wars against the United States with tribes along the coast, and Chief Joseph (Nez Perce) is well known for the wars with the U.S. soldiers on the plateau (Ruby & Brown, 1988; von Aderkas, 2005). Extended families and bands of Indians were combined to create reservations in 1855 (Ruby & Brown, 1988; von Aderkas, 2005). Ruby and Brown (1988) discuss the boarding school for AI/ANs of the PNW, and many elder AI/ANs in the region tell of the creation of the boarding school and attempts to make farmers of the AI/AN. Jefferson (2001) noted the placement of AI/AN children of the PNW into boarding schools. Loss of children to boarding schools as far away as Oklahoma, in the attempt to assimilate the AI/AN peoples, is a part of the pain and posttraumatic stress that PNW AI/ANs still recount (Strickland, Walsh, & Cooper, 2006). Coastal Indian elders tell of Indian people having been incarcerated for practicing winter ceremonies, and thus practices went "underground." In the 1970s, Amoss (1972) reported on the emergence of traditional practices, such as spirit dancing, on the coast.

The paddle to Seattle, led by the Suquamish in 1989, heralds a time of cultural resurgence with the creation of the canoe journey for coastal tribes (Port Gamble S'Klallam Tribe, 2012). Canoe-journey families now travel in groups each summer to tribes along the coast and stop at villages; feasting, gift-giving, and old traditional songs and dances are practiced (Port Gamble S'Klallam Tribe, 2012). On the plateau, the longhouses established by Smohalla remain strong along with winter ceremonies. Many are still fluent in the traditional languages on the plateau, enabling the coastal people in the process of language recovery. Language classes are provided among the tribes across the PNW region today. The current cultural and spiritual resurgence is reflected in the movements in self-determination in the management of health care and economic development. The Plateau People have experienced economic development with the harvesting of natural resources, such as trees, and with leasing of lands for farming using water from the Columbia River for irrigation; apples and peaches from the plateau region supply food for the United States. The coastal AI/AN people have established casinos and reinvested the revenues into further economic development, such as the creation of resort spa hotels and shopping malls; international trade is a part of the economic expansion for tribes in the region. Ruby and Brown (1988) suggested that the greatest war the AI/ANs of the PNW would face for the future would be learning to live with the non-Native peoples. The words of Chief Sealth (Seattle), after whom Seattle was named, reminded the Europeans who came into this land that the spirits of the Indian people would always be on this land as they walked along the silent streets of Seattle (Jefferson, 2001). Indeed, the Indian spirit and people are still culturally strong, committed to cultural values, participating in old ceremonies, singing and dancing in traditional regalia, and providing a role model of commitment to community and family values much needed in the United States today.

DEMOGRAPHIC AND EPIDEMIOLOGY DATA, TRIBES IN THE REGION, URBAN AI/ANS

In a Red Paper Project conference held in Spokane, Washington, in June 2013, Crofoot (2013) presented a paper on PNW Indians of Washington, Oregon, and Idaho. In this presentation, health data were summarized, as well as the challenges and strengths of the people.

Hoopes, Dankovchik, and Kakuska (2012) provided a report developed by the "Improving Data & Enhancing Access (IDEA-NW)" project to describe the most recent mortality data for AI/ANs in the PNW, and to provide a focus on programs that are being or have been undertaken to address some of the major concerns identified. These two reports provide a major thumbnail sketch of the major health data for AI/ANs in the PNW, and lay the foundation for understanding health disparities and steps for further action.

An introductory profile and visual imagery of each state, the AI/AN tribes, and locations of urban centers and census data provide an introduction to the discussion of the health-related data. According to the July 2010 census data, Washington state had 122,649 AI/ANs, Oregon had 66,784, and Idaho 20,034 (U.S. Census Bureau, 2012). Washington state has 29 federally recognized tribes, Oregon nine, and Idaho five. The Seattle Indian Health Board serves 238 tribes; the AI/AN Indian Clinic in Portland serves Natives from 240 tribes; and in the PNW, 38% of the AI/ANs reside in urban settings (Crofoot, 2013).

Maps obtained from websites of states and Indian people in the PNW show that Washington is composed of two major Indian populations (Figures 13.1, 13.2, and 13.3)—the Coastal Salish people of the Pacific Coast and the Plateau

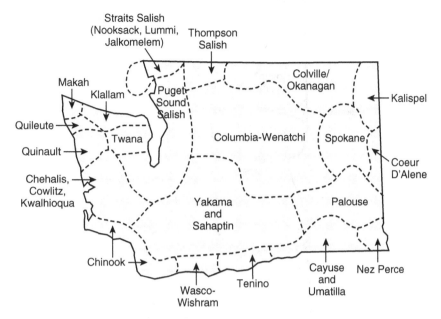

FIGURE 13.1 Map of tribes in Washington state.

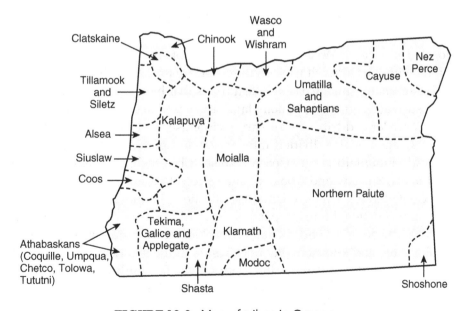

FIGURE 13.2 Map of tribes in Oregon.

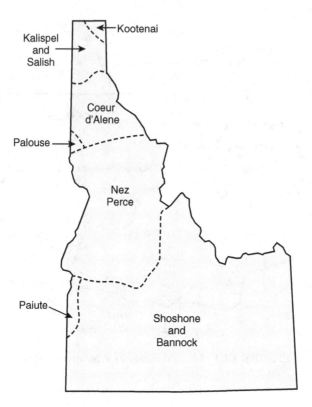

FIGURE 13.3 Map of tribes in Idaho.

People, who reside east of the Cascade mountain range that divides both Washington and Oregon. In Washington state, three large plateau tribes are located in eastern Washington, Colville, Spokane, and Yakama. These tribes, along with the Quinault tribe on the coast, are the largest in the state. Along the coast are many small Coastal Salish tribes that have no more than 1,000 members such as Suquamish, Makah, Jamestown S'Klallam, Port Gamble S'Klallam, the Confederated tribes of Tulalip, Swinomish, and Lummi. Like Washington state, Oregon is also divided into coastal and plateau tribes separated by the Cascade mountain range. Coastal Salish tribes include Clatskanie, Tillamook and Siletz, Siuslaw and Coos, to name a few. Plateau tribes in Oregon include the Confederated Tribes of Umatilla, Shoshoni, Bannock, and Northern Paiute. In Idaho, a national forest separates the northern from the southern part of the state. Flathead and Pend d'Oreille, and Nez Perce reside in the northern part of the state, and Shoshoni–Bannock reside in the southern part of the state. A part of the Northern Paiute tribe resides in the far southwest corner of Idaho as well. The tribes are divided not only by national forests and high snowcapped mountain ranges, but also by language.

The two urban centers are located in Seattle, Washington, and Portland, Oregon, which are east of the Cascade mountain range. Spokane, Yakama, and Wenatchee are medium-size cities of about 150,000 people that have hospitals and health facilities in Washington state and in Oregon. Pendleton is a small city near the "tri-cities" of southern Washington state, where hospitals are located that serve local Indian people; the city of Pendleton also has a small hospital. Northern Idaho Indian people are served by health facilities in Spokane, Washington, and in southern Idaho, the city of Boise provides hospital facilities for the region. As may be noted, the nearest large cities, which provide specialty care, diagnostic services, and trauma facilities, are located as far as 150 to 200 miles from some of the tribal reservations. Inclement weather affects access to care. In the winter months, the plateau and mountains often receive large snow accumulations, and sudden shifts in temperature result in avalanches, which often make travel through the passes impossible for several days at a time. Except for air transport provided by some of the Seattle and Portland hospitals in emergencies, travel to the major hospitals can be problematic in the winter months, which affects access to care for serious health conditions.

In considering the Indian health data for the PNW, we will first focus on the leading causes of death and the related details, which provide greater understanding of prevention that may be needed. In this respect, attention will be devoted to cancer, diabetes, unintentional injury and suicide, mental health concerns, substance abuse, and emerging issues. Although oral health and maternal child health issues are of priority for the AIHC in Washington state, attention will be directed to the overall regional concerns and state comparisons.

Indian health data for Washington, Oregon, and Idaho for 2006 through 2009, as reported by Hoopes et al. (2012), indicate that the major causes of death among AI/ANs in the PNW region were heart disease and cancer. Heart disease, the leading cause of death, was reported at 23.3%, compared with 30.1% for Whites. Cancer was listed as 19.1% for AI/ANs as compared with 23.8% for Whites. Unintentional injury and diabetes were ranked third and fourth as causes of death among AI/ANs in the PNW, suicide ranked seventh, and Alzheimer's disease ranked eighth.

The mean age for deaths among AI/ANs in Washington state was 59.4 years compared with 74.3 for Whites, 58.2 compared with 73.3 for Whites in Idaho, and 62.2 for AI/ANs compared with 75.3 for Whites. From these data, it may be noted that life expectancy for AI/ANs is considerably behind that of Whites in the region but has increased over the past 10 years (Hoopes et al., 2012).

Cancer is the second leading cause of death for AI/ANs in the PNW. AI/ANs tend to be diagnosed at a later stage than Whites (Northwest Portland Area Indian Health Board [NPAIHB], 2011). In the PNW, breast cancer represents over one in four cancers diagnosed (27.6%), lung cancer in AI/AN females is higher than for White females, and lung cancer in AI/AN males is slightly higher than in White males (NPAIHB, 2011). Prostate cancer in AI/AN males is lower than in White males. The NPAIHB (2011) reports that AI/ANs are less likely to be screened for cancer than other populations, that 38% of active Indian Health Service (IHS) patients are screened for colorectal cancer, that 40% of women have documented mammograms, and that 56% have been screened for cervical cancer.

In further examination of deaths resulting from unintentional injuries, Hoopes et al. (2012) note that men have higher rates of unintentional injuries in all three states; in Idaho, twice as many men died as women. Motor vehicle crashes accounted for a high percentage of these deaths, followed by accidental poisoning, falls, and accidental drowning. Deaths in motor vehicle crashes were higher among AI/ANs than among Whites in the region, and were associated with substance abuse such as alcohol. Washington state had the highest rates of unintentional injury deaths, followed by Idaho and Oregon. AI/ANs in Washington state also had the highest disparity when compared with White populations in Washington State. AI/ANs had a rate of 95.9 per 100,000 compared with 40.3 per 100,000 for Whites from 2006 to 2009. Motor vehicle crashes were the largest cause of unintentional deaths among AI/ANs in all three states, and were an average of 2.5 times higher than among Whites. Contributing factors noted were rural roads, distances from hospitals, time spent in cars, and substance abuse. Drug overdose related to suicide attempts was the second cause of death due to intentional injuries (Hoopes et al., 2012).

Hoopes, Dankovchik, and Kakuska further noted that there was no significant difference between AI/ANs and Whites in deaths caused by falls between 2006 and 2009; the rates among AI/ANs were only marginally higher than among Whites, and men were at a slightly higher risk. The rates of deaths resulting from falls in AI/ANs rose dramatically higher for those older than 70 years. Deaths caused by suicide accounted for about one fifth of all AI/AN injury deaths, and Idaho had the highest rate at 27 per 100,000. Oregon had the lowest rate at 16 per 100,000. The Washington state rate was 22.5 per 100,000 between 2006 and 2009. The rates for AI/ANs were 60% to 70% higher than for Whites in Washington and Oregon. Males were more likely to die than females largely because of the use of guns; in Idaho, the rates for males were four times as high as those for females. The majority of suicides occurred in AI/AN young adults ages 20 to 39 years. Roughly one half of AI/AN suicides were committed using firearms, whereas hanging ranked second as the means of death. A trend analysis of data between 1990 and 2009 showed that suicide rates in Washington state have been stable over the past 20 years (Hoopes et al., 2012).

Substance abuse remains a significant health concern. AI/ANs tend to start drinking early. Binge drinking among AI/ANs in Seattle was reported at 23.7%, 21.3% in Portland, and 26.8% in Spokane, which is considerably higher than that in the general population; increases in the use of amphetamines and prescription opiates were also reported among AI/ANs. It has been noted that AI/ANs are 58% more likely to experience serious mental health problems but are less likely to seek treatment. Depression, anxiety, posttraumatic experiences, and substance abuse are the major reported mental health concerns (Crofoot, 2013).

Crofoot (2013) further noted that mortality rates for diabetes are three times higher for AI/ANs as for the White population. The federal Indian Health Service Special Diabetes Program has had a major impact on diabetes in the PNW. Between 2007 and 2011, it was noted that there was a 6.8% increase in the proportion of patients with hemoglobin A1c (HbA1c) levels below 7.0, and a 19.5% decrease in the proportion of patients with HbA1cs over 9.5 (Urban Indian Health Institute, 2011).

In Washington state, the American Indian Health Commission (2010) noted the following health priorities: (a) maternal/infant health, (b) tobacco and other substance abuse, (c) domestic violence, and (d) women's health screening and cancer. Other health issues noted include the need for long-term care, oral health, diabetes, and mental health.

In summary, heart disease, cancer, unintentional injury, diabetes, and mental health concerns, such as suicide, rank high in priority areas of need and health disparities for AI/ANs in the PNW. Alzheimer's disease and falls are becoming a concern as AI/AN life expectancy increases. Programs and steps being taken to address some of these concerns across the life span will be considered further in this chapter.

PACIFIC NORTHWEST AMERICAN INDIAN HEALTH SERVICE DELIVERY/STRUCTURE OF HEALTH CARE

The NPAIHB (2013) estimates that over 104,000 Indian people in the PNW receive primary health care from Indian health programs. A major feature of the Indian Health Service structure in the PNW is that 74% of the management and control lies with the tribes in the region through either contracting or compacting under Title I (PL-638) of the Indian Self-Determination and Education Assistance Act of 1975, Title III, and Title V (AIHC, 2010; IHS, 2014; NPAIHB, 2013). The Indian Health Service operates six health facilities under PL-638. Two urban clinics located in Seattle and Portland—Seattle Indian Health Board and the Native American Rehabilitation Association of the Northwest, Inc.—serve the needs of urban Indians living in the region. There are no Indian Health Service hospitals (AIHC, 2010; IHS, 2014). In this discussion, we trace the laws that have contributed to the system/structure of health services delivery in the PNW, and recognize the contributions of some of the major decision-making bodies in Indian health in the region—the Northwest Portland Area Indian Health Board, the Indian Health Service, and the American Indian Health Commission for Washington State. Future concerns, initiatives, and suggestions for addressing health disparities in the region will also be included in this discussion.

Tribes provide an array of patient care, community health services as well as prevention and promotion programs either through tribal family health clinics, or by providing a form of insurance. Mental health services, drug and alcohol treatment facilities, and health counseling are also provided. Individuals and families requiring inpatient hospitalization care are referred to urban center hospitals such as Children's Hospital in Seattle; trauma victims are airlifted to urban trauma centers such as Harborview Medical Center in Seattle. The Southwest Oncology Group (SWOG) supports cancer treatment and research in both Portland and Seattle, and is linked to rural hospitals in the region. Many of the tribes provide their own family practice clinics and refer patients out to private provider specialists for prenatal and specialty care such as oncology. State public health and local health departments collaborate with tribes; some provide health provider consultants and offer programs that can be implemented in the tribal communities. The Centers for Disease Control and Prevention (CDC) funding has been provided for breast and cervical cancer education and screening. Emergency services are also provided by most tribes, and tribal personnel are trained in cardiopulmonary resuscitation (AIHC, 2010).

Within the tribes, clinics—for those providing clinic services—are staffed with an array of providers, including family practice physicians, nurse practitioners, baccalaureate and master's prepared nurses (providing direct patient care), and community health nurses (who provide home visits and health-promotion programs), social workers, dentists, pharmacists, health administrators, community health representatives (CHRs), and emergency medical technicians (EMTs). Some include alternative medicine practitioners such as acupuncture and massage therapists. For the most part, traditional healers work parallel to the Western medicine services, but the Seattle Indian Health Board employs a traditional healer/cultural specialist. The CHR program, established in 1975, has been of great value to Indian health in the PNW in that the Indian Health Service provided centralized training in the early years, and envisioned their role as one of patient advocacy/patient education, as well as offering transportation services. The NPAIHB continues to provide training for CHRs and other staff through regional conferences and the development of resources. One such example is the development of Cancer 101, a training program developed for CHRs to enhance their understanding of cancer prevention and treatment. This education program—which emerged from one of the rural tribal communities of Washington state CHRs—was further developed through a partnership involving the NPAIHB and the Fred Hutchinson Cancer Research Center, Cancer Information Service, and the Spirit of Eagles Community Networks Project. The program has been disseminated to tribal communities throughout the United States. Some clinics also provide pharmacy services. As with any rural clinic service, recruiting and retaining staff is a challenge for some. Most clinics are in the process of transitioning to computerized record systems to enhance data tracking and program planning. Patients are referred to outside specialty physicians for specialty services such as prenatal care and cancer diagnostic evaluation and treatment.

Urban Indian health is of major concern. AIHC (2010) noted that since 1990, over half of AI/ANs reside in urban settings. Urban Indians are a diverse population and have poorer health status compared with other Indians. Urban Indian programs were established under Title V in 1976 under PL 94-437 (AIHC, 2010); the majority of services provided are medical/dental and referral/other services such as alcohol and substance abuse. Services are provided on a "sliding scale" payment arrangement. Of particular concern for this population are changes needed in the Medicaid program.

DeJong (2011) traces the history of Indian health and federal laws that now support self-determination, and the AIHC (2010) further details the history as it relates to the PNW. DeJong noted that the initial legislation in Indian health was set forth in the Snyder Act of 1921, and as early as 1968, President Johnson issued a call for Indian self-determination. Two years later, Nixon also pledged support for self-determination by encouraging Congress to enact legislation with the Indian Health Transfer Act. President Ford signed into law the Indian Self-Determination and Education Assistance Act (PL-638) in 1975, which provided for greater tribal involvement in programs and in selection of health providers. The Indian Health Care Improvement Act of 1976 (PL 94-437) authorized health programs based on a community health model, and directed funding for these programs (AIHC, 2010). In the 1980s, PL 100-472 further enhanced tribal rights to control, plan, and administer health programs.

The AIHC (2010) outlined the history of laws that have influenced health service delivery in the PNW. They also note that the federal government's obligation to ensure health care for AI/ANs was set forth in the enactment of a series of federal laws, beginning with the Snyder Act of 1921. The Indian Self-Determination and Education Assistance Act of 1975 (PL-638) provided for the turnover of development for Indian health programs through contracts to tribes. The Indian Health Care Improvement Act of 1976 (PL94-437) provided support for tribal control of health programs based on a community health model. Titles I, III, and V support compacting and contracting to ensure tribal control and full responsibility for health programs. Twenty-three tribes have Title V compacts in the PNW, and 24 contracts under Title I, PL-638. The AIHC outlined three major initiatives for Washington state (2010–2013; AIHC, 2010):

1. The Commissions noted that state, tribal, and urban Indian health collaboration has been instituted at a state/tribal leader policy level to address system and policy change, and that it is necessary to align the statewide Indian health disparities efforts with the governor's five-point health care initiative for Washington state to create the infrastructure to address Indian health disparities.
2. Collaboration among agencies in the state related to American Indian health needs to be fostered.
3. Further collaboration to ensure a partnership among Washington state, tribes, and AIHC to address access to services, increased tribal provider reimbursement, and more culturally appropriate services with mechanism for evaluation needs to be developed.
4. The governor's five-point priorities for Washington state include the following: (a) evidence-based health care, (b) prevention and healthy lifestyle choices, (c) better management of chronic illness, (d) transparency in health care systems, and (e) better use of information technology.

The NPAIHB (2013) noted that since the 1920s, death rates for Indian people from infectious diseases and gastrointestinal illness have greatly decreased. In the PNW, deaths from sudden infant death syndrome have also declined significantly. Preventive programs being offered have contributed to improvements in diabetes, HIV/AIDS, cancer, and tobacco use. However, much more health improvement is needed. In outlining their 2013 legislative and regulatory priorities, the Board highlights continuing concerns. They note federal government financial issues/reductions and emphasize the moral and legal responsibilities of the federal government to ensure funding for Indian health. Because of the underfunding and the health disparities recognized for Indian people, the NPAIHB (2013) recommended that the Indian Health Service should be exempt from budget reductions. The document "Northwest Portland Area Indian Health Board 2013 Legislative and Regulatory Priorities" (NPAIHB, 2013) provides details of future recommendations for Indian health, particularly as it relates to the PNW region.

The AIHC (2010) suggested the following actions to reduce AI/AN health disparities in the PNW: (a) tribally driven assessments to determine priorities for health care services, (b) engagement of tribal communities in addressing specific disparities for the community, (c) data improvement, (d) advocacy in the system and policy arena to impact state decision making, and (e) evaluation: developing indicators and tracking systems related to social and environmental determinants of health.

In summary, the PNW has made tremendous strides in Indian health and self-determination toward the provision of health services delivery. The words of the tribal chairman of the Port Gamble S'Klallam Tribe, Jerome Sullivan, well reflect the perspectives on health care management of the AI/ANs of the PNW:

> I am proud of the strides the Port Gamble S'Klallam tribe has made over the past twenty years since we began to take over the sovereign responsibilities inherent in self-determination. Our community members are stronger, healthier, and self-sufficient. In 150 years under BIA, we could only count two college graduates in our Tribe of 1,000 men, women, and children. Today, twenty years later, we can count more than 30 bachelor degrees, two master's degrees and one law degree. We have truly "pulled ourselves up by the bootstraps" and have repeatedly shown that by Tribes running federal programs more efficiently and responsibly, great things accrue to Tribal members and families. (Port Gamble S'Klallam Tribe, 2012, p. 246)

The Northwest Portland Area Indian Health Board, Indian Health Service, and the American Indian Health Commission for Washington State are three major organizations that have emerged to support the Indian's voice in decision making in the region. Although much has been accomplished in treatment and prevention, much is still needed. It is recognized that data are greatly needed for planning; in the era of advanced technology, Indian communities will need to move forward by adopting advanced technologies. Prevention programs to address healthy lifestyle promotion and urban Indian health are but a few of the areas of concern in order to address Indian health disparities.

NURSING IN AI/AN HEALTH IN THE PACIFIC NORTHWEST

It is well recognized that there is a shortage of nurses serving AI/AN populations; recruitment is a challenge, and turnover rates are high (Fisher, Pearce,
Stanz, & Wood, 2003; Keltner, Kelly, & Smith, 2004). Although some information
points to administrative issues, lower salaries and benefits, and lack of respect as
contributors to the retention matter, limited information is available on the actual
number of nurses working in Indian health, and of those how many are Native
(Aiken, Clarke, Sloan, Sochalski, & Silber, 2002; Katz, O'Neal, Strickland, &
Doutrich, 2010). In this section, we consider the number of nurses serving in
Indian health in the PNW region, the kinds of work performed and programs
being administered, as well as education and research being undertaken by
nurses. It is suggested that nursing is making strides in partnering with tribes
and AI/AN organizations in the PNW to address the major health concerns,
as well as addressing the educational need for nurses to be well prepared in
Indian health. Some are contributing to the advancement in transcultural nursing science through research with AI/AN communities, providing outstanding
recruitment, retention, and education models, as well as much needed tribal
capacity-building models in grant writing through national training. Even so,
the shortage of nurses persists, and rural tribal communities continue to struggle
with recruitment and retention of nurses. In the spirit of tribal sovereignty and
tribal control of health evident in the PNW, some tribes are collaborating with
one other to address data management and are taking steps within the tribes to
build their workforce from within. By investing revenues gained in economic
development into education for tribal members, enhancing tribal capacity to
obtain their own health funding, and enhancing the relationships with state
government, tribes are positioning themselves to continue the efforts in eliminating Indian health disparities in the PNW. Nursing has an important role to
play in supporting tribal capacity building in health-related service delivery,
prevention/health-promotion program planning, and policy development.

In the PNW, there are 29 federally recognized tribes in Washington, nine federally recognized tribes in Oregon, and five federally recognized tribes in Idaho
(Crofoot, 2013). Health services are provided in health centers, health stations,
preventive health programs, and urban facilities (Portland Area Indian Health
Service, 2014). The Portland Area Indian Health Service operates six federal
health facilities in five tribes and the Chemawa Indian School in the region;
23 tribes operate under Title V compacts, and 24 operate under Title I contracts
(Portland Area Indian Health Service, 2014). In addition, there are two major
urban clinics serving Indian people; one is located in Portland, Oregon—
Native American Rehabilitation Association of the Northwest, Inc., and the
other in Seattle, Washington—Seattle Indian Health Board. Nurses work with
patients in the provision of direct patient care in clinics, administration of
community health nursing services, special health prevention and promotion programs, patient navigation, mental health services, school nurses in
early childhood learning centers, prenatal/postpartum programs, and social

services, to name a few. Some AI/AN nurses also work in nursing higher education recruitment and education. It is estimated that there are three to four nurses per federal tribe working in the rural tribal sector, perhaps five to seven in each urban clinic setting, and three to four in higher education, making a total of 150 and 200 nurses working in Indian health in the PNW. Of these, Katz et al. (2010) noted approximately 13% employed in the Indian Health Service, and six federally operated clinics have Native nurses. Educational preparation ranges from licensed practical nurse (LPN), associate-degree registered nurse (ADN), to baccalaureate of nursing (BSN) and graduate degrees such as the master's in nursing, doctor of nursing practice (DNP), and doctor of philosophy (PhD).

Washington State University (WSU), located in the plateau region of eastern Washington state, provides the major preparation of Indian nurses in the region (Shelton, 2008). The Native American Recruitment and Retention Program (NARR) at Washington State University Intercollegiate College of Nursing was created in 1995. The Intercollegiate College of Nursing is comprised of WSU, Eastern Washington University, and Whitman College. Eastern Washington has a number of community colleges offering nursing education from the LPN to the associate degree. This structure supports an articulation to WSU, Eastern Washington, and Whitman in which students may enter at the LPN level in their home community and advance to graduate degrees with minimal travel from their homes. As noted in a study conducted by Katz et al. (2014), although a high percentage of the Indian nurses obtaining degrees are committed to serving their home communities and often do serve in their home communities for a while, retention is a challenge. Reasons given for leaving are similar to findings from other research (Aiken et al., 2002).

As may be noted, approximately 74% of health services and programs are controlled by the tribes in the region (Portland Area Indian Health Service, 2014); the rural tribal communities thus face the same challenges as other rural clinics in recruiting and retaining well-qualified health professionals. The University of Washington School of Nursing provides the only clinical rotation experience for students to prepare them to work with tribes with American Indian faculty supervisions (Strickland, Logsdon, Hoffman, & Garrett-Hill, 2014). Both undergraduate and graduate students in community health are provided experience in two rural coastal tribal communities. Students support the tribes in community health programming in prevention and health promotion. Utilizing a framework of community engagement and program planning (Ervine, 2002), approximately 20 undergraduates experience a 4-credit clinical rotation each year provided over two quarters. They are in the field working with the tribes for 1 full day each week for 10 weeks each quarter. Master of nursing (MN) and DNP students complete three to five quarters of clinical experience for a total of 17 credits in the two tribal communities. The MN students complete a thesis or project for another six credits with the tribes, and the DNP students complete a capstone translational science research project (12 credits). Thus, the graduate students are in the field working with the tribes for 2 to 3 years per student, and provide continuity in program development. The community health nursing administrator for one of the tribes obtained a DNP in community health from the University of Washington School of Nursing; she and two Native nursing tribal members serve as field mentors for both graduate and undergraduate students. Under the research and clinical supervision of one tenured Native nursing faculty member at the University of Washington School of Nursing, undergraduates participate in research, and graduate students conduct their own research/projects. These two tribes have been undergoing cultural resurgence; the design of health-prevention programs reflects these transitions.

Health programming has been designed to build on cultural values and strengths. To address some of the major health concerns among AI/ANs in the region and in their tribal communities, emphasis has been placed on return to traditional foods; healthy food purchases; enhancement of physical activity across the life span; and the design of culturally appropriate recruitment, retention, and evaluation approaches. Intervention work is aimed at influencing individual, family, and community health behaviors, as well as the design of appropriate systems and policy change. The following are examples of MN and DNP capstone projects completed by University of Washington nursing graduate students in these two tribal clinical sites: (a) development of a culturally appropriate approach to evaluation of an Indian Health Service physical activity program designed to encourage parents to engage their children to exercise more, (b) development of culturally appropriate recruitment and retention strategies for an elder exercise program based on research evidence and tribal team perspectives, (c) development of policies to address tribal purchasing of food for tribal events, and (d) provision of a comprehensive literature review on breast cancer screening education and diabetes education programming.

In addition to working with these two tribes, some community health DNP students at the University of Washington have worked with organizations in Washington state, such as the AIHC and other local tribes, to develop policy recommendations related to maternal child health; one DNP student developed a policy recommendation along with provider training and patient education recommendations related to breast cancer survivorship. Three faculty at the University of Washington have also partnered with tribes to conduct research and build tribal capacity in research and grant preparation. Research has been conducted in women's health screening (Strickland, Chrisman, Yallup, Powell, & Squeoch, 1996; Strickland & Hillaire, 2014), suicide prevention (Strickland & Cooper, 2011; Strickland, Walsh, & Cooper, 2006), and pain conceptualization (Strickland, 2001); a proposal is under review for funding to address caregiving for elders with dementia. The National Institute of Nursing Research (NINR) funded an RC4 grant to Drs. Strickland and Logsdon to develop and provide training for tribes to conduct translational research, which is now being disseminated through the Association of American Indian Physicians, funded through the CDC. This NINR funding also supported the creation of an infrastructure and sustainable partnership between the two tribes and the University of Washington School of Nursing by providing faculty positions for a number of tribal employees and providing mentorship for students (Strickland et al., 2014).

Although the nursing profession has been working in partnerships to address many of the major AI/AN health concerns in the PNW region through the provision of direct patient care services, community health-prevention and health-promotion efforts and research, additional work is still needed. Although both the WSU Intercollegiate Nursing Program and the University of Washington School of Nursing have increased the numbers of nurses prepared to work with tribes in the region, have partnered with tribes to build tribal capacity, and have addressed health prevention and promotion of community health programs, it is recognized that only a small percentage of the current graduating nurses either go to or remain at work with tribes. Creation of sustainable infrastructure/partnerships between academic institutions/regional nursing schools and tribes/tribal organizations addressing health issues are an important step in addressing the disparities in Indian health in the PNW region. Some tribes in the region are investing in supporting nursing education for their own tribal members and establishing systems and structures to address retention. Supporting tribes in health-related research, education programming, health services delivery, and capacity building aligns with the spirit of self-determination evident among AI/AN peoples of the PNW. Figure 13.4 is a photograph of University of Washington undergraduate students serving in a clinical rotation in one tribe, and nurses working in another, Coastal Salish tribe, some of whom are tribal members.

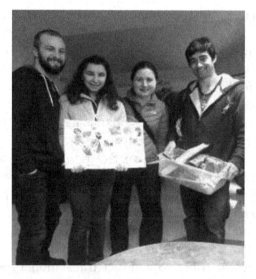

FIGURE 13.4 University of Washington student nurses in clinical rotation in a coastal tribe (*left to right*: Nate Dreesmann, Eugenyia Dokukina, Miriam Mach, Andrew Najjar).

PATIENT POPULATION CONSIDERATIONS

In addressing patient and population considerations for AI/ANs in the PNW, the focus here is on specific information that deserves scrutiny for nursing practice, especially as it relates to the design of interventions to influence health at the individual and family/community population/systems levels, and the recognition of programs that are currently being implemented. Although many health concerns have been noted for the PNW region, it is important to recognize that the AI/ANs of the PNW are culturally and spiritually strong; there is a cultural resurgence on the coast that is providing strength for the promotion of healthy lifestyles. This section is divided into cultural, spiritual, physical and mental health, and health concerns across the life span.

Culture

Strickland and colleagues (Strickland, 1999; Strickland & Hillaire, 2014; Strickland, Squoech, & Chrisman, 1999) conducted a number of studies to illustrate the importance of understanding cultural values and patterns of communication in community health nursing. In one study conducted among the Yakama people, Strickland et al. (1999) noted that although many have considered the Church as an avenue of influence in changing health behavior, the Wa'Shat Longhouse is of more value in understanding the influence of health behaviors and structures for influence. In this respect, she noted that among the Yakama people, large families are grouped along matrilineal lines, and thus the elder women of these families may be expected to be one of the best avenues of influence and the family structure for dissemination of health-related messages. Strickland et al. (1999) also noted that the talking circle pattern of communication and the arrangement of the chairs in a circle are more congruent with cultural practices and patterns of communication. Understanding patterns of communication in a group is further illustrated in Strickland (1999) as it relates to community assessment and conducting the focus group. In a recent contribution, Strickland and Hillaire (2014) outline an intervention protocol and describe the transcultural translation of evidence-based research. Each phase of the research intervention and the underlying theory are translated in this contribution. In the education intervention of this research, designed to influence women's health screening for breast and cervical cancer, the women are asked to make a commitment to the behavior change. Through focus group work in the community, it was determined that the women needed to make the commitment verbally and not in writing, as was designed in the western intervention model, and that the commitment needed to be made to the grandmothers, aunts, and community to take care of themselves for the community. This is a very different orientation than health messages often use in the Western mainstream population, which emphasizes taking care of yourself for yourself. It illustrates the value orientation to the family and tribe.

It is important to recognize that the coastal tribes are experiencing a cultural resurgence, with the return of the canoe journey beginning with the paddle to

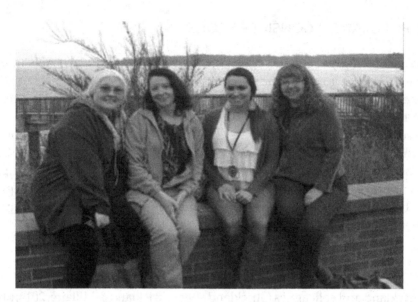

FIGURE 13.5 Nurses serving in one coastal tribe (*left to right:* C. June Strickland, associate professor University of Washington School of Nursing, Echota Cherokee; Kathy Kinsey, coastal tribal health nurse, tribal member; Renee Hummel, coastal tribal health nurse, tribal member; Barbara Hoffman, coastal tribal health nurse).

Seattle in 1989; the building of longhouses; winter dance; and naming ceremonies (Port Gamble S'Klallam Tribe, 2012). This resurgence of cultural values is also promoting family values and teamwork. To participate in the canoe journey, family members work together and participants must be alcohol and drug free. Figure 13.5 is of Dr. June Strickland, a professor in the University of Washington School of Nursing, who supervises students who have clinical rotations in the Suquamish and Port Gamble S'Klallam tribes, and three nurses employed in the Suquamish tribe.

In these examples, taken from research on tribes in the PNW, it can be seen that it is crucial to understand the cultural norms, patterns of communication, and values. Prevention of stereotyping is important. In the PNW, there is a wide range of acculturation, especially among the coastal people who intermarried with the non-Indian population early in their history. Aligning with a mentor of your gender in the community is an important step to take in gaining an understanding of culturally appropriate approaches. Note the information in the introduction to this chapter on the history of the AI/ANs of the PNW and the resources section, which contains books that provide more detail about the culture of the AI/ANs of the PNW.

Spiritual

With the arrival of the Europeans, many of the traditional ceremonies were outlawed. Even today, details of spirituality and traditional practices are greatly protected, and it is not appropriate to write about them or record information in the PNW. Both Protestant and Catholic missionaries moved into the PNW region between 1790 and 1850, and created churches and missions. Thus, both Christian religions, Protestantism and Catholicism, are practiced among the people. The Indian Shaker Church also has members among many coastal tribes (Port Gamble S'Klallam, 2012). On the plateau, the traditional religion is the Wa'Shat Longhouse (Ruby & Brown, 1988), and as with the coastal tribes, some AI/ANs are members of Protestant and Catholic churches. Sweating, spirit quests, prayers, and dancing are part of the spiritual practice of the AI/ANs in the PNW (Ruby & Brown, 1988). As was noted earlier, there has been a cultural resurgence; traditional ceremonies are being practiced along the coast, and longhouses and totems rebuilt (Port Gamble S'Klallam Tribe, 2012).

Physical Health

The major physical health concerns of AI/ANs of the PNW, as noted in the consideration of epidemiology data, are heart disease, cancer, and diabetes. Many tribes are working upstream in addressing these health matters with diet and physical activity programs.

Racial misclassification has been of concern in cancer prevention work (Hoopes, Petersen, & Vinson, 2012). Crofoot (2013) noted that greater collaboration among agencies and increased efforts have improved data-tracking systems. Targeted and culturally appropriate education programs have also had an impact in increasing breast and cervical cancer screenings. Crofoot also noted an increase in AI/AN participation in the state of Washington's breast and cervical cancer early detection programs, and increased training for providers on the latest screening and practices. Smoking rates among AI/ANs in the PNW continue to be high, contributing to cancer mortality. Efforts to prevent smoking and cancer-screening initiatives are being undertaken. "Stop smoking" campaigns provided in the THRIVE (Tribal Health: Reaching Out Involves Everyone) project and tribal efforts to enact policies related to smoking in tribal facilities are but a few of the ongoing efforts aimed at reducing smoking.

The NPAIHB Northwest Tribal Cancer Navigator Program is designed to link patients with cancer to needed services, and the Native Wellness Program of the South Puget Sound Intertribal Planning Agency (SPIPA), which provides no-cost mammograms, clinical breast exams, Pap smear tests, and cervical exams, are examples of efforts underway in the PNW region to address cancer for AI/ANs; lab indicators are greatly improving, and comorbidities are being reduced for diabetes (Crofoot, 2013). The implementation of the federal Indian Health Service Special Diabetes Program for Indians (SDPI) in tribes, urban health clinics, and the provision of coordinated diabetes screening have been recognized as having made a major contribution in diabetes and comorbidity management (Crofoot, 2013).

Mental Health

As reflected by the mental health data, substance abuse and depression are the major mental health issues pf this AI/AN population. Substance abuse is linked to high mortality related to motor vehicle crashes and suicide. Tribes in the PNW offer mental health services, including substance abuse programs. A project of the NPAIHB, THRIVE, is underway in the PNW (Hoopes et al., 2012). The NPAIHB held a regional meeting to develop a 5-year plan that is now being used to guide program planning in tribes. This project is intended to support community outreach efforts and foster a coordinated response to substance abuse. As a part of this effort, a national media campaign was developed to focus on alcohol and substance abuse among AI/AN teens and young adults (Hoopes et al., 2012). All of the campaign materials are available on the NPAIHB website. The NPAIHB is working with tribes in the PNW to address suicide as well. The THRIVE project has provided training and technical assistance to tribes in the PNW on suicide prevention. As with the substance abuse campaign, a suicide prevention campaign was also developed and has expanded to include issues related to bullying; both campaigns were funded by the Indian Health Service. Other examples of programs to address mental health are as follows: (a) Native American Youth and Family Center and the Regional Research Institute (RRI) at Portland State University, which documents culturally appropriate services; (b) NARA Northwest provides a suicide prevention program, Life Is Sacred; (c) Yakama Nation Listen Together is a youth program that addresses mental health for youth; (d) and the Confederated Tribes of Umatilla Indians (CTUIR) Yellow Hawk Clinic, which provides a suicide prevention program, Circle of Care mental health program for children, and intensive outpatient counseling (Crofoot, 2013).

Health Concerns Across the Life Span

Across the life span, the concern for infants has been sudden infant death syndrome (SIDS), but this is decreasing (Hoopes et al., 2012). Substance abuse (such as smoking among youth) and injury through motor vehicle crashes (which are often alcohol and drug related) are the major concerns for young adults. For AI/ANs ages 20 to 39 years, substance abuse and mental health issues, such as suicide and depression, are of major concern. Chronic illnesses, such as diabetes and cancer, contribute to high morbidity and health disparities for older AI/ANs. Alzheimer's disease and falls are becoming a concern for older AI/ANs as the life expectancy increases. Tribes have begun work in fall-prevention education, and some Alzheimer education is being provided (Hoopes et al., 2012).

We have focused on the health concerns for AI/ANs in the PNW, actions being taken to address them, and the cultural/spiritual considerations that provide depth to the understanding. Overall, it is recognized that there are many health disparities among AI/ANs in the PNW. There are also many agencies invested in addressing these concerns, and in the spirit of tribal self-determination, the tribes have taken a major lead in collaborating with academic institutions and federal and state agencies to address the issues. The tribes are culturally and spiritually strong, and growing in their ability to address major health concerns.

CONCLUSIONS

We traced the history of the PNW AI/ANs and noted the physical environment, demographics, and epidemiology data of this population. In the PNW, there are 29 federally recognized tribes in Washington State, nine in Oregon, and five in Idaho. It has been noted that the major health concerns/causes of mortality are heart disease, cancer, diabetes, unintentional injury (motor vehicle crashes), substance abuse, suicide, and depression. In the spirit of tribal sovereignty and self-determination, 74% of health programs and services are managed and controlled by tribes. The tribes are culturally and spiritually strong, and have experienced a resurgence of culture along the coast with the return of the canoe journey. Health services in tribes are provided in rural health clinics, or through a form of insurance in which care is provided by local providers. Two urban clinics, located in Portland, Oregon, and Seattle, Washington, serve the needs of urban Indians in the region. Hospitals in Portland and Seattle also serve the needs for specialty care, trauma services, and diagnostic evaluations not available in the rural settings and tribal clinics. Major agencies collaborating to address these concerns include the Indian Health Service, the Northwest Portland Area Indian Health Board, the American Indian Health Commission for Washington State, and academic institutions such as Portland State University, Washington State University, and the University of Washington. In considering the provision of health services and the role of nursing, it was noted that there is a major shortage of nursing services in the rural tribal communities. Nursing has created structures to increase the number of nurses prepared to provide services to Indian communities and to increase the number of Native nurses prepared to work in Indian health as well. Creation of tribal/academic partnerships and an infrastructure used to build tribal capacity for evidence-based research and education models have all been a part of this effort. Tribes have taken a leadership role in providing prevention programs and engaging in service-related research. As a result, diabetes is better managed, and greater numbers of AI/ANs are receiving the needed prevention screening in areas such as cancer. Many effective programs are being coordinated and offered throughout the region. Even so, disparities persist. Continued effort is being directed toward creating and maintaining better tracking systems for the collection of health data, addressing the health provider shortages, and addressing the leading continued causes of mortality. Nursing contributions in Indian health in the PNW provide much-needed services to the region and nationally, and also contribute to the advancement of nursing science.

CRITICAL-THINKING EXERCISE

♦ You have been recently hired as a community health nurse in a small Coastal Salish tribe of about 1,000 people. You are not an AI/AN, and have just moved to the region from the East Coast. You have never worked in a tribal community before, but you have practiced community health in a rural community for over 5 years.

♦ You have been asked to develop a plan to address the major health issues of the tribe, and to suggest the priority community health concerns you would address in the first year of work. What data would you seek? What/whom would you include in your sources of information?

♦ Whom would you involve in the planning? With what local and regional organizations/agencies would you affiliate? What challenges might you expect to encounter?

Answer:

Data: Refer to community health nursing texts on assessment, and include data such as: (a) epidemiology data; (b) demographic data; (c) existing tribally collected data; (d) perspectives on priorities noted from observations and talking to tribal administration, elders, and program administrators in the tribe. Note the strengths of the tribe as well as their concerns.

Sources of Information: Tribal website, newsletter, program documents, and reports (note sources of data listed under *Data*).

Whom to Involve in Planning? Note the structure of the tribe. Is there a tribal health committee? If so, they must be involved. Have there been any planning groups? If so, how could they be involved? Determine the lines of authority and responsibility, and program administrators who might be involved, as well as those who exercise influence both formally and informally, such as the major family groups and elders.

Local Agencies: This depends on the state in which you are working, but for any of the states in the PNW, the local agencies are the Northwest Portland Area Indian Health Board and the Indian Health Service.

Challenges: The difference in time orientation between the tribal perspectives and those of non-Indian institutions, such as the academic institutions and federal government, may pose a challenge, and available data may be limited.

STUDY QUESTIONS

♦ Consider the structure and provision of health services for AI/ANs in the PNW region. What strengths and challenges do you see in the structure?

Answer: The strengths of the structure are: (a) strong tribal control, (b) many regional agencies provide support and coordination. Challenges presented are: (a) recruiting and retaining health providers; (b) need for continued collaboration on data tracking and misclassification, and development of computerized record keeping; (c) communication between tribes and outside referral providers.

♦ Review the epidemiology data and program priorities being addressed related to health concerns for AI/ANs in the PNW. What role might nursing provide at the individual, community, policy, and structural levels in addressing needs?

Answer: The role of nursing is to: (a) provide direct patient care and prevention/promotion programs to address the health concerns, (b) enhance tribal capacity to obtain grant funding and to conduct research, (c) support development of policies to address health issues within the tribes and across the region, and (d) facilitate tribal academic partnerships for research and recruitment, and retention of health providers.

♦ If you were preparing nurses to work in rural tribal communities in the PNW, list three or four priority topics you would emphasize in the education effort.

Answer: Nursing priorities in the PNW include: (a) history, cultural values, beliefs, patterns of communication; (b) structure of tribes and health services delivery, including the laws supporting health funding and control; (c) demographic and epidemiology data; (d) program planning with an emphasis on assessment; and (e) resources, including agencies, books, and websites.

♦ Trace the history of the two major AI/AN cultural groups in the PNW region. Discuss one or two cultural strengths you have noted in this chapter that you could build on to address at least one leading health issue.

Answer: The two cultural groups are the Coastal Salish and Plateau People. The cultural values are: (a) a commitment to the tribe/community and (b) a resurgence of culture with ceremonies and return of the canoe journey, revival of language, and return to traditional foods. A leading health issue would be to address diabetes by engaging the community in the design of a nutrition program using traditional language and asking elders to serve as role models; a focus on behavior change aimed at making the changes in diet for the community and the next generation would affect the rate of diabetes in this population.

USEFUL WEBSITES

American Indian Health Commission for Washington State, Washington State Public Health website, www.doh.wa.gov

Native American Rehabilitation Association of the Northwest, Inc., http://www.naranorthwest.org/homepage-files/page 451.htm

Northwest Portland Area Indian Health Board, www.NPAIHB.org

Portland Indian Health Service, http://www.ihs.gov/Portland

Tribal websites: (Use Internet and the tribal name)

RECOMMENDED READINGS

Ashwell, R. (1994). *Coast Salish: Their art, culture and legends.* Blaine, WA: Hancock House Publishers.

Beck, M. G. (1993). *Potlatch: Native ceremony and myth on the Northwest Coast.* Seattle, WA: Alaska Northwest Books.

Brown, V. (1985) *Natives of the Pacific Coast.* Happy Camp, CA: Naturegraph Publishers.

DeJong, D. (2011). *Plagues, politics, and policy: A chronicle of the Indian Health Service, 1955–2008.* New York, NY: Rowman and Littlefield.

Jensen, D., & Sargent, P. (1986). *Robes of power: Totem poles on cloth.* Vancouver, Canada: University of British Columbia Press in association with the UBC Museum of Anthropology.

Kirk, R. (1986). *Tradition and change on the Northwest Coast.* Seattle, WA: University of Washington Press.

Liptak, K. (1991). *Indians of the Pacific Northwest.* New York, NY: Facts on File.

Ruby, R., & Brown, J. (1989). *Dreamer-prophets of the Columbia Plateau: Smohalla and Skolaskin.* Norman, OK: University of Oklahoma Press.

Ruby, R., & Brown, J. (1992). *A guide to the Indian tribes of the Pacific Northwest.* Norman, OK: University of Oklahoma Press.

Stewart, H. (1977). *Indian fishing: Early methods on the Northwest Coast.* Seattle, WA: University of Washington Press.

Stewart, H. (1979). *Looking at Indian art of the Northwest Coast.* Seattle, WA: University of Washington Press.

Stewart, H. (1984). *Cedar.* Seattle, WA: University of Washington Press.

REFERENCES

Aiken, L. H., Clarke, S. P., Sloan, D. M., Sochalski, J., & Silber, J. (2002). Hospital nurse staffing and patient mortality, nurse burn out, and job dissatisfaction. *Journal of the American Medical Association, 288*(16), 1987–1993.

American Indian Health Commission for Washington State. (2010). *Opportunities for change: Improving the health of American Indian/Alaska Natives in Washington State. American Indian Health Care Delivery Plan 2010–2013.* Retrieved from http://www.doh.wa.gov/Portals/1/Documents/1200/phsd-AIHCHealthCare.pdf

Amoss, P. (1972). *The persistence of aboriginal beliefs and practices among the Nooksack Coast Salish* (Doctoral dissertation). University of Washington Press, Seattle, WA.

Crofoot, T. (2013). *Pacific Northwest American Indian and Alaska Native health data.* Retrieved from http://saige.org/words/wp-content/uploads/2013/07/Crofoot-2013SAIGE_RedPaperColorHandout.pdf

DeJong, D. (2011). *Plagues, politics, and policy: A chronicle of the Indian Health Service, 1955–2008.* New York, NY: Rowman and Littlefield.

Ervine, N. (2002). *Advanced community health nursing practice.* Upper Saddle River, NJ: Prentice Hall.

Fisher, D. G., Pearce, F. W., Stanz, D. J., & Wood, M. M. (2003). Employment retention of health care providers in frontier areas of Alaska. *International Journal of Circumpolar Health, 62,* 423–435.

Haeberlin, H., & Gunter, E. (1952). *The Indians of Puget Sound.* Seattle, WA: University of Washington Press.

Hawthorn, H. (1965). *Cultures of the North Pacific coast.* San Francisco, CA: Chandler Publishing.

Hoopes, M., Dankovchik, J., & Kakuska, E. (2012). *Improving data and enhancing access Project (Idea-NW).* Portland, OR: Northwest Portland Area Indian Health Board. Retrieved from http://www.npaihb.org/epicenter/project/improving_data_enhancing_access_northwest_idea_nw

Hoopes, N., Petersen, P., & Vinson, E. (2012). Regional difference and tribal use of American Indian/Alaska Native cancer data in the Pacific Northwest. *Journal of Cancer Education, 27*(Suppl. 1), S73–S79.

Jefferson, W. (2001). *The world of Chief Seattle: How can we sell the air?* Summertown, TN: Native Voices.

Katz, J., O'Neal, G., Strickland, C. J., & Doutrich, D. (2010). Retention of Native American nurses working in their communities. *Journal of Transcultural Nursing, 21*(4), 393–401.

Keltner, B., Kelly, F. J., & Smith, D. (2004). Leadership to reduce health disparities: A model for nursing leadership in American Indian communities. *Nursing Administration Quarterly, 28,* 181–190.

Lewis, C. (1970). *Indian families of the Northwest Coast.* Chicago, IL: The University of Chicago Press.

Northwest Portland Area Indian Health Board. (2013). *Northwest Portland Area Indian Health Board letter to Congress and 2013 legislative and regulatory priorities.* Portland, OR: Author.

Port Gamble S'Klallam Tribe. (2012). *The strong people: A history of the Port Gamble S'Klallam tribe.* Kingston, WA: Port Gamble S'Klallam Foundation.

Portland Area Indian Health Service. (2014). *Portland area: Overseeing the delivery of health care to Native American people in the Northwest.* Retrieved from https://www.ihs.gov/Portland/

Ruby, R., & Brown, J. (1988). *Indians of the Pacific Northwest*. Norman, OK: University of Oklahoma Press.

Ruby, R., & Brown, J. (1989). *Dreamer-prophets of the Columbia Plateau: Smohalla and Skolaskin*. Norman, OK: University of Oklahoma Press.

Shelton, T. (2008). Degrees of success: Putting Native American nursing students on the path to success. *Minority Nurse, 6*, 53–56.

Strickland, C. J. (1999). Conducting focus groups cross-culturally: Experiences with Pacific Northwest Indian people. *Public Health Nursing, 16*(3), 190–197.

Strickland, C. J. (2001). Pain management and health policy in a western Washington Indian tribe. *Wiscaso Sa Review, 16*(1), 17–30.

Strickland, C. J., & Cooper, M. (2011). Getting into trouble: Perspectives on stress and suicide prevention among Pacific Northwest Indian youth. *Journal of Transcultural Nursing, 22*(3), 240–247.

Strickland, C. J., & Hillaire, E. (2014). Conducting a feasibility study in women's health screening among women in a Pacific Northwest Indian tribe. *Journal of Transcultural Nursing*. doi:10.1177/1043659614526251

Strickland, C. J., Chrisman, N. J., Yallup, M., Powell, K., & Squeoch, M. D. (1996). Walking the journey of womanhood: Cervical cancer and Yakama Indian women. *Public Health Nursing, 13*(2), 141–150.

Strickland, C. J., Logsdon, R.G., Hoffman, B., & Garrett-Hill, T. (2014). Developing an academic and American Indian tribal partnership in education: A model of community health nursing clinical education. *Nurse Educator, 39*, 188–192.

Strickland, C. J., Squoech, M. D., & Chrisman, N. J. (1999). Health promotion in cervical cancer prevention among Yakama Indian women of the Wa'Shat Longhouse. *Journal of Transcultural Nursing, 10*(3), 190–196.

Strickland, C. J., Walsh, E., & Cooper, M. (2006). Healing fractured families: Parents' and elders' perspectives on the impact of colonialization and youth suicide prevention in a Pacific Northwest American Indian tribe. *Journal of Transcultural Nursing, 17*(1), 5–12.

U.S. Department of Commerce, U.S. Census Bureau. (2012). *State characteristics: Vintage 2012*. Retrieved from http://www.census.gov/popest/data/state/asrh/2012/index.html

Urban Indian Health Institute. (2011). *Diabetes fact sheet: Native American Indian Center for the Northwest and Seattle Indian Health Board*. Seattle, WA: Author.

von Aderkas, E. (2005). *American Indians of the Pacific Northwest*. Oxford, UK: Osprey Publishing.

❖ FOURTEEN ❖

Alaska

Christopher M. Nelson

LEARNING OBJECTIVES

- To give an overview of the history of Alaska Natives and American Indians in the region
- To explain the unique health care challenges of the sub-Arctic and Arctic regions
- To examine the innovative health care delivery strategies in Alaska
- To illustrate the important roles that traditional subsistence hunting and fishing play in the lives of Alaska Natives and American Indians

KEY TERMS

- Alaska Federal Health Care Access Network (AFHCAN)
- Alaska Native
- Alaska Native corporations
- Alaska Native Medical Center (ANMC)
- Alaska Native Tribal Health Consortium (ANTHC)
- American Indian
- Community Health Aide Program (CHAP)
- Dental health aide therapist (DHAT)
- Indian Health Service (IHS)
- Inuit
- Provider deserts
- The bush
- Transcultural nursing

KEY CONCEPTS

- Alaska Native corporations
- Alaska Native identity
- Distance delivery of health care
- Subsistence hunting and fishing
- Traditional versus convenience foods

As the only part of the United States in and around the Arctic, Alaska's geography has created unique challenges that have led to a number of unique solutions and strategies for health care delivery. The initial experience of Alaska Natives has been different from American Indians in the "lower 48" as reservations and forced relocations were not a primary characteristic of the interactions between the U.S. government and the Alaska Native population.

However, the current challenges facing the indigenous population of Alaska have strong similarities to those of the lower 48, with poverty, substance abuse, and food insecurity weighing heavily on Alaska Natives. Nursing in Alaska comes with its own set of unique concerns that make for a tough and abiding set of hurdles to overcome, including provider deserts, cultural conflicts, and gender issues.

Alaska is by far the largest state, with an area of 570,640.95 square miles out of the United States' total of 3,531,905.43 square miles. The enormous distances and low population (est. 2013: 735,132) lead to challenges related to access and distance, with a population density of only 1.2 persons per square mile as compared with the average of 87.4 per square mile for the United States (U.S. Census Bureau, 2015). Many of the Alaska Natives and American Indians live in isolated villages and settlements throughout Alaska without road access to the rest of the state's infrastructure and health resources.

HISTORY OF THE AREA

Alaska has been continuously inhabited since the first indigenous people migrated across the Bering Strait from Siberia thousands of years ago. Many of those peoples continued south to eventually inhabit every corner of North, Central, and South America, whereas a substantial number remained in what is now Alaska until the present day.

In the 18th century, Russian ships appeared on the coast with merchants and Orthodox missionaries on board, ready to engage in trade with the Alaska Natives. Over the next 150 years, small numbers of Russians settled in what became known as Russian America, but their numbers never approached a thousand total residents. In 1867, the United States purchased Alaska from Russia for $7,200,000 in what was known as "Seward's Folly," as enacted by U.S. Secretary of State William Seward (U.S. Department of State, Bureau of Public Affairs, Office of the Historian, 2015).

By the time vast resources had been found in Alaska, including gold, copper, and, later, oil and natural gas, the true value of "Andrew Johnson's Ice Box" had rendered the sale by Russia into one of the best bargain land purchases in history. Compared with the American Indians in the lower 48, the reservation system of forced relocation and resettlement did not have nearly as large an impact on the local indigenous population in Alaska, with only one reservation currently remaining in the entire state (the Annette Island Reserve of the Tsimshian) after repeal of the Alaskan reservation system in 1971 (Bureau of Indian Affairs [BIA], 2015). When statehood for Alaska was obtained in 1959, federal money poured into Alaska in order to build on the existing territorial infrastructure and expand it into a state-level bureaucracy. In 1964, the Good Friday Earthquake hit Alaska on March 27 with a force of 9.2 on the Richter scale, which caused over a hundred deaths and massive destruction in Anchorage and the surrounding region (U.S. Geological Survey [USGS], Earthquake Hazards Program, 2015).

In 1968, oil reserves were discovered on the North Slope of the state, leading to a "black gold" rush that continues into the present day (Alaska Oil and Gas Conservation Commission [AOGCC], 2008). In view of the sudden urgency brought about by the discoveries (and the need for pipelines through disputed territory), President Nixon signed the Alaska Native Claims Settlement Act in 1971. The reservation system was disbanded, and the financial payment contained in the bill led to the establishment of the 13 Alaska Native Regional Corporations as agencies intended to serve as investment and development engines for the vacated tribal claim holders (Alaska Native Claims Settlement Act [ANCSA] Regional Association, 2015). Some of these corporations are counted among the largest and most successful companies in the state, with extensive land and real estate holdings, resource development investments, and recently a video game company that made a popular and critically acclaimed game incorporating the Iñupiat legend, *Never Alone* (Cook Inlet Tribal Council, 2014).

The natural gas and petroleum that started flowing out of the state in the 1970s has provided for an economy with neither state income tax nor sales tax, and the bonus of an annual dividend from the drilling tax receipts for state residents also known as the yearly "permanent fund" check (AOGCC, 2008). Some of those monies are also transferred into the Alaska Native health care system anchored by the Alaska Native Tribal Health Consortium, the Southcentral Foundation, and the Indian Health Service.

TRIBES IN THE AREA

Almost half of the 566 federally recognized tribes in the United States are found in Alaska, with 229 uniquely named tribal entities representing groups ranging in size from the population of one village to the inhabitants of an area the size of Minnesota (BIA, 2015). As the number of tribes is large, the groups are generally sorted into common language families in order to simplify discussion. These larger language groups include Iñupiat, Yup'ik, Athabascan, Tlingit, Haida, Tsimshian, Gwich'in, and Aleut, with an understanding that dialects within those categories may differ enough to be mutually incomprehensible but still have a shared origin that makes them sufficiently closely related to constitute a useful label (Figure 14.1).

As an example, the Iñupiat language has clear links with the dialects spoken by the Chukchi in Siberia through the north of Alaska across to Nunavut, Canada, and continuing further east to Greenland. (The word for the traditional treat of whale skin and blubber is "maktak" in Barrow, Alaska, "maktaq" in Iqaluit, Canada, and "mattaq" in Qaanaaq, Greenland.) Accordingly, the Iñupiat language group is used to describe the people who speak variants of that root language and who also share similar lifestyles and geographic regions. Athabascan is another large language group that stretches from eastern Alaska down to the Navajo and Apache tribes in the Southwest, but because of the

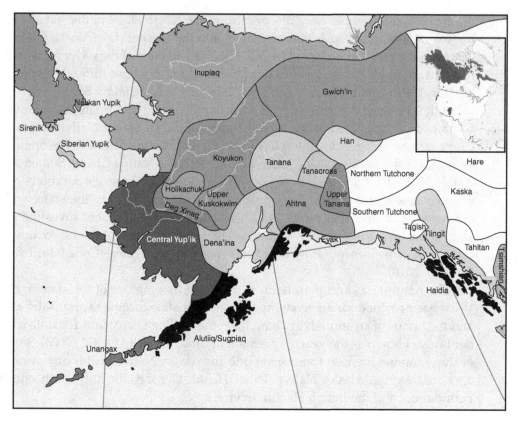

FIGURE 14.1 Indigenous peoples and languages of Alaska (UAF).

Source: Krauss, Holton, Kerr, and West (2011).

vastly different climates and geographies of the various branches of the group, it is not used as a general catch-all category (outside of the Alaskan/Canadian grouping).

These larger groups are also recognized on an international level, with the Arctic Council granting permanent participant status to the Arctic Athabaskan Council (AAC), the Aleut International Association (AIA), the Gwich'in Council International (GCI), and the Inuit Circumpolar Council (ICC). Alaska has the highest percentage of Alaska Native and/or American Indians (14.7%) as a proportion of a state's population in the country, and is home to the city with the highest AN/AI population percentage (12%): Anchorage, Alaska (Norris et al., 2012).

Because of the great diversity of dialects, geographic origins, and traditions, the Alaska Native population spans a range of identities that is as large as Alaska itself. Some of the indigenous people prefer to be called American Indian, whereas others in the same nation prefer Alaska Native, Inuit, Eskimo, or the specific tribe name. An excellent example of this phenomenon revolves around St. Lawrence Island, where residents argue over whether the proper name for the group is Siberian Yupik or St. Lawrence Yupik, with advocates for each side strenuously objecting to being labeled with the other name. Another example is that Alaska tribes can be governed by "traditional councils, Native councils,

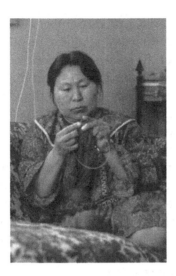

FIGURE 14.2 Knitting qiviut (musk oxen wool). Craft made at Tetlin National Wildlife refuge.
Image by S. Hillebrand, courtesy of U.S. Fish and Wildlife Service.

village councils, tribal councils, or IRA councils" (University of Alaska Fairbanks [UAF], 2015, Module 4), all of which refer to the Alaska Natives in their preferred terms (Figure 14.2).

CURRENT HEALTH PICTURE (MAJOR HEALTH ISSUES)

Like most of the lower 48, the major issues surrounding the Alaska Native and American Indian (AN/AI) population in Alaska revolve around poverty, substance abuse, and chronic diseases, including diabetes and depression. Food security is also an ongoing issue throughout the Arctic, and Alaska is no exception. Efforts to address these issues are ongoing, with innovative strategies being designed and implemented in the state that have had success in connecting rural and remote villages to better health care.

The five leading causes of death in the AN/AI population in Alaska are cancer, heart disease, unintentional injuries, diabetes, and chronic liver disease (CLD)/cirrhosis. Also appearing in the top 10 causes are chronic lower respiratory diseases, stroke, suicide, kidney disease, and influenza and pneumonia (Centers for Disease Control and Prevention, 2015). Specified in the report as other important health issues are teen pregnancy, infant mortality, HIV/AIDS, obesity, diabetes, mental health, alcohol use, and smoking.

Resources for AI/AN Patients in Region

Alaska is home to the largest indigenous-owned health care system in the world: the Alaska Native Tribal Health Consortium. Founded in 1997, the Alaska Area Native Health Service took over responsibility from the Indian Health Service in 1998 for managing health care for the AN/AI populations (Alaska Native Tribal

Health Consortium [ANTHC], 2015; Southcentral Foundation, 2014). In view of the difficulties of recruiting and retaining health care professionals to live in rural and remote areas of the state, several innovative programs have arisen to provide care that is effective for the far-flung population of the state, including the Community Health Aide Program, the Dental Health Aide Therapist Program, and the Alaska Federal Health Care Access Network (AFHCAN).

The Community Health Aide Program (CHAP) is one innovative solution to a recurring Alaskan problem: health care in isolated villages. Developed with the intention of fostering local recruitment of health care professionals who would be more likely to return to their communities, the program has two levels of training, the basic community health aide (CHA) and the community health aide practitioner (CHA/P). Although both CHAs and CHA/Ps are more limited in scope of practice than other providers, there is a parallel to the nurse and nurse practitioner levels of training, and they therefore serve similar roles in their communities (ANTHC, 2015).

The Dental Health Aide Therapist (DHAT) program is another example of innovative solution-making to address a specific problem: provider deserts. Small communities in the bush are unable to provide sufficient numbers of paying patients and income sources to dentists, and are therefore left without any dental care at all outside of fly-in visits by rotating staff. Exacerbating the lack of dental care is the reality that the visiting dentist has to triage patients on the basis of severely limited time in-village, which leads to a lack of cosmetic and preventative services. The DHAT program, much like its "sister" CHAP, recruits and trains members of a community and encourages them to return to provide dental services. Extractions, preventative care, and simple fillings are handled by DHAT using the specific training provided, allowing for visiting dentists to focus on more difficult dental situations in their limited time frames (ANTHC, 2015).

By far the largest innovative program developed for the unique Alaskan situation is the AFHCAN, a telehealth solution to address the underlying problem of the state: geography. Alaska is so large that when a state map is overlaid onto the lower 48, it stretches across the entire map from the Aleutian Islands touching California to the Alaskan Panhandle reaching into Florida, and north to south from Minnesota down to Texas (see Figure 14.3). This immense land mass has so many settlements and villages without connections to the road system that the main form of transportation is by airplane. Getting groceries using a floatplane as the shopping cart is not an exaggeration, and in-state luggage limits are nearly nonexistent, with "three free" being the state standard.

The AFHCAN system utilizes a "store-and-forward" technique that allows for transmission of health information regardless of irregularities of communications access (ANTHC, 2015). Some areas of the state have no stable Internet or cell phone connectivity, depending on satellite service that is both slow and unreliable. By connecting automatically whenever access is possible, the telehealth system provides a marvelous underlay of secure health data that aids the CHA/Ps, DHATs, and visiting providers in their work as well as allowing for guidance, diagnosis, and treatment from afar by monitoring clinicians.

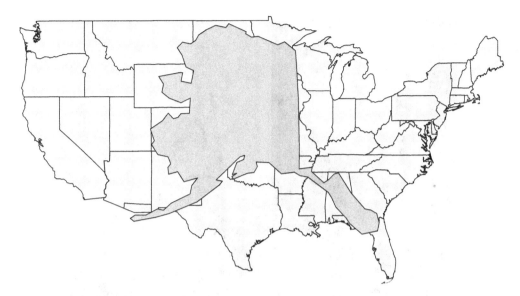

FIGURE 14.3 Alaska overlaid onto the lower 48.
Courtesy of U.S. Fish and Wildlife Service.

DESCRIPTION OF NURSING IN THE AREA

Nursing in Alaska features a wide variety of opportunities, from flight nurse into the bush and public health nursing in a rural seaside village all the way to bedside nursing in an intensive care unit at the Alaska Native Medical Center, the only level two trauma center in the state (ANTHC, 2015). With challenging weather, difficult geography, and culture clashes, recruitment and retention of nurses is an ongoing issue that impacts the level of health care delivery in the state.

Patient Population

An estimated 122,000 Alaska Natives live across the state in areas as diverse as inland valleys with winter temperatures diving below –50°F, coastal settlements on the Arctic Ocean and Gulf of Alaska, and temperate rainforests in the Alaska Panhandle (BIA, 2015).

Cultural Needs/Issues/Beliefs

Owing to the vast array of languages, tribes, and beliefs, transcultural approaches to nursing are highly valued and useful. With centuries of missionary work in Alaska by various faiths, a range of religious beliefs are held by members of the different communities as well as traditional beliefs that impact health care. A medicine bag around the neck may be gently moved to the side during an intubation, whereas an orthodox cross may be clutched in the hands of the patient. Herbs, oils, incense, drumming, songs, chants, and more are all a part of healing practice, with the Alaska Native Medical Center having a circular, domed

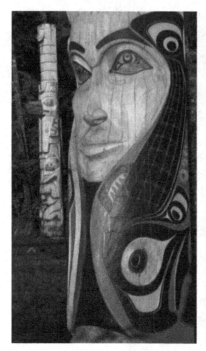 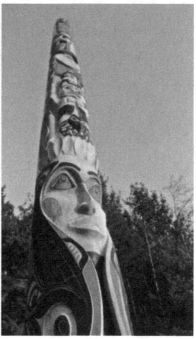

FIGURE 14.4 (*Left*): Standing beside the 80-year-old Frog Raven Pole, the brightly painted Centennial Pole is the newest totem pole in the park's collection. (*Right*): Wooch Jin Shat Kooteeya—The Holding Hands Centennial Totem Pole.

Courtesy of National Park Service—Sitka National Historic Park.

central chamber that serves as both community room and sacred space. Other examples include healing and sacred totem carvings, rattles, drums, and weavings (Figure 14.4). The key to good care is as simple as asking what the patient wants, and by allowing for those things to take place in recognition of the value they hold for the patient.

Gender issues arise in many ways, with some Alaska Native groups being matriarchal, with the eldest woman in a family in charge, and some areas with virtual segregation of the sexes in everyday life. A recent example (Alaska Dispatch News, 2014) is that of the first female hunter known to have taken a whale in Barrow, although there are stories of women in outer villages who hunted and fished long before. Nurses might not be acknowledged by members of the opposite sex or may instead be the focus of attention, depending on the origin of the patient and his or her family.

Another deeply rooted concept in the Alaska Native population is that of conflict avoidance. Community standards dictate that public disagreement is frowned on in many circumstances and is taboo in others. A patient might not feel comfortable disclosing to his or her doctor any unwillingness to take the medicine prescribed, and will simply dispose of the bottle on the way out of the clinic to avoid being disrespectful or confrontational. Young women, in particular, might not speak at all in the presence of a male provider or nurse, and simply sit silently waiting for the encounter to end.

Physical Issues

Poverty is the primary driver of food insecurity, sexually transmitted infections, and lack of access to clean water. These physical issues represent significant negative contributors to the health and well-being of the Alaska Native population and are recurring challenges that sometimes seem to defy resolution. Lack of adequate nutrition, "honey bucket" dry toileting in the absence of plumbing, and inadequate safe water supplies are all recurring issues that need to be addressed by ambitious programming.

Diabetes is endemic in the Alaska Native population, with rates that skyrocket above those in the general population, so much so that studies have investigated genetics, diet, and even cold weather as sources of the condition. With prices of fruits and vegetables reaching levels that approach the ludicrous (a half-gallon of orange juice for $22), they do not form an affordable part of the diet of residents. Rather than a food desert, the situation can be described as a food swamp: prepackaged convenience foods cost less than nutritious ingredients and draw the health of the diet level down into the depths.

Mental Issues

A difficult issue in Alaska is that of alcohol and drug addiction within the Alaska Native population. In an attempt to reduce access to alcohol, some bush villages have outlawed sales and possession by becoming "dry," with other communities choosing to become "damp," meaning alcohol is not sold in the village but is legal to own and consume. Crystal methamphetamine and other street drugs are a lingering issue that has also negatively impacted the Alaska Native population, with the recent addition of "spice," the name for various marijuana-analogues with synthetic THC that have psychoactive components that can cause psychotic breaks and catatonia.

Another uncomfortable topic is that of domestic abuse: the rates in Alaska, especially in the Alaska Native population, are many times that in the lower 48. Some bush villages have no police forces at all, which means that in the event of a rape, for example, the nearest officer might be 3 days away and will be totally unfamiliar with the community. Alcohol and drug addictions complicate the matter as well, with ongoing struggles being exacerbated by comorbidities.

Emotional/Spiritual Issues

Seasonal affective disorder and depression are overrepresented in the Alaska Native community and continue to be mental health issues at crisis levels throughout the state. As a result of these and other factors, including cultural dislocation and poverty, suicidal ideation is a recurring and difficult issue to address that cuts across gender, age, and location to severely impact communities large and small. Aggravating the issue is a strong cultural taboo in Alaska Natives against discussing suicide, which alienates those suffering from self-destructive thoughts from the very people who could offer emotional support. The tradition of not naming the dead, especially if the death was the result of suicide, stigmatizes the families and friends of the deceased as well.

Life-Span Issues (Elderly Emphasis)

High incidence of infant mortality in Alaska Native communities is matched by shortened life spans for the elders. Poverty is an ongoing problem that impacts rural and urban communities alike with negative effects that ripple through the larger state population. Older residents of the area also show serum titres of various zoonotic diseases that they were exposed to in the past, with unknown impacts on their life spans.

Elders are given pride of place in many of the Alaska Native communities, with first choice of food, great respect being shown by all, and specialized services that attempt to make life easier for them. (Reserved parking spaces near the doors of the community buildings are a perfect example of how the elders are protected by the community, especially in areas with brutal cold winters.) Specialty agencies have been set up by the Alaska Native Tribal Health Consortium and the Southcentral Foundation to research the special health needs and concerns of the elders.

Conclusion and Nursing Implications

In the final analysis, nursing in Alaska is fraught with challenges related to the enormous distances in the state, the diversity of the state population, and the need for culturally sensitive care.

THE NORTHERN NATIONS: FROM SIBERIA TO GREENLAND

When discussing the Arctic of Alaska, it is helpful to remember that the Iñupiat and Yupik groups found there are closely related to peoples ranging from Siberia across the top of North America all the way to Greenland (Figure 14.5).

The governing situations for the various peoples illustrate a wide range of rights and privileges:

The Chukchi and Nenets peoples of Russia are called "small minority language groups" by the government rather than "indigenous peoples," possibly to prevent claims under the United Nations Declaration of the Rights of Indigenous Peoples, and therefore are not able to govern themselves.

The North Slope Borough of Alaska's Iñupiat has vast mineral wealth from the reserves of oil and natural gas that have been developed in their region, and are a federally recognized tribe with all the rights and privileges associated with that status.

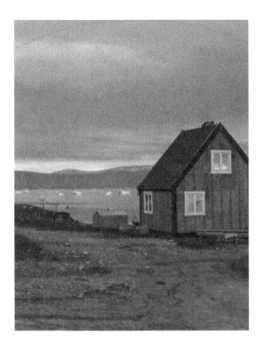

FIGURE 14.5 Qaanaaq, Greenland.
Photo by Chris Nelson.

A group of Inuit, Metis, and First Nations peoples of Northern Canada have been organized into the Territory of Nunavut within the federal system, with largely sovereign self-government.

Northern Quebec has a group of settlements described as Nunavik, although there are no regional governments or powers associated with the name. The three Greenlandic regions (linked to the West, East, and North Greenlandic languages) have become the semiautonomous nation of Greenland within the Kingdom of Denmark. Danish is no longer a national language, with Kalaallit (West Greenlandic) now serving as the only official language and self-government except for some powers vested with Denmark (foreign relations, military, etc.; Figure 14.6).

SUBSISTENCE AND TRADITIONAL FOODS

Throughout the Arctic region, food insecurity is an ongoing hazard, especially in the case of indigenous peoples. Although the North Slope Borough has unique and extensive financial resources from its developed oil and natural gas reserves and uses snowmobiles, whereas Qaanaaq, Greenland, has an average annual income of under $10,000 and uses dogsleds, the residents of both places must supplement their diet with subsistence hunting and fishing (Figures 14.7–14.9).

The cost of food is prohibitive, with milk costing more per ounce than gasoline, and whatever meager fruits and vegetables have survived the journey

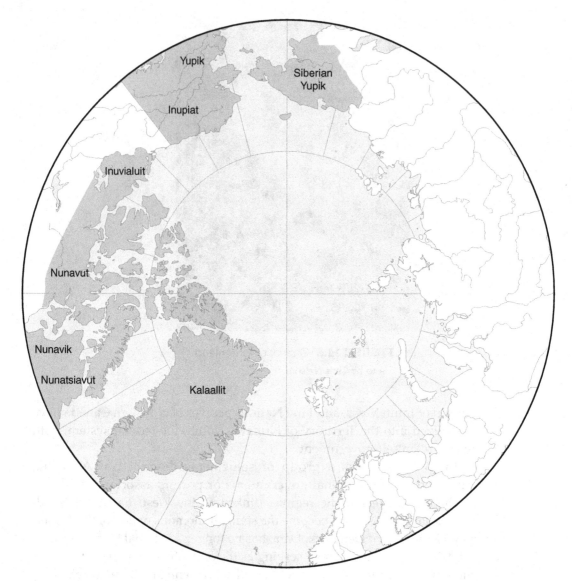

FIGURE 14.6 Northern Nations.

Courtesy of Karl Musser via Creative Commons Attribution—Share Alike 3.0 license.

to the north being priced at scandalous levels. Accordingly, the peoples of the Arctic continue to hunt and fish to supplement their diets, and that is reflected in the wide variety of foods they eat:

- Whale: bowhead and beluga in Barrow, narwhal in North Greenland
- Walrus
- Seal
- Polar bear
- Caribou/reindeer
- Musk oxen
- Arctic hare

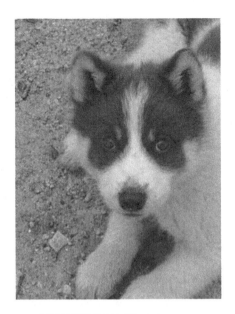

FIGURE 14.7 Sled dog.
Photo by Chris Nelson.

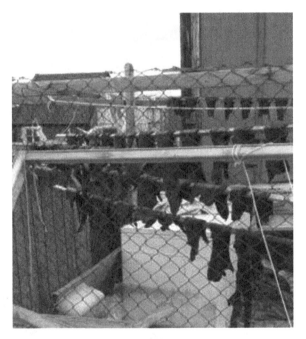

FIGURE 14.8 Narwhal drying.
Photo by Chris Nelson.

- Birds: geese, migrating species
- Salmon/trout
- Berries: salmonberries, bog blueberries, lowbush cranberry, blackberry
- Edible plants: wild rhubarb, sea weeds and beach greens, Eskimo potato, sourdock (Jones, 2010; Unger, 2014)

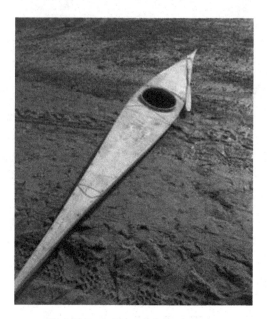

FIGURE 14.9 Sealskin kayak.

Photo by Chris Nelson.

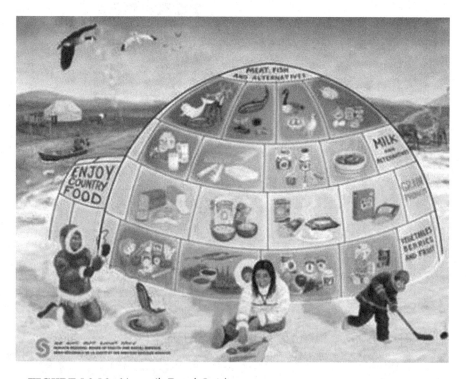

FIGURE 14.10 Nunavik Food Guide.

Courtesy of the Nunavut Regional Board of Health and Social Services, Canada.

The Canadian government published an inclusive new food guide ("the food igloo") that showed traditional foods as being part of a good diet for Nunavik in north Quebec (Figure 14.10).

CRITICAL-THINKING EXERCISES

♦ Imagine that you are a member of a federally recognized tribe consisting of one village in the bush of Alaska, and that you have had to travel to Anchorage for an emergency appendectomy. What questions and concerns might you have for your nurse?

♦ If your Alaska Native patient is not responding to your questions, what might you do to elicit a response? Some ideas might include having a provider of the opposite sex ask the questions, or reaching out to an elder in the family. Do you have any other ideas?

STUDY QUESTIONS

♦ How would you approach a new Alaska Native patient? Would your approach differ according to their tribal background, age, or sex? If so, how?

♦ A female elder in your care is nearing the end of her life. She is from the Tlingit nation and has numerous relatives of various ages and both genders in the room. You have to decide whom you approach for decision making. Whom do you choose and why?

♦ Food insecurity is a part of poverty all across the United States, disproportionately impacting Alaska Natives and American Indians. What forms of subsistence hunting and fishing have you heard of in your region?

USEFUL WEBSITES

♦ Alaska Native Heritage Center, www.alaskanative.net
♦ Alaska Native history, education, laguages, and cutlures, www.alaskool.org
♦ U.S. Fish and Wildlife Service, Alaska Native Affairs, www.fws.gov/alaska/external/nativeamerican.html

RECOMMENDED READINGS

American Indian/Alaska Native Suicide Prevention. (www.sprc.org/aian)
National Resource Center for American Indian, Alaska Native, & Native Hawaiian Elders. "Voices of our elders." (www.uaa.alaska.edu/elders/)

REFERENCES

Alaska Dispatch News. (2014, October 2). Whaler makes history as Barrow's first known woman to take a whale. Retrieved from http://www.adn.com/article/20141002/whaler-makes-history-barrows-first-known-woman-take-whale

Alaska Native Claims Settlement Act Regional Association. (2015). *ANCSA timeline*. Retrieved from http://ancsaregional.com/interactive-history/

Alaska Native Tribal Health Consortium (2015). *Opening doors to better health: ANTHC 2014 annual report*. Anchorage, AK: Author.

Alaska Oil and Gas Conservation Commission. (2008). *Fifty years of service to Alaska*. Juneau, AK: Alaska State Government.

Bureau of Indian Affairs. (2015). Indian entities recognized and eligible to receive services from the United States bureau of Indian affairs. Department of the Interior. *Federal Register 80*(9), 1942–1948.

Centers for Disease Control and Prevention. (2015). *National vital statistics system*. Retrieved from http://www.cdc.gov/nchs/nvss.htm

Cook Inlet Tribal Council. (2014). *Never alone* (Kisima Ingitchuna). Anchorage, AK: Upper One Games, LLC.

Jones, A. (2010). *Plants that we eat (Nauriat Nigiñaqtuat): From the traditional wisdom of the Iñupiat elders of Northwest Alaska*. Fairbanks, AK: University of Alaska Press.

Krauss, M., Holton, G., Kerr, J., & West, C. T. (2011). *Indigenous peoples and languages of Alaska*. Anchorage, AK: Alaska Native Language Center and UAA Institute of Social and Economic Research. Retrieved from https://www.uaf.edu/anlc/resources/anlmap/

National Resource Center for American Indian, Alaska Native, & Native Hawaiian Elders. (n.d.). *Voices of our elders*. University of Alaska-Anchorage. Retrieved from http://elders.uaa.alaska.edu

Norris, T., Vines, P. L., & Hoeffel, E. M. (2012). *The American Indian and Alaska Native population: 2010*. Washington, DC: U.S. Department of Commerce, Economics and Statistics Administration, U.S. Census Bureau.

Southcentral Foundation. (2015). *Alaska Native people shaping health care*. Retrieved from www.southcentralfoundation.com

Unger, S. (2013). *Qaqamiigux: Traditional foods and recipes from the Aleutian and Pribilof Islands*. Anchorage, AK: Aleutian Pribilof Islands Association.

University of Alaska Fairbanks. (2015). Federal Indian law for Alaska tribes. Tribal Management Course (TM 112). Retrieved from https://tm112.community.uaf.edu/unit-4/modern-tribal-governments-in-alaska/

U.S. Census Bureau, U.S. Department of Commerce. (2015). *USA QuickFacts*. Retrieved from http://quickfacts.census.gov/qfd/states/00000.html

U.S. Department of Health and Human Services, Office of Minority Health. (2015). *Profile: American Indian/Alaska Native*. Retrieved from http://minorityhealth.hhs.gov/omh/browse.aspx?lvl=3&lvlid=62

U.S. Department of State, Bureau of Public Affairs, Office of the Historian. (2015). *Purchase of Alaska, 1867*. Retrieved from https://history.state.gov/milestones/1866-1898/alaska-purchase

U.S. Geological Survey, Earthquake Hazards Program. (2015). *The great Alaska earthquake and tsunami of March 27, 1964*. Retrieved from http://earthquake.usgs.gov/earthquakes/events/alaska1964/

FIFTEEN

Northern Great Plains

Margaret P. Moss and Donna M. Grandbois

LEARNING OBJECTIVES

- Recognize the unique population numbers found in the Plains. These states have some of the highest percentages of American Indians in the country, or American Indians are the largest minority in a state, and/or most American Indians are found on reservations—and the implications that these have for determinants of health in this region.
- Distinguish the impact of dichotomous worldviews, health belief systems, and culturally compatible health care professionals
- Plan for care of traditional American Indians in the Plains Area by gaining a better understanding of culture in the region

KEY TERMS

- Four medicines
- Great Plains
- Indian Health Service administrative areas
- Smudging
- Sun dance
- Sweat
- Wounded Knee

KEY CONCEPTS

- Health disparity
- Historical trauma
- Indigenous worldview
- Overlapping cultures

The Great Plains is one of the largest regions in America and cuts a sizable swath across the middle of the country (please refer back to area map at the beginning of Part II of this text). This chapter focuses on the Northern Plains, where a majority of Plains people live and where health disparities are among the greatest in the United States. The Northern Great Plains region typically includes the states of North Dakota, South Dakota, Nebraska, and Iowa. The Indian Health Service (IHS) covers this region, as does the Great Plains Tribal Chairman's Health Board, which is involved in public health and health care provision.

The IHS is divided into 12 administrative/geographical areas of the United States—Alaska, Albuquerque, Aberdeen, Bemidji, Billings, California,

Nashville, Navajo, Oklahoma, Phoenix, Portland, and Tucson—with each service unit providing health care to a unique group of tribes located within these specific regions. This text uses nine geographic cultural areas versus the 12 administrative areas of the IHS, so there is, necessarily, overlap of areas.

The Aberdeen Area Office headquarters, located in Aberdeen, South Dakota, has formally changed their name to the Great Plains Area IHS, effective January 10, 2014, indicating to all stakeholders that it will take time to complete all the required name change updates (IHS, 2014). The Great Plains Area Office provides health services to approximately 124,443 American Indian (AI) people who reside within 17 service units located on 16 reservations (see Figure 15.1).

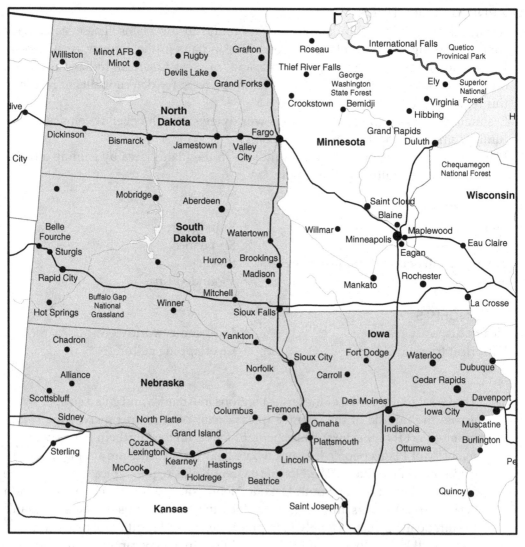

FIGURE 15.1 Great Plains Area for Indian Health Service.

Source: IHS (2015a).

The terms *American Indian/Alaska Native* (AI/AN), *American Indian* (AI), and *Native American* (NA) will be used interchangeably throughout this chapter. Additionally, reference may be made to Native or Indian.

There are eight service units in South Dakota, four in North Dakota, three in Nebraska, and one in Iowa. Service units are the next lower administrative unit under each Area Office, in this case the Great Plains Area. In addition to reservation-based service units, health care services are provided at three nonreservation service units located in Rapid City, South Dakota; Trenton, North Dakota; and Norfolk, Nebraska. The service unit in Trenton, North Dakota, is affiliated with the Turtle Mountain Band of Chippewa Indians, who live in Belcourt, North Dakota.

The Great Plains Area Office also provides health services to approximately 6,000 AIs who are not counted in the user population of the area, and who do not reside within a service unit. However, they do meet the IHS eligibility criteria for health services provided by IHS or tribally operated direct care facilities. The largest concentrations of the nonservice unit-eligible patients are found in the urban areas of Aberdeen and Sioux Falls in South Dakota, and Bismarck and Grand Forks in North Dakota. Additionally, although approximately 3,917 Indians live in Fargo, the state's largest metropolitan area (North Dakota Indian Affairs, 2011), there are no IHS service units located there to provide services. North Dakota currently has no federally qualified health clinics that specifically serve Indian people, and no Title V funding for their health care needs.

For the purposes of this chapter, Montana and Minnesota will also be included in the Northern Great Plains region because many of the tribes overlap into these states. For example, many Turtle Mountain Chippewa hold trust land in Montana. Montana is part of the Billings Area IHS Unit, which provides health services to more than 70,000 AI people in Montana and Wyoming, according to Billings Area Director, Anna Whiting Sorrell. Although approximately 79,572 Native Americans live in Montana (U.S. Census Bureau, 2010), some are either not eligible for services, are geographically isolated from IHS facilities, or prefer to seek health care elsewhere.

Minnesota is served by the Bemidji IHS Service Unit. This service unit also includes Michigan, Wisconsin, Indiana, and Illinois, and is home to 34 federally recognized tribes numbering over 110,000 Indian people, with 108,857 calling Minnesota home (Annual Estimate, U.S. Census Bureau, 2014). For reasons similar to Montana, not all Native Americans receive care at Bemidji IHS facilities. As this area was largely covered under Chapter 8, Minnesota will not be a major focus here.

A PUBLIC HEALTH PERSPECTIVE IN THE NORTHERN GREAT PLAINS REGION

The Great Plains Tribal Chairman's Health Board (GPTCHB), established in 1986, is a nonprofit organization serving what was formerly the Aberdeen Area of the IHS. Their stated mission is to "provide quality public health support and health care advocacy to the tribal nations of the Great Plains by utilizing effective and culturally credible approaches" (GPTCHB, 2015a para 1). The vision of the GPTCHB is that all tribal Nations and communities in the Great Plains will reach optimum health and wellness through lasting partnerships with health organizations, and embrace culturally significant values that are empowered by tribal sovereignty. They advance this vision through the formation of tribal partnerships, utilizing a public health framework, to collaborate with tribes to improve the health of the AI people by providing public health support and health care advocacy.

The GPTCHB is the designated organization to provide consultation for the Great Plains Area Office. They represent 18 tribal communities in the four-state region of North Dakota, South Dakota, Nebraska, and Iowa. Both the IHS and the Great Plains Tribal Chairman's Health Board maintain extensive records, data, and documentation of the Indian people they serve, so both are excellent resources for population-specific information.

The Northern Plains Tribal Epidemiology Center (NPTEC) is a component of the GPTCHB, and is one of 12 tribal epidemiology centers funded by the IHS's Division of Epidemiology and Disease Prevention to assist in improving the health of AI/ANs. For a more in-depth look at each tribe served by the GPTCHB (Table 15.1; GPTCHB, 2015b), see their website at http://gptchb.org/.

This chapter will provide a brief history of some of the states, indicating the tribes that reside within each state's boundaries, the current health status of the AIs who live in the states comprising the Northern Great Plains region, some of the resources available to them, or the lack thereof, as well as a description and discussion of the disparity of Native nurses and culturally appropriate nursing services in these states. Patient population will be discussed with reference to physical, mental, emotional, and spiritual issues. Finally, the need for more NA nursing students and nurses will be addressed, as well as the need to create a safe, validating learning environment for students that is synchronous with indigenous cultures and worldviews.

SNAPSHOT OF SOME OF THE NORTHERN GREAT PLAINS STATES

North Dakota

A unique feature of North Dakota is that its largest minority population is American Indians (North Dakota Indian Affairs Commission, 2011). North Dakota is still a sparsely populated, rural state with a total population of 672,591 for all races. Currently, 42,996 AIs (including those reporting AI/AN in combination with other races) call North Dakota home—which is 6.4% of the total population (U.S. Census Bureau, 2010)—with 3,917 living within the Fargo–Moorhead Metro area, which is the largest city in the state. The North Dakota Indian Affairs Commission website (www.nd.gov/indianaffairs/?id=37) indicates that more AI people live on the states' four reservations (19,963 or 54.6%—counting those reporting as one race) than those who live off (16,628 or

TABLE 15.1 Great Plains Tribal Chairman's Health Board Membership List

Cheyenne River Sioux Tribe—Cheyenne River Reservation: www.sioux.org

Crow Creek Sioux Tribe—Crow Creek Reservation: www.crowcreekconnections.org

Flandreau Santee Sioux Tribe—Flandreau Reservation: www.fsst.org

Lower Brule Sioux Tribe—Lower Brule Reservation: www.sdtribalrelations.com/lowerbrule.aspx

Mandan, Hidatsa, and Arikara Nation (Three Affiliated Tribes)—Fort Berthold Reservation: www.mhanation.com

Oglala Sioux Tribe—Pine Ridge Reservation: www.oglalalakotanation.org

Omaha Tribe of Nebraska—Omaha Reservation: Omaha-nsn.gov

Ponca Tribe of Nebraska—Ponca Service Delivery Area: www.poncatribe-ne.org

Rosebud Sioux Tribe—Rosebud Reservation: www.rosebudsiouxtribe-nsn.gov

- Sac and Fox Tribe of the Mississippi in Iowa/Meskwaki Nation—Meskwaki Settlement: www.meskwaki.org

- Santee Sioux Tribe of Nebraska—Santee Reservation: www.santeedakota.org

- Sisseton-Wahpeton Oyate of the Lake Traverse Reservation: www.swo-nsn.gov

- Spirit Lake Tribe—Spirit Lake Reservation: www.spiritlakenation.com

- Standing Rock Sioux Tribe—Standing Rock Reservation: www.standingrock.org

- Trenton Indian Service Area http://www.ndstudies.org/resources/IndianStudies/turtlemountain/historical_trenton.html

- Turtle Mountain Band of Chippewa Indians—Turtle Mountain Reservation: tmbci.kkbold.com

- Winnebago Tribe of Nebraska—Winnebago Reservation: www.winnebagotribe.com

- Yankton Sioux Tribe—Yankton Reservation: www.yanktonsiouxtribe.com

Source: GPTCHB (2015b).

45.4%—counting those reporting as one race), *which is different than other states*. Additionally, the AI population (one race) increased by 16.8% from 2000 to 2010, whereas the AI population (one race alone or in combination with one or more other races) increased by 22.1% from 2000 to 2010.

The following are the four tribes in North Dakota: the Turtle Mountain Band of Chippewa Indians; the Mandan, Arikara, and Hidatsa Nation; the Spirit Lake Nation; and the Standing Rock Sioux Tribe, which straddles the states of North and South Dakota. The Sisseton–Wahpeton Oyate Nation also overlaps into South Dakota, but is usually considered one of the tribal groups in South Dakota. The Trenton Indian Service Area, located in the northwest corner of North Dakota, and the northeast section of Montana are affiliated with the Turtle Mountain Band of Chippewa Indians. Trenton has its own governing structure, covering an area that spans approximately 6,200 square miles.

The economic picture in North Dakota is seen through the following statistics from North Dakota Compass, a social indicators project founded by the Center for Social Research at North Dakota State University and Wilder Research. For example, the data for North Dakota show that

- The gross domestic product grew by 9.7%, the highest growth rate for all 50 states since 2009.
- Per capita output is the third best in the nation for working-age adults (16–64) at $104, 809.
- The median household income was $55,759, although Whites averaged $27,000 more than AI/AN households, when averaging data between 2011 and 2013.
- It is second in the nation for yearly percent age of job change, posting 4.4% job growth from July 2014 to July 2015 (North Dakota Compass, 2015).

The economics for North Dakota are some of the best in the United States as a result of the activity of the Bakken Formation, which is producing a million barrels of oil a day (U.S. Energy Information Administration, 2013). Unfortunately, this brings with it many health and welfare issues for North Dakota's Native population.

Oil

A current reality in the northwestern part of the state is an ongoing oil boom. The Bakken Formation covers much of the outer northwest quadrant of North Dakota. There are also areas in Montana and Canada under which this formation lies. Fracking is the means used to extract oil and gas versus drilling into a reservoir. This North Dakota oil field is the largest oil field in the United States (Mason, 2014). This has had a great impact on Fort Berthold especially, where the Three Affiliated Tribes of North Dakota (the Mandan, Hidatsa, and Arikara Tribe) are located. Multiple health and wellness impact problems are on the rise, including drug use, prostitution and sex trafficking, murder, assault, rapes, lack of housing and food for the huge influx of people, and the setting up of "man-camps" (Horwitz, 2014). There have been multiple deaths from the nonstop oil trucks on small reservation roads and only about a 18 tribal police covering just under 1 million acres.

The enrolled individual members of the tribe are not seeing the profits in any real measure from the immense number of barrels of oil being produced. It is a stark example of poverty within riches. These concerns transcend health, health care, safety, security, and welfare. There is an impact on all domains of the person.

Health Care

Health care services consist of 19 Indian Health Service Units and tribally managed service units to provide health care to a four-state region. The Area Office's Service Units include seven hospitals, eight health centers, and several smaller health stations and satellite clinics. The IHS website indicates that each facility incorporates a comprehensive health care delivery system by providing inpatient and outpatient care, and conducts preventive and curative clinics. Tribal involvement is a major objective, with several tribes assuming management of their own health care programs through contractual arrangements with the IHS (IHS, 2015a).

Urban Indians living in the metropolitan areas of North Dakota are especially hard hit because there are virtually no health care provisions in place for them, either through the IHS, Urban Indian health centers, or clinics, although they mirror the same disparities experienced by other tribal groups across the country. Further impacting this dire situation is the fact that Title V Maternal and Child Health funding is not available for North Dakota's urban Native people. Nationally, AI/AN infant mortality rates in 2007 to 2009 were 26% higher than the U.S. all-races rate (6.6%) for 2008. Essentially, urban AIs have greater need, but much less or no access to services (IHS, 2015b).

South Dakota

This state is notable for having one of the highest population percentages of AI/ANs in the United States. South Dakota has nine federally recognized Nations and reservations within its borders. These are: (a) the Cheyenne River, (b) Crow Creek, (c) Flandreau Santee, (d) Lower Brule, (e) Pine Ridge, (f) Rosebud, (g) Sisseton Wahpeton, (h) Standing Rock, and (i) Yankton Nations (see map at www.sdtribalrelations.com/maptribes.aspx; South Dakota Department of Tribal Government Relations [SDDTGR], 2015). Additionally, nonreservation areas, such as Rapid City, have high concentrations of AI/ANs.

Population

- The total population estimated for South Dakota in 2014 was about 853,000.
- The percentage of AI/ANs, reporting as one race, was 8.9% for 2013 as compared with 1.2% in the United States—*this is one of the largest percentages of AI/ANs in a state,* where the norm is 1% or less (U.S. Census Bureau, 2015).

Not only are state percentages high for AI/ANs in South Dakota, but there are about twice as many AI/ANs by number as found even in North Dakota.

Indian Health Service health care for AI/ANs in South Dakota is still under the aegis of the Aberdeen Area Office (now Great Plains) as in North Dakota. The Aberdeen offices for the Administrative Region are based in South Dakota. South Dakota facilities include the Cheyenne River Sioux Tribe–Eagle Butte Hospital, the Fort Thompson Indian Health Center, the Great Plains Area Youth Regional Treatment Center for youth age 13 to 17, Lower Brule Indian Health Center, Pine Ridge Hospital, Rapid City Indian Hospital, Rosebud Hospital, Woodrow Wilson Keeble Memorial Health Care Center, and the Yankton Service Unit. Some are hospitals, some are clinics run by service units, or satellite health care services.

Two well-known reservations in South Dakota are the Pine Ridge and Rosebud Lakota reservations. Pine Ridge will be highlighted here. The people of Pine Ridge are the Oglala Lakota. Both historic and fairly modern conflicts occurred at the Wounded Knee site on the Pine Ridge reservation, the first being in 1890, the Battle of Wounded Knee, where 200 to 300 men, women, and children were killed by U.S. soldiers in what is often referred to as the Wounded Knee Massacre (Greene, 2014). The book, *Bury My Heart at Wounded Knee: An Indian History of the American West*, has become an American classic (Brown & Sides, 2007). This book told of these events for the first time from the Indian perspective, facing east, where the influx of Europeans came from (Brown & Sides, 2007). Usual histories were told by Europeans heading/facing/conquering the west. Brown felt it important to change perspectives in every way.

In 1973, there was the Wounded Knee Incident, a 71-day armed stand-off between Indian activists and the federal government. Well-known American Indian Movement (AIM) activists, such as Russell Means and Dennis Banks, were a part of this incident. A U.S. marshall was paralyzed, two AIs were killed, and another was unaccounted for until a halt was called (The Learning Network, 2015).

With these types of ongoing conflicts between the Lakota and the U.S. government, historical trauma has played a major role in the health and welfare outcomes for these people. *Historical trauma* refers to the unresolved grief of atrocities visited upon your ancestors that effects on you today (Brave Heart, 1995). These can and do hit all four domains of health—physical, spiritual, mental, and emotional. Further, with alcoholism, accidents, poverty, housing, employment, and education challenges, this particular reservation has some of the worst health outcomes and life expectancies of AI/ANs in the nation. Youth suicides have assumed epidemic proportions, life expectancies are the worst in the nation, and, in fact, in the Western Hemisphere, variously reported as being in the 40s and 50s (males at the lower end; Kavanagh, Absalom, Beil, & Schliessmann, 1999; McLeigh, 2010).

Over 10 years ago, the U.S. Commission on Civil Rights (2004) published a devastating report on AIs that included statistics on Pine Ridge, where unemployment was at 80%, and two out of three people were living beneath the poverty level. In comparison, from the same report in 2004, the national poverty rate was 7.5%. This is a huge discrepancy. Little has changed in the ensuing 11 years.

Health Disparity

In 2015, there are still unimaginable disparities in predictors of health. Suicides in South Dakota are double for AI/ANs as compared with non-Hispanic Whites (NHW); death from unintentional injuries is almost four times greater for AI/ANs, diabetes has trebled, and infectious diseases—influenza and pneumonia—are over 2½ times greater (Office of Women's Health [OWH], 2012; see Table 15.2).

TABLE 15.2 South Dakota Health Disparities Comparing AI/AN (Largest State Minority) and Non-Hispanic White Death Rates per 100,000

STATE		NON-HISPANIC WHITE	AMERICAN INDIAN/ ALASKAN NATIVE	HEALTHY PEOPLE 2020 NATIONAL TARGET	STATE RANK
South Dakota	Population (2012) (all ages)	84.8	9.5		
South Dakota	All cause	678.7	1,317.2	+	17
South Dakota	Heart disease	151.7	205.9	+	17
South Dakota	Coronary heart disease	118.1	173.0	100.8	32
South Dakota	Total cancer	168.4	242.8	160.6	22
South Dakota	Colorectal cancer	17.0	*	14.5	35
South Dakota	Lung cancer	44.5	63.5	45.5	20
South Dakota	Stroke	39.7	52.1	33.8	29
South Dakota	Chronic obstructive pulmonary disease (age 45 & over)	123.8	193.1	98.5	30
South Dakota	Diabetes-related	72.3	266.4	65.8	38
South Dakota	Influenza and pneumonia	14.9	40.0	+	28
South Dakota	Unintentional injuries	37.3	126.8	36	40
South Dakota	Suicide	15.5	31.0	10.2	45
South Dakota	Diagnosed high blood pressure (2011)	28.6	39.9	26.9	23
South Dakota	Obesity (2012) (age 20 & over)	27.7	36.9	30.6	27
South Dakota	No leisure-time physical activity (2012)	21.2	30.0	32.6	23
South Dakota	Smoking currently (2012)	19.4	53.1	12	37
South Dakota	Eats 5+ fruits and vegetables a day (2009)	15.2	16.5	+	53
South Dakota	Cholesterol screening in past 5 years (2011)	71.3	63.2	82.1	39

(continued)

TABLE 15.2 South Dakota Health Disparities Comparing AI/AN (Largest State Minority) and Non-Hispanic White Death Rates per 100,000 (*continued*)

STATE		NON-HISPANIC WHITE	AMERICAN INDIAN/ ALASKAN NATIVE	HEALTHY PEOPLE 2020 NATIONAL TARGET	STATE RANK
South Dakota	Routine check—up in past 2 years (2012)	78.3	76.9	+	34
South Dakota	Dental visit within the past year (2012)	73.2	59.5	+	9
South Dakota	Health insurance coverage (2012; ages 18–64)	86.4	89.6	100	9

Optimism

At the center of all of the devastating numbers are people. A return to traditionalism, and/or the continued use and practice of indigenous ways is important in maintaining health and optimism in the face of so many negative social and structural determinants of health. A pictorial of some of the context and practices of Pine Ridge can be found in the "Useful Websites" section at the end of this chapter.

Iowa

The Winnebago Hospital (WBH) is part of the Great Plains Area Office, IHS, and is located in Winnebago, Nebraska, which is 20 minutes south of Sioux City Iowa and a 1-hour drive from Omaha, Nebraska. The WBH serves tribally enrolled members in the tri-state area that includes Nebraska, Iowa, and South Dakota. These tribes are the Winnebago Tribe, Omaha Tribe, and the Santee Sioux Tribe. There were approximately 14,043 Native Americans and Alaska Natives (AI/AN) living in Iowa in 2011, with the AI population expected to increase to 17,300 by 2040 (State Data Center of Iowa). Nearly half, or 44.8%, of the total AI/AN population live in Woodbury, Polk, and Tama counties, whereas another 38.5% live in the five urban cities of Sioux City, Des Moines, Davenport, Cedar Rapids, and Council Bluffs, according to the 2010 Census. As many as 2,254 AI/ANs (20.3%) live in Woodbury County, more than in any other Iowa county, making it more diverse than the state as a whole. The Regional Workforce and Economic Development Status Report (June 2013) found that Iowa is the least racially diverse state among the benchmarks referenced in the statewide report (Kansas, Minnesota, Missouri, and Nebraska), and is far less racially diverse than the nation as a whole. The report cites statistics to show that the State of Iowa has over 91% of its population reporting as White, compared with 74.1% nationwide. For a more in-depth snapshot of Iowa please refer to the Iowa Data Center (2012).

Montana

Montana is a sparsely populated state with nearly 1 million residents living in a geographical area of nearly 146,000 square miles. The metropolitan areas of Montana consist of only seven cities with more than 20,000 residents, and only 15 cities with 5,000 to 20,000 residents (The Census and Economic Information Center [CEIC], 2014). American Indians tend to live in the more rural areas of the state, with only 18% living in one of the seven cities of 20,000 or more as indicated in the 2010 Census, and only 5% living in cities of 5,000 to 19,999, compared with 36% and 11%, respectively, of White residents.

With the majority of Montana's AI population living in rural, more isolated areas of the state where employment, health insurance, and access to most resources are more likely to be limited, it is not surprising that more than one third of AI residents live below the federally defined poverty level, compared with only 13% of White residents. American Indian residents experience almost three times the unemployment rate that prevails among White residents, and more than twice as many lack health insurance coverage.

The culture of poverty that exists for Montana's AIs is responsible for poorer health, higher disease rates, lower life expectancy, and greater difficulty obtaining health care. Nearly 40% of Montana's AIs are uninsured and are ineligible for Indian Health Service care because they do not live on a reservation and/or are not a member of a federally recognized tribe. According to a recent news release in the *Montana Gazette* (May 25, 2014), many who do have access to IHS do not receive comprehensive health care; instead, they must deal with severe underfunding and understaffing, as well as long wait lists and rationed care. Because many AI people are unable to receive needed care, life span as well as quality of life are severely compromised. For example, White men in Montana live 19 years longer than AI men (until 75 years of age compared with 56 years of age). White women live 20 years longer than AI women (until 82 years of age compared with 62 years of age). In addition, for all but suicide, the mortality rates for each of the leading causes of death were lower for White residents than for AI residents. American Indian elderly often have a cultural/spiritual tenet against suicide as they must follow the path laid out for them (Moss, 2000), as opposed to the White population, in which suicide among the elderly is significant.

The leading cause of death and the biggest killer of adults in Montana is cardiovascular disease, with 11% of White residents and 14% of AI residents reporting a diagnosis of coronary artery disease, a history of heart attack, or a history of stroke. More than a quarter of Montana's residents reported being diagnosed with high blood pressure, and more than a third reported being diagnosed with high serum cholesterol. Additionally, being overweight or obese increased the risk factors for nearly two thirds of White respondents and more than three quarters of AI respondents. Smoking compounded these risk factors incrementally for AIs, who had substantially higher smoking rates than White residents.

According to the Montana Central Tumor Registry Annual Report (2010), cancer is the second leading cause of death in Montana, with an average of

5,000 new cases diagnosed each year (Department of Public Health and Human Services, Montana, 2010). The most common types of cancer are lung (15%), breast (14%), and colorectal cancer (10%), which mirror the incidence nationally, accounting for more than half of all newly diagnosed cancers. American Indian residents of Montana, because of a higher prevalence of smoking, have substantially higher incidence rates of lung cancer than White residents. American Indian residents also have higher incidence rates of colorectal, kidney, liver, and stomach cancers. Higher incidence rates of colorectal cancer may be attributed to notably lower participation in screening. The higher incidence rate of liver cancer may be caused by a higher prevalence of cirrhosis of the liver and hepatitis for AI patients.

Federally Recognized Tribes of Montana

- Assiniboine and Sioux Tribes, Fort Peck Indian Reservation
- Blackfeet Tribe, Blackfeet Indian Reservation
- Chippewa–Cree Indians, Rocky Boy's Reservation
- Confederated Salish and Kootenai Tribes, Flathead Reservation
- Crow Tribe
- Fort Belknap Indian Community, Fort Belknap Reservation
- Northern Cheyenne Tribe, Northern Cheyenne Indian Reservation

Minnesota

The American Indians of the Northern Great Plains in Minnesota overlap with those of the Northeast Woodlands area and will not be discussed in depth in this section, although some of the tribes and their practices are found in both areas.

The federally recognized tribes of the Great Plains are:

- Lower Sioux Indian Community
- Minnesota Chippewa Tribe, including
  - Bois Forte Band (Nett Lake)
  - Grand Portage
  - Leech Lake
  - Mille Lacs band
  - White Earth
- Prairie Island Indian Community
- Red Lake Band of Chippewa Indians
- Shakopee Mdewakanton Sioux
- Upper Sioux Community
- Crossing state Lines—Ho-Chunk Nation of Wisconsin

Health Resources

A number of public health care programs include funding specifically set aside to meet the needs of American Indians in Minnesota. For example, the state

Consolidated Chemical Dependency Treatment Fund formula includes allocations for American Indians living on and off reservations. The federal Alcohol, Drug Abuse, and Mental Health block grant includes an allocation for AI services. The state law establishing community health boards authorizes special grants to these boards to provide services to American Indians living off reservations. These grants are administered by the Minnesota Department of Health and are awarded on a competitive basis. Current grantees serve the Bemidji area: Duluth, Minneapolis, and St. Paul.

NORTHERN GREAT PLAINS OVERALL

"Problems at the U.S. Department of Veterans Affairs medical centers get much attention, but similar stories of neglect at IHS clinics go virtually unnoticed" ("Resolve problems at the IHS," 2014, para 1).

Montana has had a higher poverty rate than the adjacent states of Idaho, North Dakota, South Dakota, and Wyoming since 2000 (Haynes & Young, 2011). AI/AN males suffer inordinately from a combination of increased burden of illness and lack of utilization of health care services. Programs targeted at anomie, loss of traditional male roles, violence, and alcoholism are among the most urgently needed. American Indian/Alaska Native males' death rates exceed those of AI/AN females for every age up to 75 years, and account for six of the eight leading causes of death. Accidents, suicide, and homicide are epidemic among AI/AN males. "Paradoxically, AI/AN males account for only 37.9% of outpatient visits, versus 62.1% for females, and only 47% of hospitalizations excluding childbirth" (Rhoades, 2003, p. 774).

As we have learned in previous chapters, the mortality rates for AI/AN due to alcoholism, tuberculosis, diabetes, injuries, and suicides, are all negatively disproportionate to rates seen in the United States for all races. This hold true on the Great and Northern Plains. "In trying to account for the disparities, health care experts, policymakers, and tribal leaders are looking at many factors that impact upon the health of Indian people, including the adequacy of funding for the Indian health care delivery system" (Indian Health Service, 2015c, para 6). For a discussion on American Indian public health disparities and regional differences in health, please see the presentation of AI physician Dr. Donald Warne at Public Health Live @ www.youtube.com/watch?v=Wk1PdA_CJ-Y

WORLDVIEW AND HEALTH PERSPECTIVE

In order to provide care for an indigenous person, is it imperative to know his or her worldview and understand how to respond to questions such as: How do you walk upon the earth? What relationships are vital to your well-being? How do you view life? What is the meaning of life? What are your perceptions and beliefs surrounding death? What does it mean to be sick? What does it mean to die? Why do some tribal groups refuse to talk about death? Is it because they know that our thoughts and words hold enough power to bring about manifestation? What does it mean when something is sacred? Is our health and well-being considered sacred, and is our connection to the land and Mother Earth a sacred relationship? Can effective nursing care be provided to a person if the caregiver has no knowledge and/or respect for people who hold a vastly different worldview? Did anyone ever ask?

The next sections will discuss some of the practices and beliefs that keep the AI/AN people going, bolster their resilience, and maintain traditions.

NATIVE NURSES CARING FOR THEIR OWN

A Native nurse, connected to the indigenous worldview, is intrinsically going to focus on the heart or spirit of her or his patient. He or she will know that the physical manifestation of all illness is basically an expression of what is out of balance there. This imbalance or disconnection resides at or within the core of the problem, and the patient can be guided back to the heart/soul connection and be able to voice not only what is broken, but how it broke, and what it will take to fix it. The effective AI/AN nurse will be able to blend aspects of indigenous healing and tenets of professional nursing care to bring about optimum spiritual, emotional, and physical and mental health outcomes.

NURSES CARING FOR AI/AN PATIENTS ON THE PLAINS

As within the other cultural groups, there are histories, environmental and social circumstances, beliefs, and practices that all play into the population's health and well-being. This is true of the Plains Area. By now you have seen that the Plains covers a great expanse in the middle of the country and overlaps with almost every other area (refer to the cultural area map at the beginning of Part II). This chapter focuses on the northern areas of the Plains, but tribes of the Great Plains, their practices, cultures, and languages overlap into almost all other areas.

The same federal policies and, later, state policies have affected how, where, and when AI/ANs receive care in the Great Plains areas. There are, as you have read, many IHS facilities, such as hospitals, clinics, and health stations, throughout the Plains. Nurses may encounter issues that are unique to this area and some that are shared with the general AI/AN population when caring for AI/ANs of the Northern Great Plains, whether on the reservation, in border towns, or in more urban areas (Figure 15.2).

Throughout this text, we have discussed the four domains of the person and the physical, mental, spiritual, and emotional aspects of health. Indigenous cultural/religious/medicine practices carried on in the Plains are equally identifiable from each other in many cases. In thinking about parts of the person, practices and environment should not be separated from the whole or from each other.

Some of the cultural practices found in this vast area may have been indigenous to the Plains or may have been adopted over the centuries. Therefore, nurses practicing in this region would be wise to have at least an understanding of some of the practices they may encounter that may have health implications before, during, and after contact with the health care system. Practices

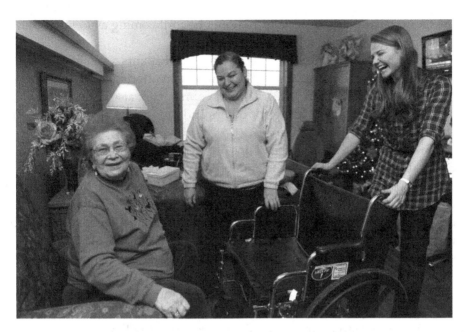

FIGURE 15.2 Caring for a tribal elder. Pictured is Ms. Louise Crosby, Dr. Donna Grandbois's mother, with two nursing students—Sharon Whitebear (*middle*) and Elizabeth Uglestad (*right*).
Courtesy of Donna M. Grandbois.

may include the Sun Dance (and flesh offerings), sweats, smudging, the four medicines, and Wiping of the Tears.

Over 13 years ago, the American Association of American Indian Physicians voted unanimously to approve "a resolution acknowledging and supporting Native American traditional healing and medicines *as part of the spectrum of health care* appropriate for Native Americans" (U.S. Commission on Civil Rights, 2004, p. 40; emphasis ours). Some of these practices or concepts have been discussed in previous chapters. They are laid out here in the context of the Plains.

Certainly not unique to the Plains but prominent in this area is the Sun Dance ceremony that occurs in the summer, usually around the solstice. To participate in a Sun Dance is a commitment. In some instances, this is a 4-year commitment to dance each of those years. During a Sun Dance, the participant will go to the designated grounds, fast during this time, pray, and abstain from alcohol. He or she will be there for 4 days. This may include participation that involves piercing in the pectoral region for males, and if females, piercing in the shoulders. It is important to understand what Sun Dance participants are going through physically, spiritually, mentally, and emotionally.

Nurses in the area may encounter a patient who presents to the health care system during Sun Dance as a result of dehydration, low blood sugar, or asthma (from smoking a pipe or fires in the area). Following these religious practices, either soon or thereafter, nurses may notice scars on patients that would have resulted from the piercings. It is likely that nurses coming into this area may not be familiar with either the practice or any health implications (see Box 15.1). Participants and leaders often had to hide this practice until 1978 and the emergence of the American Indian Religious Freedom Act (AIRFA, 1978), and, therefore, some of the older participants, especially, may not be forthcoming as to what they were participating in that led to the health encounter.

There may also be flesh offerings from participants, or helpers, in which a small part of the flesh is given to the Creator as an offering at the tree designated for the Sun Dance (Figure 15.3). This, of course, may also result in an injury or scarring. Offering up suffering for others and one's body to the Creator are the spiritual bases for the Sun Dance.

Sweats are also used on the Plains. Every sweat is different, even within one reservation. A sweat lodge is a rounded, low structure with an area in the center for stones (called the grandfathers) that have been heated to extreme temperatures on a fire outside and then brought in (Figure 15.4). Sweats are used for purification, talking to the Creator in direct connection, and being close to the ancestors. They can occur once a week or more or less often. There may be sweats for women only, men only, or both genders. Prayer and songs are key to the sweats. Some songs are meant only for the sweat.

During the sweat, a person will be on the outside watching the door and helping. Participants may need to leave or may wish to return. Participants sit in a circle in the structure around the fire to pray. It will become extremely hot, and participants stay in for varying amounts of time. They can be in there for an hour or more. Various indigenous medicines can be used, depending on the

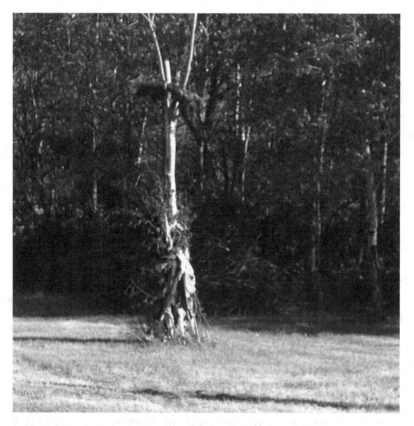

FIGURE 15.3 Sun Dance grounds 2015—tree of life.

BOX 15.1 Sun Dance Patient/Case Study

Ms. B, tribal elder of the Turtle Mountain Band of the Chippewa Tribe had committed to dance. It was her third year. She helped with cooking for other community members and helpers, but she herself was fasting. She was a 65-year-old diabetic female, was intensely religious, and had fully committed to completing the ceremony. It was a spiritual need.

Around the fourth and last day of the ceremony, Ms. B. started sweating and shaking and had to seek help for low blood sugar. Still on the grounds of the Sun Dance, she was given traditional medicine—maple syrup. This did relieve her, yet she finally needed to go to the clinic as she became dehydrated. She had been able to complete her religious/spiritual commitment, which to her was the most important thing.

Nurses practicing in the Plains cultural area should be aware of the cultural practices needed for spiritual and emotional health but that may impact physical health, which is seen as less important, especially to elders.

What might the nurse taking care of Ms. B ask in order to fully understand what she had just completed and what other problems may result?

leader and his or her particular gifts. However, because of the smoke from the fire, the heat, the enclosed dark area, and the time factor, there may be physical/mental implications. If participants have asthma or high blood pressure, or are elderly, young, or anxious, care must be taken in deciding whether to participate and for how long. Nurses practicing in this region should be aware of the processes and conditions.

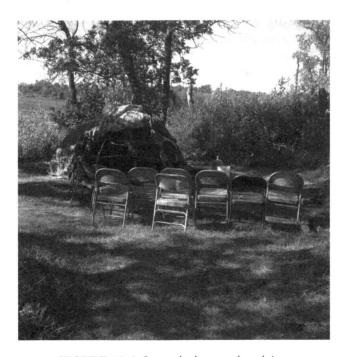

FIGURE 15.4 Sweat lodge on the plains.

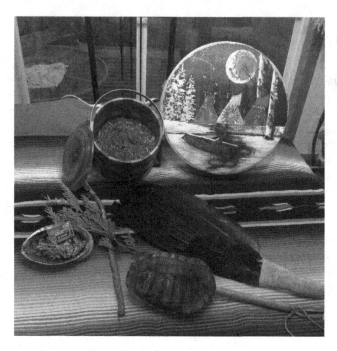

FIGURE 15.5 Smudging tools and the four medicines.

The four medicines: (1) cedar, (2) tobacco, (3) sage, and (4) sweet grass will play into the practices and traditions and everyday life of many on the Plains. For example, they will be used in the sweats or for smudging. In smudging, a vessel (maybe a shell) is used to hold one or more of the medicines (Figure 15.5). These are burned in the shell to produce smoke. The participant is then "washed" with the medicinal smoke by bringing it toward his or her body and washing it over his or her head and torso using a waving motion of the arms and hands. This can be done alone or with someone guiding the smoke, usually with a feather.

Nurses working in this cultural area may encounter a Native patient who has cedar in her or his shoes. This is a protective measure, and likely not something seen in the general population. Most traditional or culturally active persons will offer tobacco. This will be given to elders as a mark of respect and honor, or outdoors as a token of thanksgiving, or for other reasons as appropriate. Tobacco is also used in pipe ceremonies. People smoke to talk with spirits and the Creator. But again, some of these practices may have implications for asthmatics. Nurses need to be aware, as once again, patients may not necessarily want to talk in depth about the traditional practices.

The Wiping of the Tears is a ceremony focusing on emotional and spiritual well-being (in addition to the always connected mental and physical wellness). A medicine man will pray and sing with you as you call on or pray to the ancestors to help heal the participant experiencing physical pain, but, more often, spiritual and emotional pain. Such ceremonies have been held annually at the Wounded Knee site, at the site of the World Trade Center, with returning veterans, and in individual ceremonies.

In many IHS facilities, there may be procedures in place to allow for smudging and use of traditional medicine. Usually, the patient can ask for this. Many nurses in the IHS are not Natives or even from the area, and may not be familiar with cultural and religious or other indigenous practices.

NEED FOR MORE NATIVE AMERICAN NURSING STUDENTS

"While African Americans, Hispanic Americans, and Native Americans represent more than 25 percent of the U.S. population, they comprise fewer than 9 percent of nurses, 6 percent of physicians, and only 5 percent of dentists" (Cooper & Powe, 2004, p. 21). The Plains area does have more programs for Native nurses than the rest of the country. These are in tribal colleges, at the University of North Dakota, and North Dakota State University, to name a few. However, the student numbers, especially at the tribal schools, can be quite low. Some of these programs are discussed in Chapter 18 on nursing education.

There is also a need to prepare Native nurses in areas outside of Indian country. Continuity between providers and patients assists in better communication, flow of processes, and, in some cases, health outcomes (Cooper & Powe, 2004).

Non-Native nurses necessarily play a role in the care of AI/AN patients, especially now that 78% of AI/ANs are off reservation. Therefore, incorporating AI/AN cultural, historical, and political concerns that affect health outcomes and health care access into nursing programs can only assist in "closing the gap" on some of the more egregious disparities suffered by AI/ANs in the United States.

NANAINA

A word about the National Alaska Native American Indian Nurses Association (NANAINA). Although not specific to the Plains, this region of the country has high percentages and numbers of AI/ANs, and it is important to recognize that there exists an association of Native nurses. Their mission is stated thusly: "NANAINA unites American Indian/Alaska Native (AI/AN) nurses and those who care for AI/AN people to improve the health and well-being of AI/AN people" (NANAINA, 2015, para. 3). This would be an organization where nurses, Native (full members, students, or retired) and non-Native (associate), can learn about best practices and share research and scholarship. It is led by Native nurses with an interest and commitment in carrying out the mission (see more at http://nanainanurses.org/).

CONCLUSIONS

The Great Plains area is unique to the country and nursing in several ways. It is an expanse that goes through the middle of the country, touching many of the other Native cultural groups save Alaska and California. There are urban areas that will also include any Alaska Natives who have come to the "lower 48." Therefore, overlap of cultures, languages, histories, and origins will be a feature of this area.

This chapter focused on the Northern Plains to capture many unique features of the population in this area. Some of these are that North Dakota and South Dakota have AI/ANs as their largest minority population, in contrast to the national level, where AI/ANs are usually the smallest minority, around 1%. In South Dakota, about one in 10 people is Native. This is a large Native population as compared with many other states. In North Dakota, most AI/ANs are on reservations, whereas nationally most AI/ANs live off reservations.

These statistics will have implications for health provision by nurses. First, nurses will be more likely to encounter a Native patient in the Dakotas than they would if practicing in many other parts of the United States. Therefore, nurses should be aware of some of the unique practices of the people they may encounter, which might have health implications. They also need to know not just health outcomes, which are at times staggering for this population, but the context of life and history of this population.

Nursing schools in the Plains (and elsewhere) should have targeted coursework on the unique features of AI/ANs and their implications for nurses. In the

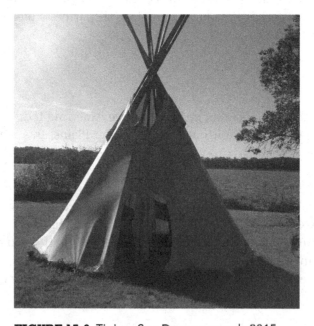

FIGURE 15.6 Tipi on Sun Dance grounds 2015.

Plains, nurses should at least be familiar with the Sun Dance, sweats, smudging, the four medicines, and ceremonies such as the Wiping of Tears. Nurses, as advocates for all of their patients, need to be at the forefront in making sure their AI/AN patients can feel free to request assistance in participating in those practices that are culturally appropriate within a health care setting (smudging, prayers, fasting, visits by traditional healers), or assistance in how best to safely participate in these practices outside of the health care setting (if they have asthma, high blood pressure, anxiety, diabetes, or are elderly, for example).

American Indians often hold a holistic, spiritually grounded worldview that stipulates that a multidimensional connection exists among all aspects of life, and their ability to heal must be supported by a health care system that incorporates these beliefs (Figure 15.6). Nurses can be at the forefront of this advocacy need.

STUDY QUESTIONS

◆ Name three ways in which AI/AN population statistics found in the Northern Plains states are different from populations found nationally. What would be the impact on nursing?

◆ Go to the recommended website, Photographs of Pine Ridge by Aaron Huey. Discuss what you found most surprising about the context of life for this tribe. How will that affect their health, either positively or negatively?

◆ As a nurse, how would you go about advocating permitting (in house) or assisting in access to a traditional indigenous practice for your patient as "part of the spectrum of health care appropriate for Native Americans."

USEFUL WEBSITES

Agency for Health Care and Quality National Healthcare Disparities Reports, 2003–2010 http://www.ahrq.gov/qual/measurix.htm

Center for Rural Health, University of North Dakota, http://ruralhealth.und.edu/

Great Plains Tribal Chairman's Health Board (GPTCHB), http://gptchb.org/

Institute of Medicine Report of Unequal Treatment: Confronting Racial and Ethnic Disparities in Health Care, Report Briefs and Slide presentations, http://www.iom.edu/Reports/2002/Unequal-Treatment-Confronting-Racial-and-Ethnic-Disparities-in-Health-Care.aspx

NANAINA, http://nanainanurses.org/

National Cancer Institute, http://surveillance.cancer.gov/statistics/types/race_ethnic.html

Northern Plains Tribal Epidemiology Center (NPTEC), http://nptec.gptchb.org/

Photographs of Pine Ridge by Aaron Huey, http://www.slate.com/blogs/behold/2014/02/20/aaron_huey_photographs_the_pine_ridge_reservation_in_south_dakota_in_his.html

Racial and Ethnic Disparities in North Dakota, http://www.national-consortium.org/~/media/Microsites/Files/National%20Consortium/06012012-ND-Commission-to-Study-Racial-and-Ethnic-Bias-in-the-Courts.ashx

RECOMMENDED READINGS

Eschiti, V. S. (2004). Holistic approach to resolving American Indian/Alaska Native health care disparities. *Journal of Holistic Nursing*, 22(3), 200–208.

Grandbois, D. M., Warne, D., & Eschiti, V. (2012). The impact of history and culture on nursing care of Native American elders. *Journal of Gerontological Nursing, 38*(10), 3–5.

McGibbon, E., Etowa, J., & McPherson, C. (2008). Health care access as a social determinant of health. *Canadian Nurse, 104*(7), 22–27.

Moss, M. P. (2005). TOLERATED ILLNESS™ concept and theory for chronically ill and elderly patients as exemplified in American Indians. *Journal of Cancer Education, 20*(S1), 17–22.

REFERENCES

American Indian Religious Freedom Act, Pub. L. No. 95-341, 92 Stat. 469 (1978).

Brave Heart, M. Y. H. (1995). *The return to the sacred path: Healing from historical trauma and historical unresolved grief among the Lakota* (Unpublished doctoral dissertation). Smith College, Northampton, MA.

Brown, D., & Sides, H. (2007). *Bury my heart at Wounded Knee: An Indian history of the American west.* New York, NY: Macmillan.

Census and Economic Information Center (CEIC). (2014). *Population demographics.* Montana Department of Commerce. Retrieved July 27, 2015, from http://ceic.mt .gov/Population/PopulationProjections.aspx

Cooper, L. A., & Powe, N. R. (2004). *Disparities in patient experiences, health care processes, and outcomes: The role of patient–provider racial, ethnic, and language concordance.* Retrieved July 29, 2015, from http://www.commonwealthfund.org/programs/ minority/cooper_raceconcordance_753.pdf

Department of Public Health and Human Services, Montana. (2010). *Tumor registry.* Retrieved July 27, 2015, from http://dphhs.mt.gov/publichealth/cancer/ tumorregistry

The Great Plains Tribal Chairman's Health Board. (2015a). *Mission, vision, values.* Retrieved July 11, 2015, from http://gptchb.org/mission-vision-values/

The Great Plains Tribal Chairman's Health Board. (2015b). *Member tribes.* Retrieved July 11, 2015, from http://gptchb.org/member-tribes/

Greene, J. A. (2014). *American carnage: Wounded Knee, 1890.* Norman, OK: University of Oklahoma Press.

Haynes, G., & Young, D. (2011). *Montana poverty report card, December 2011.* Montana Department of Public Health & Human Services, Montana State University Extension. Retrieved July, 1, 2014, from http://www.montana.edu/wwwextec/countydata/ statewidereportdec2011.pdf

Horwitz, S. (2014). Dark side of the boom. *The Washington Post.* Retrieved July 11, 2015, from http://www.washingtonpost.com/sf/national/2014/09/28/dark-side-of- the-boom/

Indian Health Service. (2014). *Tribal leader letters from Yvette Roubideaux, newsroom.* Retrieved July 27, 2015, from http://www.ihs.gov/newsroom/triballeaderletters/

Indian Health Service. (2015a). *Great Plains area.* Retrieved from https://www.ihs.gov/ greatplains/

Indian Health Service. (2015b). *Trends in Indian health 2014 edition.* Retrieved July 23, 2015, from https://www.ihs.gov/dps/index.cfm/publications/trends2014/

Indian Health Service (2015c). *Disparities.* Retrieved from https://www.ihs.gov/ newsroom/factsheets/disparities/

Iowa Data Center. (2012). *Native Americans in Iowa: November, 2012.* Retrieved from http://www.iowadatacenter.org/Publications/aian2013.pdf

Kavanagh, K., Absalom, K., Beil, W. J., & Schliessmann, L. (1999). Connecting and becoming culturally competent: A Lakota example. *Advances in Nursing Science, 21*(3), 9–31.

The Learning Network. (2015). *Standoff at Wounded Knee comes to an end, May 8, 1973—The New York Times*. Retrieved July 8, 2015, from http://learning.blogs.nytimes.com/2012/05/08/may-8-1973-standoff-at-wounded-knee-comes-to-an-end/?_r=1

Mason, J. (2014). *Oil production potential of the North Dakota Bakken*. Retrieved July 27, 2015, from http://www.researchgate.net/profile/James_Mason12/publication/265289072_Oil_Production_Potential_of_the_North_Dakota_Bakken/links/5438d38f0cf2d6698bdeda8e.pdf

McLeigh, J. (2010). What are the policy issues related to the mental health of Native Americans? *American Journal of Orthopsychiatry, 80*(2), 177–182. doi:10.1111/j.1939-0025.2010.01021.x/full

Moss, M. P. (2000). *Zuni elders: Ethnography of American Indian aging* (Unpublished doctoral dissertation). Texas Medical Center, Houston, TX.

National Alaska Native American Indian Nurses Association. (2015). *About us—Mission*. Retrieved July 29, 2015, from http://nanainanurses.org/

North Dakota Compass. (2015). *Economy—Overview*. Retrieved July 8, 2015, from http://www.ndcompass.org/economy/#.VZyxgEbe8Zy

North Dakota Indian Affairs Commission. (2011). *Statistics and data*. Retrieved July 27, 2015, from http://www.nd.gov/indianaffairs/?id=37

Office of Women's Health. (2012). *State profile*. Retrieved July, 29, 2015, from http://www.healthstatus2020.com/disparities/ChartBookData_list.asp

Resolve problems at the IHS [Editorial]. (2014, July 30). *Rapid City Journal*. Retrieved from http://rapidcityjournal.com/news/opinion/editorial-resolve-problems-at-the-ihs/article_e3d82830-ddd4-525c-8984-f96109a5e6d1.html

Rhoades, E. R. (2003). The health status of American Indian and Alaska Native males. *American Journal of Public Health, 93*(5), 774–778.

South Dakota Department of Tribal Government Relations. (2015). *Location of reservations*. Retrieved July 8, 2015, from http://www.sdtribalrelations.com/maptribes.aspx

U.S. Census Bureau. (2015). *South Dakota: QuickFacts*. Retrieved July 8, 2015, from http://quickfacts.census.gov/qfd/states/46000.html

U.S. Commission on Civil Rights. (2004). *Broken promises: Evaluating the Native American health care system*. Washington, DC: Author.

U.S. Energy Information Administration. (2013). *Bakken oil production forecast to top 1 million barrels per day next month—Today in energy*. Washington, DC: Author. Retrieved July 28, 2015, 2015, from http://www.eia.gov/todayinenergy/detail.cfm?id=13811

SIXTEEN

Urban American Indians

Lisa Martin and Margaret P. Moss

LEARNING OBJECTIVES

- To be able to describe what factors help form urban Indian identity
- To compare and contrast social context for urban Indians with those in Indian country
- To identify differences in access to care for Urban American Indians and those in Indian country
- To distinguish between where services are needed and where services are available for urban Indian elders
- To be able to identify three conditions that are part of the environment of most American Indian adolescents today
- To be able to state two reasons why Type 2 diabetes is occurring earlier in life and give three examples of possible health complications adolescents face with early diagnosis
- To be able to describe three areas to include in the development of culturally respectful health care for American Indian adolescents

KEY TERMS

- Assimilation
- Belmont report
- Blood quantum
- Cultural safety
- Holism
- Linear
- Mobilization
- Oppression
- Relational
- Reservation
- Stressor
- Tribal enrollment
- Type 2 diabetes

KEY CONCEPTS

- Critical theory
- Migration and remigration
- Mixed-methods research
- Modern diet
- Patterns of residency
- Relocation and assimilation programs
- Tribe-specific data
- Worldview

This chapter, which is the last in Part II, provides nurses with needed information on the 10th and final "cultural group" in this text—*urban* American Indians (UAI). It was important to add this nongeographic yet "place-oriented" population of American Indians and Alaska Natives (AI/ANs) so the nurse can understand both the shared and distinguishing characteristics and issues that may impact health and acquisition of health care for UAI. The importance of looking at this group apart from their natal, indigenous, or familial root places stems from the fact that now 78% of AI/ANs live off reservations (U.S. Census, 2012), with a large proportion of these individuals considered to be residing in urban settings. Others may live off the reservation in rural, suburban, frontier, or other census designations besides urban.

The chapter introduces the special issues of UAI, their shared histories with other AI/ANs, and federal policies especially impacting UAI. There is a discussion on UAI elders and urban migration, followed by a focus on adolescents and issues around type 2 diabetes in particular. Adolescents are greatly impacted in cities owing to poor school outcomes, lack of health services, inner city food deserts, and isolation from cultural roles and relationships, to name just a few issues.

Adolescent reflections are provided at the end of the chapter so the nurse may consider the adolescent health experience in more detail and in the adolescents' own words. Developmental and cultural considerations can improve overall health and well-being, and are considered the best practice to promote health and healing for the next generations of AI/ANs. And finally, recommendations are offered for moving this mostly forgotten yet exponentially growing UAI health agenda forward.

WHAT IS *URBAN*?

An urban area is defined following each decennial, 10-year collection of census data, and is currently defined as a "continuously built-up area with a population of 50,000 or more" (U.S. Census Bureau, n.d.). Those persons who live in these areas are considered the urban population. In terms of AI/ANs, according to the 2010 Census, the place with the most AI/ANs was New York, NY, with 112,000 UAI, followed by Los Angeles with 54,000 UAI (U.S. Census, 2012). The top 12 U.S. cities with UAI total almost 500,000 AI/AN (Figure 16.1). According to Weaver (2012, p. 470), "Native people are invisible in large, multicultural cities."

Historically, American Indians/Alaska Natives had been found mostly on reservations, pueblos and trust lands, that is, in "Indian country" following the reservation period in the mid-1800s, as previously described in Chapter 3. It was not until the 1990 Census that more than half of the AI/ANs were proven to be off reservation. Therefore, the urban influx has been recent, and significant, but the response of the health care system, Congress, and the Indian Health Service (IHS) has not kept pace. With the inadequate funding provided to IHS by Congress, few dollars can be allotted to the IHS overall, and even fewer are

NUMBER UAI

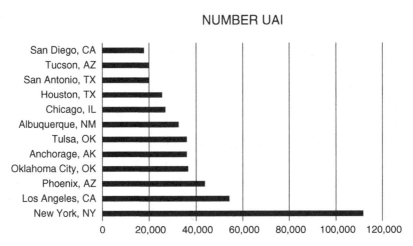

FIGURE 16.1 Top 12 U.S. cities with urban American Indians per the 2010 Census.

allotted to urban care. *This must change.* Change in the decades-long inadequate funding for IHS will be discussed in greater detail in Chapter 17.

Off reservation, UAI do not have easy access to their seats of government (Weaver, 2012). And they have very little political voice in cities (Weaver, 2012), where they now usually represent less than 1% of the population. They lose the land-tied practices and medicines important in all four domains of health. They may have to embrace new practices and medicines, without their history. All of these issues and more play into the identity of the UAI.

URBAN IDENTITY

According to Martinez, "Urban American Indians possess tribal identities, a strong intertribal identity, and familiarity with multicultural city populations. Urban Indians also have a connection to homelands where they visit relatives, and attend events and ceremonies" (2014, p. 1). American Indians/Alaska Natives moved to cities both voluntarily and as a result of federal relocation programs initiated in the 1950s that promised jobs and housing. These promises often fell short of expectations. Many AI/ANs were then trapped with no money or transportation back to their homes. The programs were largely on the East and West Coasts, and larger cities in the Midwest—which is why there are so many UAI now in New York, Los Angeles, and in Chicago.

Some moved to the city for reasons apart from these programs, such as for educational opportunities, participation in the armed forces, or different employment opportunities.

One distinct difference between reservation-based and urban populations is the intertribal connection found in the city. Although there are certainly members of other tribes on any given reservation, in cities this is the norm. Nurses working with urban populations should get to know the intertribal organizations and resources available in their areas.

A list of *regional* intertribal organizations can be found at www.ncai.org/tribal-directory/tribal-organizations, for example, Affiliated Tribes of the Northwest Indians, Alaska Inter-Tribal Council, Great Lakes Intertribal Council, and Intertribal Council of the Five Civilized Tribes.

Cities themselves have intertribal organizations. For example, in Minneapolis, MN, there is an elder-specific organization, Intertribal Elder Services Inc. There is also the Minneapolis American Indian Center (MAIC), which is in the center of the city's AI/AN community and is one of the oldest of these centers (Figure 16.2). The MAIC "provides educational and social services to more than 10,000 members of the community annually. It preserves and supports American Indian cultural traditions through the arts, youth and intergenerational programs" (MAIC, 2015, para. 1).

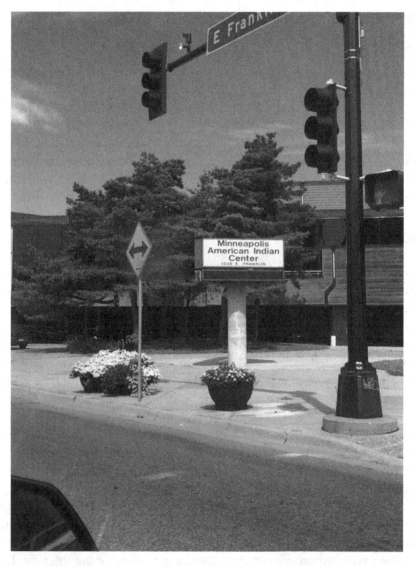

FIGURE 16.2 Minneapolis American Indian Center.

Urban American Indians tend to fall into several pockets of interaction. They may be completely isolated from all contact with other UAI in their environment. They may live in neighborhoods with many UAI families. Or they may be involved with an American Indian Center in their city or other AI/AN focused group (Martinez, 2014).

Misidentification

As discussed in the Overview of this book, misidentification has been a problem for data surrounding AI/AN, and this difficulty only increases in urban settings. More important, this is one area in which nurses can make an immediate impact just by asking each of their patients how the patient identifies rather than guessing or assuming. American Indians/Alaska Natives are more likely than any other racial group to be racially misclassified, for example, in cancer registries and in death records (Jim et al., 2014). This results in underestimates of the incidence of cancer and incorrect documentation by race for cause of death (Jim et al., 2014).

The misidentification problem increases once patients are outside of Indian country or counties with high concentrations of AI/AN. In cities, although the raw numbers may be high, concentrations remain low by percentage. In New York, although there are over 100,000 UAI, that is comprises a fraction of the other of 8 million people.

BARRIERS TO CARE IN URBAN AREAS

It will be important for nurses to understand the living context of urban Natives. There are few AI/AN-specific resources for health in cities. Many UAI have no formal membership, that is, enrollment, in their heritage tribes. Therefore, they will not be able to access IHS services, either direct services or contract care. Contract services are what would normally be available in most cities (as opposed to direct IHS care services), especially in the East, where there are no IHS hospitals and few clinics. However, any patient needing services outside of the IHS would have to be approved by his or her tribe first. This approval may be difficult to obtain, and nurses need to know that UAI patients may then have to wait for care, if they are enrolled, until they can return to the reservation to get care where cost is not a factor. This is the current context in 2015. Unfortunately, not much has changed in the almost 34 years since Shannon & Bashur wrote, "In comparison to Indians living on reservations, urban Indians have generally been neglected and few among them receive benefits from the Indian Health Service or other federal or state programs" (1982, p. 571). The other scenario is waiting indefinitely for care. This causes health problems that could have been mitigated to become worse, sometimes irreversibly.

In the New York City example, as mentioned the largest number of UAI live there, abouttwice as many as in the next largest city, and yet no urban Indian clinic, no health services specific to UAI, are found there. There is, however, the

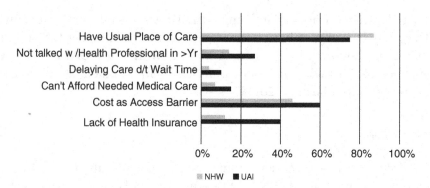

FIGURE 16.3 Barriers to care for UAI as compared to NHW by percentage.

American Indian Community House (AICH), which provides education, referrals, counseling, and social programming. The AICH is in lower Manhattan and may not be easily accessible to those in all five boroughs. Urban AI/ANs in New York City come from tribes all over the nation. They may be across country from any tribally specific services for their members.

As AI/ANs often live at higher poverty levels, have lower Western educational attainment, less employment and, therefore, less employment-based insurance coverage, they will need greater case management for health and health-related resources. Issues around education gaps are noted in Chapter 18. High school graduation rates of AI/ANs lag behind all groups and can be as low as 25% in some urban areas. Some of the significant disparities noted in the literature on UAI as compared with non-Hispanic Whites (NHW) are found in Figure 16.3 (Rutman, 2013).

Not only are there disparities in health (outcomes), but disparities persist as a result of structural issues such as getting access to and paying for care in urban areas (structure and process). Playing into the realities of barriers to care today for UAI are the same histories that have affected America's indigenous people nationwide.

DIFFERING WORLDVIEWS AND HISTORICAL CONTEXT

As has been argued throughout this text, the goal of the European colonization period was to acquire greater and greater expanses of North American territory—territory that had previously been the home to AI/ANs. In the effort to acquire the desired land, AI/ANs and their way of life were viewed as an obstacle.

From Christopher Columbus and the early colonists' first encounter with American Indians in North America, profound differences in worldview were obvious. The term *worldview* originates from the German word *weltanschauung*. In German, *welt* can be translated as *world* and *anschauung* as *view* or *outlook*. Worldview is a concept fundamental to German philosophy and epistemology, and refers to a wide-world perception (Husserl, 1970). The term is selected in reference to its broad appeal and inclusiveness of individual, community, and global perspectives. An individual's worldview comprises a framework of ideas and beliefs through which he or she interprets the world and interacts with it. As individuals construct a worldview, others can see a worldview operating at a community and systems level, or from the subconscious realm (van Manen, 1997).

The relationship between the predominant worldview of American society and the worldview of American Indians has been referred to in numerous ways. In health care and nursing literature, the worldview of the predominant American society is often referred to as a "Western" or "linear" view, whereas that of American Indians has been referred to as "relational" or "holistic" (Plumbo, 1995). Key characteristics of each perspective can be seen in Table 16.1.

Shared aims between the Western and relational worldviews are difficult to ascertain. Inherent in each view are opposing beliefs and priorities, which have evolved to the present time and offer little common ground. The linear and relational worldviews consist of unique priorities, and the differences lend great insight into the struggling relationship between the U.S. federal government and American Indian tribes, which has existed from the first encounter with the early colonists and persists today.

For the past century, oppression has been a predominant characteristic associated with American Indian life experiences in this country, manifested as historical trauma. Oppression can be understood better when references regarding worldview are understood. Finding ways to integrate these different worldviews, and sharing and incorporating unique elements offered by different disciplines and various systems of knowledge are necessary (Aerts et al., 1994) to achieve collaboration and integration essential to progress toward improved health for American Indians.

Beginning in the early 1900s, assimilation became a focus of U.S. policy in order to bring American Indians into a Western or linear worldview. Leclerc (2008) observed the following with regard to assimilation policies that began with the removal of cultural language:

> A policy of assimilation is one that uses strong measures to accelerate the downsizing of one or more linguistic minority group(s).The ultimate goal of such policies is to foster national unity based on the idea that a single language in the country will favor that end. (p. 256)

TABLE 16.1 A Comparison of Western and Relational Worldviews

CHARACTERISTICS OF THE WESTERN OR LINEAR WORLDVIEW	CHARACTERISTICS OF THE RELATIONAL OR HOLISTIC WORLDVIEW
Based in Western European and American thought	Based in tribal cultures
Based on logic	Can include illogical relationships
Cause must occur before effect.	Obtaining balance among many factors in one's life
Interventions are logically targeted to a symptom or cause.	Interventions utilize the cycle of nature, spiritual forces, balance, and achieving harmony.

In order to prevail over the vast American Indian population at that time, colonists and then the United States government pursued an approach of assimilation for expansion and territory acquisition. The goal was to remold the Indian's system of values into the mainstream society's ways of thinking (Scasz, 1999). Assimilation equaled disappearance of the "Indian problem."

The early assimilation and displacement period in American history brought destruction to the American Indian population that was no less than genocidal in scale. The sustained influx of Europeans brought new diseases, as well as removal of Indian livelihoods, languages, and ways of life. Reservations became holding areas for tribal communities and were often places of intense suffering owing to poverty, starvation, and disease.

At this time, education for AI/ANs, was considered essential to achieving assimilation policy objectives. Off-reservation schooling, often using the boarding school mechanism, was initiated. This off-reservation schooling resulted in the removal of American Indian children from their families without cultural support and often forbidding children from practicing the culture, language, and Indian way of life. Also within this period began the shift from the traditional American Indian diet to the modern diet, or one of primarily processed, high-fat, high-carbohydrate foods (King, n.d.). Today, the modern diet is considered a major contributor to the increasing levels of type 2 diabetes among American Indian youth (King, n.d.).

Removal from cultural ties, histories, and roles has been both mandated and voluntary. Each resulted in varying degrees of success in urban areas. In the remainder of the chapter, the focus is on arguably two of the most affected groups within the UAI populations, the elders and the adolescents. Nurses who gain an understanding of these two groups will necessarily incorporate families, women and children, communities, and end-of-life issues into their skill sets. Our aim is to gain a greater understanding of this most underrepresented of populations in health care—the AI/AN. And the most underserved of these are the urban American Indians.

URBAN INDIAN HEALTH CARE—THE "U" IN THE I/T/U HEALTH SYSTEM

There does exist a network of urban Indian health centers and professionals, as noted Chapter 5. (Please see the clickable map of urban Indian health organizations found under "Useful Websites" at the end of this chapter.) However, these urban Indian health centers are not available in every urban area and funding is usually an issue. Often, they serve as referral, counseling, and educational centers, but provide no medical care.

Some cities, such as Minneapolis, MN (in Hennepin County), do have clinics that provide health care to UAI. They work on a sliding-scale basis and provide basic medical, dental, and mental health/counseling services. Hennepin County also has prescription medication help with copays as long as the patient can prove residency in the county and prove tribal enrollment.

Of course, this assumes some sort of prescription benefit either from the state or through insurance and enrollment in a tribe. However, as discussed, many UAI do not have employment, insurance, or tribal enrollment.

These centers and urban networks, nonprofits, and clinics try to overcome inordinate health issues, environmental conditions, and poverty with very few resources. Some health indicators, show the situation of UAIs in comparison with that of Non-Hispanic Whites in the urban setting as follows: accidental deaths—38% higher; diabetes—54% higher; liver disease and cirrhosis—126% higher; and alcohol-related deaths—176% higher (Annie E. Casey Foundation [AECF], 2008). This same report—Urban Indian America—also states that urban Indian women receive less prenatal care than *even their reservation counterparts*, and infant mortality numbers are worse for UAI populations as well (AECF, 2008).

In terms of economic stability factors, the data show the adverse position of the UAI in increased poverty rates (20.3% vs. 12.7% for NHW), higher unemployment rates (70% higher than NHW), and homelessness (300% higher for UAI than for non-Indians; AECF, 2008). Home ownership is lower (46% vs. 62%) and issues such as lack of plumbing, phones and kitchen facilities are major concerns.

Nurses need to recognize these realities when they ask patients to call for appointments, fill their prescriptions, take their medications, refrigerate their insulin, or keep their feet clean when they may lack the basic necessities to carry out these discharge orders. Nurses working with these populations must ask about the circumstances, ability, environment, and community resources available for the patient to carry out the needed care. This was discussed in Chapter 1 in the context of a holistic view, family as client, and environmental concerns.

In keeping with the holistic theme, traditional (indigenous) ways of caring for ailments other than the physical include how to approach mental health issues, which are also characterized by huge gaps in care and disparities in occurrences in UAI (Hartmann & Gone, 2012). Using traditional approaches in concert with Western approaches in urban areas can be one way to mitigate outcomes, but there have been issues for this population. Hartmann and Gone found the following tensions in this approach:

1. Traditional healing protocols versus the realities of impoverished urban living
2. Multitribal representation in traditional healing services versus relational consistency with the culture keepers who would provide them
3. Enthusiasm for traditional healing versus uncertainty about who is trustworthy
4. The integrity of traditional healing versus the appeal of alternative medicine (2012, para. 1). Success in resolving these tensions would likely hit all four domains in some way— mental, spiritual, emotional, and physical. These tensions must be resolved at the community level, where it is important to recognize the membership of the community, resources, and trust-building successes with practitioners.

In addition, Wendt and Gone (2012) found that UAI viewed urban clinics as a vital place to be among other American Indians that enabled them to feel connected to the following:

1. Native culture
2. A place where one feels at home and welcome
3. A place in which health services are delivered in an especially intimate and hospitable manner

THE PUSH-AND-PULL FACTORS OF MIGRATION AND URBAN LIFE FOR AMERICAN INDIAN/ALASKA NATIVE ELDERS

> Probably nowhere is the gap between Indian and Western views of medicine greater than in the minds of Indian elders. . . . elders are most likely to embrace traditional values and to face linguistic, cultural, and other barriers to the utilization of health services. (John & Baldridge, 1996, p. 1)

Current AI/AN migration appears to be mostly voluntary within a multiepoch history of movement, which has included primitive, involuntary, and voluntary migrations. The complexities surrounding AI/AN migrations originate in the distinctive status of these people who hold dual citizenships and reside concurrently in both of their nations when reservation based. This "nation within a nation" phenomenon in the United States is peculiar to its indigenous population (Deloria & Lytle, 1998). Migration from the reservation to U.S. urban centers *is* movement of AI/ANs from their nation of origin to their nation of destination. This represents at once internal and external migration defined as movement between and within (a) nation(s).

Dual citizenship epitomizes the unique nature that discriminates AI/ANs from all other minority groups in that they hold this within the boundaries of the United States. Many issues surround tribal nationality, sovereignty, and indigenism for AI/AN elders. These are in addition to issues shared with all other U.S. minority groups, which are, by definition, exotic to the United States. And yet in aging and other health-related issues, AI/AN elders are simply labeled as minorities.

Huge gaps exist between the circumstances of AI elders and those of all others across races in their age brackets. Yet the literature is almost nonexistent in regard to their needs, beliefs, health decisions, or aging behaviors. Concerning these, some of the most comprehensive findings of this group are two decades old. These Americans are among those with the poorest health outcomes. They have the shortest life span of all other U.S. elders 65 and over, the highest mortality rates, and the lowest health utilization rates (Administration on Aging [AoA], 1996). American Indian elders are among the poorest ethnic groups, with 81% reporting not being in the labor force, 84% having an income less than $20,000—the highest percentage of poverty for any ethnic group—and one in eight having less than a 5th-grade education (U.S. Census, 1993). There have been few focused research or practice efforts in their direction. They are often isolated, live in dismal conditions, and do not "fit" with generally accepted theories on aging, as noted through previous research and practice during 25 years of contact (Moss, 2000).

During fieldwork in the U.S. Southwest, Moss noted that the tribe with which she was conducting ethnographic work on aging had historically centered itself around a middle village in clan groups (Moss, 2000). The clans, likewise, were centered around families. The family groups were centered around the elders. This centering of families, clans, and the village was all by design. Upon removal of certain members through movement or migration, the structure (whether family, clan, or village) lost a measure of integrity.

In the 1970s, in an effort to create low-income housing for the tribe's growing population, government subdivisions were added outside of the village area. Younger people in the families reportedly took advantage of the low-cost housing and a chance to start their own families. The movement represented less than an 8-mile range from start to finish. The unforeseen impact on the elders was in some cases devastating, with repercussions continuing today. There was, concurrently, an impact on those who had moved (Moss, 2000).

According to Sowell, "What migrations have meant has not been merely a relocation of bodies but, more fundamentally, a redistribution of skills, experience, and other human capital" (1996, p. 38). Grandparents were traditionally the teachers of the grandchildren; they were major caretakers of the grandchildren and set the rules in the households for all. They provided the blessings and spiritual guidance for the household as well as doing the cooking and performing other tasks. When the younger parents and their children moved away, there was a great loss of role and family connection for the elder. This had far-reaching implications that extended even into their spirit world, which in turn affected their health and well-being.

Those who had moved found increased incidence of alcohol use, spousal abuse, child neglect, and a host of social issues that come with breaking traditional family units bound by intact rules and rituals. Therefore, it was found that if a move of a few miles within the boundaries of Indian lands could cause such disruptions, migrations out of the boundaries and into distant urban centers also caused upheavals.

It is recognized that migration among indigenous peoples has been occurring since their initial trek across the Bering land bridge around 15,000 BCE (there are alternative theories of migration into North America; however, timeframes remain about the same). Those first migrations were representative of primitive migration wherein people went in search of food and shelter following the trails of animals they hunted (Flanders, 1998). Around 1250 ACE—1540 ACE, there were significant shifts in the Southwest Pueblo IV period. According to Spielmann (1998), through migration, the entire Pueblo world's demographic shifted east from the "Four Corners" region, causing dramatic demographic, social, economic, and political reconfigurations. Perhaps a parallel can be drawn today wherein the AI/AN demographic has shifted not in direction but in locality, that is, from reservation to urban center.

Examples of urban migration are both forced and voluntary. Forced migrations affect UAI elders today, including drafts of AI/AN veterans in World War II, the Korean War, and the Vietnam War. One AI/AN elder wrote of his successes when he left the reservation to go into the service. Although successful in the service, in athletics, and other valued areas of the White world, when he returned to his reservation, none of it was any use to him as an Indian person (Wyaco, 1998).

American Indians have been allowed citizenship only since 1924, well within the cohort of elders alive today (Deloria & Lytle, 1998). As of the writing of this book, elders in their 90s may have been born without citizenship rights. Those in their 60s, 70s, and 80s know that their parents or older siblings were not citizens. This leads to trust issues. Nurses need to be aware that trust issues are a major concern for AI/AN elders seeking care, and to also understand why.

Additionally, forced migration can be seen in the removal of children to "Indian schools" and through adoption and foster care through the mid-20th century (Swinomish, 1991). With the Indian Child Welfare Act of 1975, the practice of allowing other races to adopt and remove children from their traditional upbringing has been largely halted. Again, the children and/or the parents involved in this form of removal are alive today and either approaching middle adulthood or older. Therefore, whether by choice or circumstance, by 1990, 62% of an estimated 2 million AIs resided in off-reservation areas (Baldridge, 1995).

Another aspect of migration exists in remigration (Moss, 2001). From previous research, data suggest that many elders who have migrated return to the reservation in their later years (Moss, 2000). In Minnesota, one tribe was known to have 100% of all elders over 85 years old within their tribal land (M. Snobl, personal communication, May 1, 2000).

The implications of AI/AN migration between urban and reservation areas lie in an understanding of who migrates and why, how old they are when they migrate, whether or not they remigrate and why, as well as an understanding of the consequences of migration. Many AI/AN elders remigrate to their tribal lands in their middle-old or old-old years. For those planning for the UAI elderly population, then, to have services for frail AI elderly in urban centers may not be a priority. Conversely, the old-old reside mainly on tribal lands, and therefore congregate meal centers should not be the major model funded for tribal elders. Rather, they will need long-term and skilled care.

Urban elder centers would do well to have programming appropriate for the young-old (65–70 years) and the middle-old (70–75 years). The programming should include the four domains of health—physical, mental, emotional and spiritual. Sweats, smudging, and herbal use should be incorporated as appropriate. Urban centers will recognize the intertribal nature of their clientele and adapt and intersperse traditions into care offered.

If younger AI/ANs are in the cities, either by the process of migration or by birth as one of the first, second, or third generations of AI/AN people to be born off tribal lands, but return to the tribal lands as elders, there will be implications for acceptance for these returning Natives. People migrating, either coming back or moving, to their tribal lands for the first time likely bring with them money as well as changed attitudes, causing resentments (Sowell, 1996). There will undoubtedly be an adjustment or readjustment period requiring other more tailored services. A discussion of this aspect of migration is currently lacking in the literature.

The shifting of the AI/AN populations away from reservations, pueblos, and trust lands has had and will have an impact on elders who remain on the reservation, elders who have migrated to urban areas, and those who remigrate. Elders must then make decisions based not only on their health needs but also on their roles in and relationships with family and community. One such relationship is with the youth.

LIFE IN THE URBAN SETTING FOR AI/AN ADOLESCENTS

The historic oppression and trauma experienced by AI/ANs continues today and has an impact on AI/AN adolescents. The impact is manifested in lower health status and challenging life circumstances facing adolescents. The health of the current generation of AI/AN adolescents is in crisis, with poor health indicators, family breakups, and continued discrimination against the Indian way of life. All of these aspects disproportionately affected AI/AN youth.

It is important for nurses to take into consideration AI/AN history toward urban living and mobilization when caring for AI/AN adolescents. Patterns of residency for AI/ANs have evolved through the history related to their relationship with the U.S. government. Historical perspectives documenting this period in history reveal a direct link with elements of assimilation policy; from boarding schools and relocation; to the devastating social, economic, and health conditions that AI/ANs face today.

A common experience in the lives of AI/AN adolescents is frequent mobility and relocation. Many teenagers move between the reservation, a rural area, and an urban community as a lifestyle. The frequent geographic transitions play a prominent role in life and contribute to the social, economic, and environmental stressors that challenge normal adolescent development. Such stressors increase the likelihood of poorer health outcomes (Schulz et al., 2006) and the ability to successfully manage health needs. Understanding urban-based AI/AN adolescents' daily experiences is of importance in informing researchers and health providers on: (a) how and where adolescents live, (b) how their experiences may contribute to a higher prevalence of disease, and (c) measures to prevent disease in current and future generations.

Kulis, Wagaman, Tso, and Brown (2013) found that urban American Indian adolescent identity had three dimensions: (1) identification, (2) connection, and (3) culture/spirituality. Identification referred to tribal and ethnic heritage. Connection referred to reservation ties. And finally, culture referred to the adolescent's involvement in traditional cultural and spirituality practices. Nurses practicing with this population should learn to ask about these dimensions to determine whether the youth feel connected to their respective communities. Knowing this will assist in finding best practices to determine whether Western medicine, traditional medicine, or a mix, should be used for best outcomes.

STATE OF KNOWLEDGE ON AMERICAN INDIAN ADOLESCENT HEALTH CARE

Overall, knowledge about health care for AI/AN adolescents is in its formative stages and represents two domains. The first is the positivist paradigmatic perspective employing quantitative research methods primarily used in medicine. The second is the constructivist paradigmatic perspective utilizing qualitative methodologies. Convenience sampling, purposive sampling, and cross-sectional sampling that includes several tribal communities is a frequent approach to research.

A large number of research studies have been designed to conduct secondary analyses on the longitudinal study of the Pima Indian tribe in central Arizona that focused on type 2 diabetes. These analyses are important for the future development of clinical case definitions and diagnostic criteria for further medical research on type 2 diabetes in AI/AN adolescents. Specific recommendations on creating collaborative, tribal-supported research endeavors, however, are absent in both knowledge domains and need to be addressed in order to make culturally appropriate efforts in this area.

Who Is an Adolescent?

Just as there are misidentification issues for UAIs, there are also issues around the definition of the adolescent age group. From the variety of terms used in referring to adolescents, it is clear that the state of knowledge is in its formative stages. For example, some authors use the term *youth* to refer to the age range of 10 to 14 years, *child* for the age range of 5 to 10 years, or *adolescents* for the age range of 15 to 19 years (Acton et al., 2002). Other authors use no specific age range in reference to the terms *child, children,* or *youth*, which could encompass various ages within childhood and adolescence. Using a variety of terms to define adolescence prevents direct comparisons between studies. Therefore, development of a standardized terminology would advance knowledge development.

UAI Adolescents and Type 2 Diabetes

Whereas there is a growing appreciation of the complexities of factors contributing to early onset of type 2 diabetes and other diseases, research has offered little in terms of insights into the daily experiences of AI/AN adolescents (Joe, 1994). Future health research on AI/AN adolescents must consider the complex historical origins and development of disease in order to understand its growing prevalence. Therefore, to increase the overall health of AI/AN adolescents, it is important to consider AI/AN history in the United States. There are historical contributions to health status at the present time, and history can illuminate factors affecting AI/AN youth today.

Prior to World War II, diabetes was not a topic of concern for AI/ANs, and chronic diseases like type 2 diabetes were rare or nonexistent (Dixon & Roubideaux, 2001). Events contributing to the recent development of type 2 diabetes in AI/AN youth date back to the early 1880s—the beginning of the

United States' assimilation policy era with colonization efforts by European settlers at that time.

HEALTHY PEOPLE 2020

Healthy People 2020 (U.S. Department of Health and Human Services, Office of Disease Prevention and Health Promotion, 2014a) is a comprehensive national initiative that provides a framework for disease-prevention and health-promotion efforts in the United States. It includes national health objectives designed to identify the most significant preventable threats to health, and establishes national goals to reduce those threats. Healthy People 2020 is designed to achieve these overarching goals: (a) to attain high-quality, longer lives free of preventable disease, disability, injury, and premature death; (b) to achieve health equity, eliminate disparities, and improve the health of all groups; (c) to create social and physical environments that promote good health for all; and (d) to promote quality of life, healthy development, and healthy behaviors across all life stages. Healthy People 2020 goals are addressed by several health topics and objectives, one of which is diabetes.

The goals of the Healthy People 2020 diabetes focus are to address Westernization of diet, which is a diet high in fat and processed foods as well as total calories, and has been associated with a greater number of overweight persons in the United States when compared with the situation a decade ago, especially within high-risk racial and ethnic groups. Healthy People 2010 (U.S. Department of Health and Human Services, Office of Disease Prevention and Health Promotion, 2014b) documented diverse and complex factors contributing to the increasing presence of diabetes in adolescents: obesity, improper nutrition (including increased ingestion of fats and processed foods), and lack of physical activity are occurring in persons under age 15 years and may explain the increasing diagnosis of type 2 diabetes in adolescents.

- Increased television watching associated with diminished physical activity may also contribute to the emergence of type 2 diabetes in youth.
- Personal behaviors are influenced by beliefs and attitudes, and these are greatly affected by community and cultural traditions.
- In many racial and ethnic communities, fatalism, use of alternative medicine, desirability of rural living conditions, lack of economic resources, and other factors will influence significantly both the availability of health care and the capabilities of persons with diabetes in handling their own care.
- Thirteen percent of the total U.S. population speaks a language at home other than English.
- Cultural and linguistic factors affect interactions with health care providers and the larger health system (Healthy People (2014).

The degree to which diabetes prevention strategies recognize and incorporate these traditions will greatly determine a program's effectiveness. Current research utilizing Healthy People 2020 priorities for diabetes is timely, and will lend insight and help to achieve these overall goals.

The state of knowledge about the health of urban-based AI/AN adolescents is evolving. Important to framing the next generation of research on type 2 diabetes in urban-based AI/AN adolescents is exploration and testing of theoretical perspectives based on the constructivist or critical theory paradigmatic perspective, which is underrepresented in the literature. There is a need for mixed-method research specific to adolescents to include behavioral considerations, family, and the tribal community. Research based on the critical-theory perspective would be beneficial for knowledge development and allow for the inclusion of culturally specific factors for the AI/AN adolescent, family, tribal community, and include the adolescents' perspectives on living with this disease.

In general, adolescents can experience health care differently than adults. Adults often have a learned understanding or interpretation of meaning that directs their interpretation of the health care experience. A learned understanding or interpretation may also be influenced by cultural and social expectations. In comparison, adolescents experience health care with or without fewer learned associations. What is currently available in the science of health care with AI/AN adolescents is limited in voices of or expression of adolescent experiences in living with disease.

HEALTH CARE AVAILABLE TO URBAN-BASED AMERICAN INDIAN ADOLESCENTS

In general, most health professionals do not realize the historical meaning that diabetes has for AI/ANs. Type 2 diabetes is increasingly diagnosed in AI/AN adolescents, and there is a great need for primary and preventive health care in this area. Although research continues to emerge, three important gaps in the literature on urban youth living with type 2 diabetes are noted here:

- Despite advancing empirical and descriptive studies in the field of diabetes research, diagnosis rates in AI/ANs continue to be higher than those of any other population in the world.
- Extant literature on type 2 diabetes in AI/AN adolescents does not convey what is known about adolescents' experiences in living with this disease.
- There are few health programs specific for AI/AN adolescents living with type 2 diabetes.

THE INDIAN HEALTH SERVICE

The IHS is a federally funded branch of the U.S. Department of Health and Human Services. It came into existence through treaty negotiations in the 1800s between leaders of Indian nations and the U.S. government in order to provide health care and services in exchange for acquiring land. The IHS is currently responsible for the delivery of health services to all federally recognized AI/ANs through a system of facilities and programs located within the IHS, tribal (T), and urban (U) areas. The existence of the IHS/T/U, or I/T/U, has been outlined in past treaties, judicial determinations, and Acts of Congress (USDHHS, 2011).

American Indian health facilities that comprise the I/T/U provide general health care services for eligible AI/ANs in the United States. Each type of facility may not offer identical services, and some services may be available only at certain facilities. Usually, available services may include, but are not limited to, emergency health care, dental care, immunizations, primary care, behavioral health care, and children's health care (Arizona Healthcare Cost Containment System, 2011).

The I/T/U facilities and programs are considered "prepaid" with the land ceded by American Indian tribes in greater than 800 ratified treaties and presidential executive orders. Therefore, tribal members using I/T/U health programs are not charged for services (Urban Institute, 2014). In terms of providing adolescent-specific health care, the IHS is not fully funded by the federal government to fulfill its mission. Therefore, age-specific diabetic health care and coordination that are needed to support adolescents with type 2 diabetes may not be available in all areas. In addition, diabetes-specific health care becomes even more challenging to obtain and maintain when the adolescent is frequently mobile or relocating. And, finally, urban Indian health care funding represents less than 1% of the total IHS budget. The huge shortfall that exists for Indian health care overall is critically low for urban care (USDHHS, 2015).

Over successive generations, the I/T/U organizations continue to develop the capacity to serve traditionally medically underserved communities of AI/ANs in the United States, and are considered essential health care providers by the communities they serve. Many facilities provide health care in the most remote locations in the United States, where such services would otherwise not be available. Furthermore, the unique cultural background of AI/ANs requires providers in the I/T/U network to understand the language, community norms, unique health needs, and the means of incorporating traditional AI/AN healing, ceremonies, and practices in all areas of health care.

There are increasing numbers of AI/AN adolescents with type 2 diabetes with a shortage of health care available through the IHS to serve them. There is a gap in the literature on health care for uninsured AI/AN adolescents, namely, for those adolescents in rural, urban, or federally nonrecognized tribes not served by the IHS. Tribal communities are not uniform in verifying an individual's AI/AN heritage for tribal enrollment. Tribal communities typically use the blood quantum or percent age of AI/AN heritage (PIH) as verification of AI/AN ancestry as a requirement for tribal membership. The mission of the IHS is specific to meeting the health care needs of all AI/ANs, and federal funding of the IHS played a major role in the quality and quantity of services available to American Indian communities, including American Indian adolescents. The incidence of urban disease is not well represented in the literature, and further developments in this area would contribute greatly to understanding the scope, nature, and present health in urban-based adolescents.

IMPLICATIONS FOR ETHICAL PRACTICE WITH AMERICAN INDIAN ADOLESCENTS

In 1978, the Belmont report presented three principles for the ethical conduct of research in the United States: respect for persons, beneficence, and justice (The National Commission for the Protection of Human Subjects of Biomedical and Behavioral Research, 1978). In research and health care with adolescents, special consideration of these principles is necessary.

For adolescents, the respect for a person's principles balances adolescent participants' independent decision making and continued special protections. Continuation of special protections is important in research with adolescents in order to address their emerging cognitive capacity to consent to research participation (Society for Adolescent Medicine [SAM], 2003). The principle of beneficence is applied through extending and maximizing the benefits of research to adolescents by their inclusion in studies either as individuals or in groups. The principle of justice focuses on including and promoting the participation of groups, such as AI/AN adolescents, who have been historically excluded from participation in research. Another important consideration in the implementation of the principle of justice is the researcher's preparedness to work with the AI/AN adolescents' culture, environment, and community to access all of the direct or indirect benefits that the research may provide.

Within the theoretical and data-based literature, it is a matter of concern that details on the consideration of these ethical principles and researcher preparedness to work with AI/AN adolescents and their communities are minimally addressed. Although existing federal policies have occurred because of the recommendation of the Belmont report to include women, minorities, children, and adolescents in research (SAM, 2003), knowledge of methods of inclusion of AI/AN adolescents continues to develop. In future efforts focused on the health of AI/AN adolescents, the Belmont report's ethical principles of respect for persons, beneficence, and justice could be used as a framework for discussing knowledge development and best practices in working with adolescents and their communities.

Nursing research has utilized the principle of justice to consider the concept of *cultural safety* in nursing practice with diverse cultural populations. Studies based in Africa, Canada, and New Zealand (Anderson et al., 2003; Polaschek, 1998; Smye & Browne, 2002; Spence, 2001) have explored cultural safety based on postcolonial discourse aimed at understanding power relationships in nursing service delivery (Smye & Browne, 2002). Within the discourse, nursing sets up systems that enable the less powerful to genuinely monitor the attitude and service of the powerful to create useful and positive change (Polaschek, 1998).

Cultural safety is designed to focus attention on the idea of "life chances," which Smye and Browne (2002) describe as health services, education, and decent housing within an environment where it is safe to be born of a different racial or ethnic group. Cultural safety is not about cultural practices, but rather about recognition of the social, economic, and political position of certain groups within society, such as the indigenous people of New Zealand, the aboriginal people of Canada (Smye & Browne, 2002), and AI/ANs. Cultural safety focuses on nursing with less powerful populations in a society and prompts nurses to "think critically about ourselves, our patients and to be mindful of our own social, cultural, economic, and historical location" (Anderson et al., 2003, p. 196). The ideas represented in the concept of cultural safety have ethical significance, relate to the concept of social justice, and have implications for future nurses and other health practitioners who will work with AI/AN communities.

In the United States, research involving cultural safety can positively affect nursing practice by preparing nurses to consider the relational worldview and use it to create new approaches to quality and comprehensive health care for AI/AN communities. From now on, the profession of nursing will increasingly be called on to provide culture-specific health care in a society of growing numbers of languages, family structures, and values. To address this challenge, future research can move forward by including ideas represented in cultural safety and in the Belmont principles.

URBAN-BASED AMERICAN INDIAN ADOLESCENT HEALTH CARE: AN EXAMPLE WITH TYPE 2 DIABETES

The specific challenges that urban-based American Indian adolescents face in accessing health care support require an approach that allows exploration and description of the adolescents' experiences and includes their voice and perspectives. Adolescent experiences with health care can reveal supporting social and family structures that are instrumental in achieving future health goals, as well as research and programmatic efforts. To consider this topic further, a few assumptions about the ability to provide health services to urban-based AI/AN adolescents are listed here, using the example of those living with type 2 diabetes.

Assumptions

- Urban-based AI/AN adolescents have similar experiences related to living with type 2 diabetes.
- Living with type 2 diabetes in an urban area is different from the experience of living with the disease in a reservation community.
- Social and economic realities affect the urban-based adolescent's experiences in living with type 2 diabetes.
- The unstructured health interview can allow the adolescent to share valid, vivid, and useful recollections of everyday life with type 2 diabetes.

• The opportunity to share perspectives on health provides adolescents with the opportunity to reflect on their own voice and experience, contributing to development and growth.

More than ever before, AI/AN adolescents are being diagnosed with type 2 diabetes, the adult form of this disease, with limited knowledge available on how to provide culturally and developmentally appropriate prevention and intervention strategies. Thus, an increasing number of adolescents will likely develop life-changing health complications because of early diagnosis. When type 2 diabetes occurs earlier in life, serious health complications associated

TABLE 16.2 Complications of Diabetes

COMPLICATION	RISK AND OUTCOME
Heart disease and stroke	In adults 20 years of age and older, approximately 65% of deaths among people with diabetes were caused by heart disease and stroke, with the risk of stroke two to four times greater than that in adults without diabetes (Centers for Disease Control [CDC] National Center for Chronic Disease Prevention and Health Promotion, 2011).
Blindness, end-stage renal disease	Diabetes is the leading cause of new cases of blindness among adults aged 20 to 74 years of age, and is the leading cause of end-stage renal disease, accounting for 44% of new cases (CDC National Center for Chronic Disease Prevention and Health Promotion, 2011).
Nervous system disease	Nervous system disease occurs in about 60% to 70% of people with diabetes and often results in impaired sensation to the feet or hands and other nerve problems like carpal tunnel syndrome (CDC National Center for Chronic Disease Prevention and Health Promotion, 2011).
Amputations and dental disease	Amputations and dental disease occur more frequently among people with diabetes, and among young adults, those with diabetes have about two times the risk of dental disease as those without diabetes (CDC National Center for Chronic Disease Prevention and Health Promotion, 2011).
Birth defects and hyperglycemia in newborns	Poorly controlled diabetes before conception and during the first trimester of pregnancy can cause severe birth defects and hyperglycemia among newborns (CDC National Center for Chronic Disease Prevention and Health Promotion, 2005).
Ketoacidosis and coma	Uncontrolled diabetes can often lead to a biochemical imbalance that can cause life-threatening events such as diabetic ketoacidosis and coma (CDC National Center for Chronic Disease Prevention and Health Promotion, 2011).

with the disease may also develop earlier in life (see Table 16.2). This trend presents a stark contrast to the early 1900s, when the disease was practically absent in the population. In some areas, diabetes prevalence rates have soared to over 50%, especially for AI/AN adults over the age of 35 (Joe, 1994).

In a southwestern U.S. tribal community, Pavkov et al. (2006) found that adolescents diagnosed with type 2 diabetes before the age of 20 had a substantially increased risk during middle-age adulthood of kidney failure requiring dialysis, and a significantly higher rate of early death. In the community, there was a crucial need to learn about the prevention of type 2 diabetes in current and future generations of AI/AN adolescents as early diagnosis threatened to impact productive years and longevity (Indian Health Service [IHS], 2007).

In response, research initiatives with AI/AN communities are beginning to reveal a broader scope of factors associated with the disease. Factors include gender, age, diet, activity level, as well as genetic susceptibility related to AI/AN ancestry, social and economic conditions, migratory patterns, and the effects of modernization. In the future, understanding the degree to which these factors contribute to the occurrence and management of the disease in adolescents will be necessary to create solutions toward disease prevention earlier in life. With continued research, it is possible to discover new methods of prevention and disease management as the diagnosis occurs at earlier ages.

FUTURE HEALTH CARE FOR AMERICAN INDIAN ADOLESCENTS

There are important areas to be considered in order to actualize the goals of diabetes prevention in AI/AN adolescents. Prevention and treatment during adolescence is challenging because the developmental milestones that are part of this period of life. Grey (2005) found a common reluctance in adolescents to adhere to the recommended diabetes treatment and management, as well as a marked vulnerability among adolescents to poorer outcomes in diabetic metabolic control, because of the necessity of family involvement in daily disease management, or the potential for family conflict in this area. Many AI/AN adolescents, their families, and cultural communities are geographically fragmented, absent, or not available for needed support.

To address these challenges, more research focused on the period of adolescence is needed to understand adolescent needs, how to incorporate the family environment (Grey, 2005), as well as AI/AN adolescents' perspectives and experiences in living with type 2 diabetes. Lastly, it is difficult to reverse obesity, which often occurs concurrently with the diagnosis of type 2 diabetes. Improving health care for AI/AN adolescents requires health care professionals to obtain specialized knowledge on AI/AN culture, history, and the similarities and differences between tribes and their beliefs, values, and practices.

The most recent U.S. Census cannot provide the total number of AI/AN adolescents in the age cohort of 12 to 19 years; therefore, epidemiologic evidence of type 2 diabetes using census data approximates true occurrence. The U.S. Census and IHS data include AI/ANs from federally recognized tribal communities, but not from federally unrecognized tribal communities. Recognition of all tribal communities in the United States, including those not registered with the federal government, and a revision in the federal definition of who is American with Indian heritage are changes that are needed in order to bring health improvement and services to all AI/AN adolescents (Bierman, Collins, & Eisenberg, 2002).

With the increased mobility of AI/AN adolescents in society, use of health services varies according to the type of health insurance used; the status of the adolescents' residency; mobility among rural, reservation, and urban areas; the ability to afford copayments; and available family support. In order to improve health care for AI/AN adolescents, clinical practice guidelines are needed that incorporate the unique circumstances of adolescents in urban areas who are mobile between different communities. Steps toward improved health care also need to include recognition of the historical effects of the relationship between AI/AN tribes and the U.S. government. It is now essential to focus on building trust in relationships so increased participation of AI/ANs in census surveys, health care, and other institutional settings is realized.

As our society begins to confront the full challenge of type 2 diabetes appearing earlier in life, more research is needed to understand adult versus adolescent disease experiences (American Diabetes Association, 2000; Bennett, 1999; Hannon, Rao, & Arslaniain, 2005; Pavkov et al., 2006). In order to acquire further knowledge about adolescents living with type 2 diabetes and other diseases in urban communities, it is important to talk directly with AI/AN adolescents and their communities to learn of their experiences and perspectives. Adolescents' experiences and stories of life in their own words can assist in directing revised policy and funding for culturally appropriate health care programs. Such programs can lessen the impact of serious complications for adolescents diagnosed early with this disease and improve their overall health status and health outcomes for life.

FUTURE APPROACHES TO AMERICAN INDIAN ADOLESCENT HEALTH CARE

A successful approach to guiding health care in AI/AN communities would allow the inclusion of the holistic and spiritual context of the adolescent, including cultural components and social/economic circumstances. The Four Winds Model for Native Nutrition (Conti, 2002) based on the beliefs of the Oglala Sioux tribe in South Dakota is an example of model development in this area. Conti demonstrated that dramatic change in the availability of food, diet composition, the amount of physical activity, and lifestyle in AI/AN communities most likely contributed to the health disparities that currently exist. This culturally specific nutrition model provides a prescriptive approach for returning to a traditional diet comprising traditional and contemporary foods. Lowe and Struthers's (2003) conceptual model of nursing with AI/ANs is another example of an approach to guiding nursing practice in AI/AN communities within a holistic or relational worldview.

Christopher (2005) discussed the following seven areas for effective, culturally appropriate, and ethical research with AI/AN communities:

1. Understand the impact of historical relations between the U.S. government and AI/ANs on the present-day attitude of the AI/AN people, especially in regard to research.
2. Acquire knowledge of the issues specific to tribes, and avoid the common mistake of grouping all tribes together.
3. American Indian/Alaska Native individuals and communities must be invited to be involved and to share their perspectives.
4. Communities must get information back and have access to data collected from them.
5. Communities must receive benefits from research and program efforts.
6. The importance of addressing assets and broader social issues must be recognized.
7. The needs of the community must be placed above other interests.

These areas can lead to the creation of collaborative approaches with AI/AN populations, and contribute to greater benefits of health care to AI/AN adolescents and their communities.

With the exception of two region-specific studies (Dabelea et al., 1998; Lee et al., 2004), a gap identified in the literature is data on specific tribal communities. With the U.S. health care system underprepared to serve individuals with chronic long-term illnesses like type 2 diabetes, future tribe-specific research may be a way to reveal innovative primary, secondary, or tertiary care approaches to this problem. Tribe-specific data can lead to tribe-specific interventions. Such interventions could direct the development of research that empowers adolescents with type 2 diabetes to engage in prevention and disease-management strategies within their own tribal community.

A national perspective on all AI/AN adolescents living with type 2 diabetes is needed. Secondary literature sources report on a broader range of knowledge, including socioeconomic indicators, insurance use, level of education, and family status. A literature review of these sources would contribute to a national perspective on AI/AN adolescents with type 2 diabetes and could be instrumental in evaluating descriptive and demographic sources and trends. This perspective would be useful for a comparative analysis of the current status of AI/AN adolescents.

CONCLUSIONS

Urban American Indians share the same histories with all other AI/ANs. This includes all the policies discussed in Part I of this book from the reservation to the self-determination eras. However, some policies led to migration to cities, beginning in the 1950s and increasing until more AI/ANs were off reservation than on as of the 1990s. Relocation programs, adoption, fostering and boarding schools, and termination of tribes are some of the policies that specifically led to the increase in UAI.

Important for the nurse to understand is the lack of funding for this group via the IHS mechanism. There are few programs aimed at AI/ANs in cities with actual direct care. There are American Indian Centers and nonprofits that refer, counsel, and educate. Urban American Indians have barriers to care that far exceed those for people belonging to the urban dominant culture.

Urban elders feel a pull to move back to reservations where they can receive care in their spiritual and emotional domains, even though services are lacking for physical elder care. The cities have physical care in the form of long-term care and assisted living, for example, but no programs that also cater to the specific needs of intertribal clientele.

Finally, methods of developing collaborative relationships are essential to join in partnership with urban-based AI/AN adolescents and their communities. The Canadian First Nation's recommendations to serve AI/AN youth support research and program approaches to embrace the adolescent, family, and community in future efforts with type 2 diabetes in adolescents. The Canadian First Nation's community recommends: (a) involvement of AI/AN youth in the development of research, programs, and services accessed by youth; (b) family and community perspectives in the design of future research and programs addressing type 2 diabetes with AI/AN adolescents; and (c) AI/AN history and traditions (National Indian & Inuit Community Health Representatives Organization2000).

Urban communities need nurses who are committed to understanding the issues of AI/AN widely, and UAI specifically, and who can incorporate ideas of holism through an intertribal perspective.

ADOLESCENT REFLECTIONS

The following are adolescent reflections on living with type 2 diabetes. Read and discuss what insights the reflections provide in terms of AI/AN adolescent health care practice, education, policy, and research.

• It runs in our family. My mom has it. I went with her to her classes to know more about it, and so if anything happens, 'cause she's a type 2 diabetic too. And she takes pills, so we gotta make sure everybody does, family members. My two brothers, me, my boyfriend and my dad went with her to the classes to know more about it.

- It (type 2 diabetes) was affecting [name of reservation removed] like, there were—how would I say that? Like how I lost my motivation, lot of people I noticed too that they just lost their motivation, you know.
- Type 2 diabetes is hard to live with. When I started giving my own shots [on the reservation], [name removed] he showed me how, right through his shirt. He was like, this is how you do it. My grandpa, he had diabetes. When I got diagnosed, he was at the hospital, I guess. My mom would always call my grandpa, and, [name removed] ain't taking her insulin, and did this—I don't know. It's a hassle. My grandpa had complications of diabetes that led to his death. And—yeah.

- If I did change every thing, it would eventually come back, because it runs in my family, you know. It's like in the traits of our family of all the ladies, you know, somebody—there's something wrong with so many in all the females, and I don't know, it's just—. You know my grandma has cancer, and my auntie has thyroid problems, and then she's—it's scary. The diabetes comes early, but they started getting sicker with cancer and thyroid problems when they're older. And, I don't know, it just seems like—I'd always talk to my mom and I had told her, you know, I feel like I'm gonna be one of them persons out of my aunties and my grandmother, that's gonna be one of 'em that gets sick just like them. And she's like, no, no, no, that won't happen to you. I said yeah. They started out like me, started out with diabetes, and end up going on to a lot of other things.
- It feels like everybody's—I don't know, like, I have no friends that have diabetes, and it's like I'm the only one. And I'll go to my doctors and they'll be like well, you can meet people with diabetes, and it's mostly elders. And so I get really frustrated because elders is not the same as kids. Elders, they have a different mind-set, and they're on top of their stuff. While kids are still growing up and still wondering—you know what I'm saying? Wondering what to become if their diabetes or whatever is in the way. I don't know. It's really, really frustrating. Sometimes I just feel like giving up.
- The only thoughts I have is I wish it would go away, or I'd rather be dead than have this and live with this. That's like my thoughts. Every morning when I wake up I—I think that there's no point in—like what am I getting up for? I understand there's school—you know what I'm saying? I'm in that kind of—I don't know—that kind of state.
- I: Can you say more about what you were thinking or feeling in that regard?

    R: Just that I have to really be careful what I do now. Especially when I get older. If I can get it under control, and possibly go away. But if it doesn't, then I gotta really watch what I do. Because, you know what I'm saying, is that, if I really did die or something, then that <would>—I don't know. That doesn't scare me. People always tell me—cause I kinda don't care for my diabetes. And as I'm getting older now, it's kind of catching up to me, like my legs are hurting. If I just sit there, my back hurts a lot. And like, I just hate when people tell me to take my insulin, or did you check your blood sugar? It's like, leave me alone. You know what I'm saying? And it gets really hard, and depressing, and it just—I wish I could do my diabetes my way. But you have to follow doctor's orders and—I know people are scared.

• After I started noticing changes too, is that I didn't have much energy no more like I used to. I wasn't motivated on running and jogging. 'Cause I used to jog and I used to lift weights and stuff. I was tired, and I'd just do one set, you know, work out, and I'd just be tired. Usually I don't get tired like that. Another thing too that kept me kinda healthy too, that which I'm still doing right now is I'm going to pow-wows and dancing and stuff like that. It kept me in shape and healthy and stuff. One thing I was worried about that was—after I started noticing, 'cause I haven't danced in about a year when I start noticing those symptoms. And my grandma passed away too, so I was kinda going through some stuff. And I got out of shape and start drinkin' pop and stuff like that. One thing I noticed too, I couldn't dance no more 'cause I was so outa shape. I'd spin around too fast and I'd almost black out and stuff. So after that I just quit dancing.

• Think they [blood sugars] got high 'cause of how I was eating. 'Cause it seems like when you eat certain foods or drink certain things it makes it like go super high. And they say when your sugars go high that's when you feel like you ain't got no energy, you know. Just makes you feel like really run down. I didn't really believe that until I felt that way that day. That's how I knew. And I don't know, my grandma said when she feels like that she eats something sweet, but that doesn't work for me. I don't think it does. I don't think she takes her medicine like I do.

• Well, I think you get diabetes from eating too much sugar and all that, and eating too much. Well, now I'm working out, but I played football. I think you just get it from eating too much and not exercising that good. I used to be a heavy pop drinker a lot. I used to drink a lot of pop, like most every day. Like any kind of pop I'd drink, and I used to make my tea with a lot of sugar and stuff, and I—I always used to be healthy before, and I could do all kinds of stuff—run, and I could do back-flips and all that. And I—like later on down the road I would know that it'd affect me, and I heard about people getting diabetes, and I never thought that'd happen to me. Like, right now it's like, like—cause see I just—like I think I still like get those stars in my vision and stuff like that. It's like whenever I jump up too fast or something like that.

• Yeah, and my grandmother, too. She kind of thought about it, [about] buying a whole bunch of stuff, like pop, and like a whole bunch of sugar stuff—a lot of stuff she gets me. Sometimes it's sugar free and only like 100 calories [potato chips]. I remember she got those once. But she only gets stuff that I'm available to eat. And if I get a pop, it's like a treat to me. The hardest part is not being able to eat the stuff that I want.

I: What did you have to give up that you used to eat?

R: Pop, a lot of chips, … kind of a lot of sugar stuff.

I: And what do you eat now, compared to what you used to?

R: Well, I have breakfast, lunch and dinner, but I'm only allowed to have like one snack per day.

- It started off when I got pregnant with my baby, and I got diabetes when I was pregnant with her. And then after, it never went away. It just stayed with me. And ever since then I been on medicine, and I'm taking medicine, and going to the doctor regularly, but I don't know, it just seems different from—you know, it seems like from when before I had (child's name). I felt different. But now it's just, I feel—I don't know, I feel sick sometimes from it I guess. Oh, my face got really tingly, and I was sweating all the time and just feelin' sick. And I didn't know what was wrong, and I went in and they checked my sugars and they were like super high. So, they put me on medicine, and it seems like as soon as they did I felt better.

- I: Okay, when you think about this in your life, what effect do you think diabetes will have in your life, in the years to come?

R: I don't know, like, with it when you get older and they say if you don't take care of yourself it can make you blind, and there's certain types you can lose your fingers and toes, you know. If you don't take care of yourself. And that's just what scares me. 'Cause there's a lot of my family members that did get sick off of it, you know.

I: When you think of your future, what do you think about in living with diabetes?

R: I think that I won't make it past 25. But, when I was younger I used to think well, I'm not going to make it past 15, and now look I'm 19, and I don't know.

STUDY QUESTIONS
♦ What seems to be of most importance in living with type 2 diabetes for the adolescent?
♦ Are community and family experiences from the reservation or urban area a component of the adolescents' reflections?

♦ Does the adolescent share memories of a past relative or a community member on the reservation who had lived with type 2 diabetes?

♦ What do you find most insightful in these reflections?

♦ What direction for AI/AN health care is evident from the reflections?

USEFUL WEBSITES

♦ American Indian Community House in NYC, http://www.aich.org/services/health//

♦ *Federal Register* list of U.S. urban areas and urban clusters, http://www.gpo.gov/fdsys/pkg/FR-2012-03-27/pdf/2012-6903.pdf

♦ National Indian Council on Aging, www.nicoa.org

♦ Urban Indian Health Organizations: clickable map, http://www.uihi.org/urban-indian-health-organization-profiles/

REFERENCES

Acton, K. J., Burrows, N. R., Moore, K., Querec, L., Geiss, L. S., & Engelgau, M. (2002). Trends in diabetes prevalence among American Indian and Alaska Native children, adolescents and young adults. *American Journal of Public Health, 92*(9), 1485–1490.

Administration on Aging. (1996). *Home and community-based long-term care in American Indian and Alaskan Native communities: Final report.* Washington, DC: Author.

Aerts, D., Apostel, L., DeMoor, B., Hellemans, S., Edel, M., Van Belle, H., & Van der Veken, J. (1994). *World views: From fragmentations to integration* [Translation of L. Apostel & J. Van der Veken [1991] with some additions]. Brussels, Belgium: Academic and Scientific Publishers, VUB Press.

American Diabetes Association. (2000). Type 2 diabetes in children and adolescents. *Diabetes Care, 23*(3), 381–389.

Anderson, J., Perry, J., Blue, C., Browne, A., Henderson, A., Khan, K. B., . . . Smye, V. (2003). "Rewriting" cultural safety within the postcolonial and postnational feminist project: Toward new epistemologies of healing. *Advances in Nursing Science, 26*(3), 196–214.

The Annie E. Casey Foundation. (2008). *Urban Indian America.* Retrieved from http://www.aecf.org/search?q=urban+indians

Arizona Healthcare Cost Containment System. (2011). *Prevention services accomplishments 2011.* Retrieved from http://www.azdhs.gov/documents/prevention/reports/prevention-services-accomplishments-2011.pdf

Baldridge, D. (1995). *Mapping Indian elders.* Albuquerque, NM: National Indian Council on Aging.

Bennett, P. H. (1999). Type 2 diabetes among the Pima Indians of Arizona: An epidemic attributable to environmental change? *Nutrition Reviews, 57*(5), S51–S54.

Bierman, L. N., Collins, K. S., & Eisenberg, J. M. (2002). Addressing racial and ethnic barriers to healthcare: The need for better data. *Health Affairs, 21*(3), 91–102.

Centers for Disease Control and Prevention—National Center for Chronic Disease Prevention and Health Promotion. (2011). *National diabetes fact sheet—National estimates.* Retrieved from http://www.cdc.gov/diabetes/pubs/pdf/ndfs_2011.pdf

Christopher, S. (2005). Recommendations for conducting successful research with Native Americans. *Journal of Cancer Education, 20*(Suppl.), 47–51.

Conti, K. (2002, October). *The four winds model for native nutrition: Finding wicozani through our tradition.* Presentation conducted at the meeting of the University of

Pennsylvania Schools of Nursing and Medicine and the Lenape Nation of Pennsylvania, Tribal Host, Philadelphia, PA.

Dabelea, D., Hanson, R. L., Bennett, P. H., Roumain, J., Knowler, W. C., & Pettitt, D. J. (1998). Increasing prevalence of Type 2 diabetes in American Indian children. *Diabetologia, 41*, 904–910.

Deloria, V., & Lytle, C. (1998). *The nations within: The past and future of American Indian Sovereignty.* Austin, TX: University of Texas Press.

Dixon, M., & Roubideaux, Y. (Eds.). (2001). *Promises to keep: Public health policy for American Indians and Alaska Natives in the 21st century.* Washington, DC: The American Public Health Association.

Flanders, S. (1998). *Atlas of American migration.* New York, NY: Facts on File.

Grey, M. (2005, April). *Clinical research: From efficacy to effectiveness to translation.* Paper presented at the meeting for the Midwest Nursing Research Society on Advancing the Clinical Research Enterprise: Translation and Dissemination, Cincinnati, Ohio.

Hannon, T. S., Rao, G., & Arslaniain, S. (2005). Childhood obesity and type 2 diabetes. *Pediatrics, 116*(2), 473–479.

Hartmann, W. E., & Gone, J. P. (2012). Incorporating traditional healing into an urban American Indian health organization: A case study of community member perspectives. *Journal of Counseling Psychology, 59*, 542.

Husserl, E. (1970). *The crises of European sciences and transcendental phenomenology.* Evanston, IL: Northwestern University Press.

Indian Health Service. (2007). *Type 2 diabetes and youth: Acting now for future generations.* Retrieved from http://www.ihs.gov/MedicalPrograms/Diabetes/index .cfm?module=resourcesFactSheets_Youth07

Jim, M. A., Arias, E., Seneca, D. S., Hoopes, M. J., Jim, C. C., Johnson, N. J., & Wiggins, C. L. (2014). Racial misclassification of American Indians and Alaska Natives by Indian Health Service contract health service delivery area. *American Journal of Public Health, 104*, S295–S302.

Joe, J. R. (1994). The perceptions of American Indian adolescents with diabetes. In J. R. Joe & R. S. Young (Eds.), *Diabetes as a disease of civilization: The impact of culture change on indigenous peoples* (pp. 329–356). Berlin, Germany: Mouton de Gruyer.

John, R., & Baldridge, D. (1996). *The NICOA Report: Health and long-term care for Indian elders.* Retrieved from http://moon.ouhsc.edu/rjohn/longterm.pdf

King, G. (n.d.). *Type 2 diabetes: The modern epidemic of American Indians in the United States.* Retrieved from http://www.as.ua.edu/ant/bindon/ant570/Papers/King/ king.htm

Kulis, S., Wagaman, M. A., Tso, C., & Brown, E. F. (2013). Exploring indigenous identities of urban American Indian youth of the southwest. *Journal of Adolescent Research, 28*(3), 271–298.

Leclerc, J. (2008). *Politiques d'assimiation in l'aménagement linguistique dans le monde.* [Assimilation of policies in language planning in the world]. Quebec City, Quebec, Canada: Université Laval, TLFQ.

Lee, E. T., Begum, M., Wang, W., Blackett, P. R., Blevins, K. S., Stoddart, M., … Alaupovic, P. (2004). Type 2 diabetes and impaired fasting glucose in American Indians aged 5–40 years: The Cherokee study. *Annals of Epidemiology, 14*(9), 696–704.

Lowe, J., & Struthers, R. (2003). Nursing in the Native American culture and historical trauma. *Issues Mental Health Nursing, 24*(3), 257–272.

Martinez, D. (2014). Urban American Indians. *Social Science Research Network.* doi: 10.2139/ssrn.2476142

The Minneapolis American Indian Center. (2015). *The heart of urban Indian country*. Retrieved from http://www.maicnet.org

Moss, M. P. (2000). *Zuni elders: Ethnography of American Indian aging* (Doctoral dissertation). University of Texas-Houston, Health Science Center, Houston, TX.

Moss, M. P. (2001, October). *Mapping the impact of population migration on American Indian elders* (Abstract No. 28322). Paper presented at American Public Health Association (APHA) 129th Conference., Atlanta, GA.

The National Commission for the Protection of Human Subjects of Biomedical and Behavioral Research. (1978). *The Belmont report: Ethical principles and guidelines for the protection of human subjects or research* (DHEW Pub. No. [OS] 78-0012). Washington, DC: U.S. Government Printing Office.

National Indian & Inuit Community Health Representatives Organization. (2000). *Youth and diabetes*. Retrieved from www.niichro.com

Pavkov, M. E., Bennett, P. H., Knowler, W. C., Krakoff, J., Sievers, M. L., & Nelson, R. G. (2006). Effect of youth-onset type 2 diabetes mellitus on incidence of end-stage renal disease and mortality in young and middle-aged Pima Indians. *Journal of the American Medical Association, 296*(4), 421–426.

Plumbo, M. A. (1995). Living in two worlds or living in the world differently. *Journal of Holistic Nursing, 13*(2), 155–173.

Polaschek, N. (1998). Cultural safety: A new concept in nursing people of different ethnicities. *Journal of Advanced Nursing, 27*(3), 452–457.

Rutman, S. P. (2013). *Barriers to and use of health care among American Indians and Alaska Natives in urban areas: Findings from the national health interview survey (2006–2009)*. Paper presented at the 2013 Council of State and Territorial Epidemiologists (CSTE) Annual Conference.

Scasz, M. (1999). *Education and the American Indian: The road to self-determination since 1928.* Albuquerque, NM: University of New Mexico Press.

Schulz, L. O., Bennett, P. H., Ravussin, R., Kidd, J. R., Kidd, K. K., Esparza, J., & Valencia, M. E. (2006). Effects of traditional and western environments on prevalence of type 2 diabetes in Pima Indians in Mexico and the U.S. *Diabetes Care, 29*(8), 1866–1871.

Shannon, G. W., & Bashshur, R. L. (1982). Accessibility to medical care among urban American Indians in a large metropolitan area. *Social Science & Medicine, 16*, 571–575. doi:10.1016/0277-9536(82)90310-0

Smye, V., & Browne, A. (2002). "Cultural safety" and the analysis of health policy affecting aboriginal people. *Nurse Researcher, 9*(3), 42–56.

Society for Adolescent Medicine. (2003). Guidelines for adolescent health research: A position paper of the society of adolescent medicine. *Journal of Adolescent Health, 33*(5), 396–409.

Sowell, T. (1996). *Migrations and culture*. New York, NY: Basic Books.

Spence, D. (2001). Prejudice, paradox, and possibility: Nursing people from cultures other than one's own. *Journal of Transcultural Nursing, 12*(2), 100–106.

Spielmann, K. (Ed.). (1998). The Pueblo IV period: History of research. In *Migration and Reorganization: The Pueblo IV Period in the American Southwest* (Anthropological Research Papers No. 51). Tempe, AZ: Arizona State University.

Swinomish Tribal Community. (1991). *A gathering of wisdoms*. LaConner, WA: Swinomish Tribal Mental Health Project.

Urban Institute. (2014). *A national roundtable on the Indian Health System & Medicaid Reform.* Retrieved from http://www.urban.org/research/publication/national-roundtable-indian-health-system-medicaid-reform

U.S. Census Bureau. (2012). *The American Indian and Alaska Native population: 2010.* Retrieved from http://www.census.gov/prod/cen2010/briefs/c2010br-10.pdf

U.S. Census Bureau (n.d.). The urban and rural classifications. Retrieved from http://www2.census.gov/geo/pdfs/reference/GARM/Ch12GARM.pdf.

U.S. Department of Health and Human Services. (2011). *Testimony on the Indian Health Care Improvement Act by Michael H. Trujillo, M.D., M.P.H., M.S.* Retrieved from http://www.hhs.gov/asl/testify/t000308c.html

U.S. Department of Health and Human Services. (2015). *FY2015 budget in brief—IHS.* Retrieved from http://www.hhs.gov/about/budget/fy2015/budget-in-brief/ihs/index.html

U.S. Department of Health and Human Services, Office of Disease Prevention and Health Promotion. (2014a). *Healthy People 2020.* Retrieved from http://www.healthypeople.gov/2020/leading-health-indicators/2020-LHI-Topics

U.S. Department of Health and Human Services, Office of Disease Prevention and Health Promotion. (2014b). Healthy People 2010. Retrieved from http://www.healthypeople.gov/2010

van Manen, M. (1997). *Researching lived experience.* London, Ontario, Canada: University of Western Ontario.

Weaver, H. N. (2012). Urban and indigenous: The challenges of being a Native American in the city. *Journal of Community Practice, 20,* 470–488.

Wendt, D. C., & Gone, J. P. (2012). Urban-indigenous therapeutic landscapes: A case study of an urban American Indian health organization. *Health & Place, 18,* 1025–1033. doi:10.1016/j.healthplace.2012.06.004

Wyaco, V. (1998). *A Zuni life. A Pueblo Indian in two worlds.* Albuquerque, NM: University of New Mexico Press.

Policy, The Future of Nursing, and Indian Country

*I*n Parts I and II, the reader was introduced to history and cultural areas as they pertain to patients in Indian country, narrowing from a national, historical view to regional perspectives. In Part III, the reader is reintroduced to a broader context. Here, the reader explores funding as a major component of increasing care options and access in Indian country. The reader learns about mandatory versus discretionary funding, which impacts not only the patients but those who care for them. And, finally, the future of nursing is discussed with a focus on educational and differences that the AI/AN population "bring to the table" as compared with the population at large.

SEVENTEEN

Indian Health Funding: Time for Change

Marilynn Malerba and Margaret P. Moss

LEARNING OBJECTIVES
♦ Understand the impact of a federal health program that has a mandatory versus a discretionary budget as designated by Congress
♦ Distinguish how funding impacts federal health programs directly and indirectly
♦ Discuss how funding issues relate to health disparities gaps

KEY TERMS
♦ Discretionary budgets
♦ Mandatory budgets
♦ Sequestration

KEY CONCEPTS
♦ The "PayGo" rule
♦ Treaties as supreme laws of the land
♦ Underfunding

Since first contact with European immigrants, American Indians/Alaska Natives (AI/ANs) have endeavored to protect their traditional ways of life, well-being, land bases, populations, and forms of government. The policies of the United States toward its first peoples have undergone many changes: treaty-making, reorganization, assimilation, relocation, termination, re-recognition and currently, self-determination and self-governance.

The trust and treaty responsibility of the U.S. government for the provision of health, education, and general welfare for the people of our First Nations is well documented by our U.S. Constitution (U.S. Const. art. I, § 3), treaties, legislation, and canons of construction for Indian law. These rights recognize the major contributions of millions of acres of land, mineral rights, waterways, and natural resources by AI/AN governments. Why, then, does federal policy continue to severely underfund Indian Health, resulting in diminished health status and quality of life with a life expectancy below that of mainstream America for our first peoples?

BACKGROUND

The trust and treaty relationship between the American Indians/Alaska Natives (hereafter referred to as Indians as appropriate to legal terms) and the U.S. government is well established in the U.S. Constitution, treaties between the Indian Tribes and the U.S. government, federal law, case law, and the canons of construction that govern the interpretation of written documents such as treaties (Wilkinson, 1988). Many treaties were negotiated in the 1700s with the Continental Congress. Treaty-making continued until 1871, with approximately 380 treaties negotiated (Wilkinson, 1988), at which time the federal government ended this policy of relations with Indian Tribes. The U.S. Congress implemented some of its powers by passing the Indian Trade and Intercourse Act of 1790 (Act to Regulate Trade and Intercourse with Indian Tribes, 1790). This Act articulated the federal government's role in setting policy to implement the various components of such treaties in recognition of its treaty responsibilities.

The more than 240 pre-federal American Indian treaties point to early motivations for treaty making as an effort to establish peaceful relations between the ever-increasing numbers of European immigrants and the local tribes in the east. The tribes were attempting to protect their homelands, people, and sacred sites. The European immigrants wished to establish communities in which to live, while ensuring that the tribes would not bear arms against the colonists when fighting for independence from England began (Staley, 2012).

Later, treaties focused on the ceding of indigenous lands, the establishment of land bases for tribes, as well as the ongoing provision of goods and services. Many of the treaties contained similar language such as the one negotiated in 1895 with the Assiniboine and Gros Ventre:

> For and in consideration of the conveyance, cession and relinquishment hereinbefore made, the United States hereby covenants and agrees to advance and expend . . . such sums, or so much therefore as may be necessary in any one year, shall be expended in the purchase of cows, bulls, and other livestock, goods, clothing subsistence, agricultural implements; in providing employees, in the education of Indian children, in procuring medicine and medical attendance, in the care and support of the aged, sick and inform, helpless orphans . . . and in such other ways as may best promote their civilization and improvement.
> (Deloria & DeMallie, 1999 p. 383)

Tribes then began to be considered dependent sovereigns or wards of the federal government and, as such, were accorded special protections under the Marshall trilogy (*Cherokee Nation v. Georgia 1831, Johnson v. M'intosh 1823, Worcester v. Georgia 1832*).

Thus, treaties should be viewed as positive substantive rights , which can be interpreted to mean a second party is required to provide an entitlement (Stone,

2002). This relationship gets translated into practice by statute law, formal legal rule, or administrative law. Bergman et al. (1999), quote Senator Daniel Inouye regarding the trust responsibility of the United States to provide for the health of Indians: "Over 100 years ago, the Indian people of this nation purchased the first pre-paid health care plan, a plan that was paid for by the cession of millions of acres of land to the United States" (Inouye, 1993, p. 601).

There is a "swinging pendulum" of law and legal decisions known as Federal Indian Law: varying between recognizing Indian Tribes as nations with inherent sovereignty with solemn treaty rights and at other times abrogating treaties with solemn promises neglected and broken by state and federal governments alike (Silvern, 1999).

INDIAN HEALTH SERVICE

Against the backdrop of this history, the Indian Health Service (IHS) is considered. The War Department was initially charged with federal health services for Indians in 1824, primarily for the purpose of containing contagious diseases (Bergman, 1999). This responsibility transferred to the newly established Bureau of Indian Affairs in 1849. The 1921 Snyder Act authorized funds for "the relief of distress and conservation of health (and) for the employment of physicians… for Indian Tribes" (Snyder Act, 1921, Section 13, p. 1).

In 1928, the Institute for Government Research published the Merriam Report (Committee on Indian Affairs United States Senate, 1928) describing the deplorable conditions on Indian reservations and attributing those conditions to failed federal policy and administration of Indian affairs (Wilkins, 2009). Specifically referenced were the poor health and social living conditions that the AI/ANs were experiencing. In response, Congress shifted policy to formally recognize Indian tribes, ushering in a new era of dealing with tribes as governmental entities with the passage of the Indian Reorganization Act in 1934 (Cornell & Kalt, 2008; Indian Reorganization Act, 1934).

More recent federal law passed for the health care of Indians is the Indian Health Care Improvement Act initially passed in 1976 (Indian Health Care Improvement Act, 2000) and permanently reauthorized by the Patient Protection and Affordable Care Act, as amended (Patient Protection and Affordable Care Act, 2011). This Act recognizes the relationship between the federal government and the American Indian people, and the need to eradicate the severe health inequalities experienced by AI/ANs. As partially cited, the Indian Health Care Improvement Act states:

The United States Congress finds the following:

(1) Federal health services to maintain and improve the health of the Indians are consonant with and required by the Federal Government's historical and unique legal relationship with, and resulting responsibility to, the American Indian people. (Indian Health Care Improvement Act, 2000, Section 1601 [1])

The provision of Indian health care services is an exchange between two sovereigns, not an entitlement program. Tribes have ceded much to the United States prior to its formulation and up to the current day, creating certain treaty rights and trust responsibilities agreed on by both parties. The federal government has a responsibility to uphold these rights and responsibilities.

FEDERAL BUDGETS: DISCRETIONARY VERSUS MANDATORY

Why is IHS chronically underfunded at 57% level of need, and (b) Why is this budget a nondefense discretionary line item in the federal budget? As a discretionary line item, Congress has the ability to erode the federal trust responsibility to tribes by diminishing or eliminating funding for this service. Could this not be considered a modern-day termination policy of the United States (Westmoreland & Watson, 2006)?

The way IHS is funded puts the service and health status for all served at risk. Indian health funding resides in the nondefense discretionary budget in contrast to the entitlement or mandatory Medicare, Medicaid, Children's Health Insurance, and Social Security programs. Clearly, parity is diminished by the assigning of discretionary versus mandatory funding status to a program. Entitlement (mandatory) budgeting is established through legislation, under which services are provided to recipients deemed eligible by establishing legislation. Mandatory budgeting increases with population growth, inflation, and new technologies, thus providing the same or improved level of care to recipients without any further congressional action. If this does not occur, there are private rights of action available to recipients (White, 1998).

In contrast, with the exception of the Special Diabetes Program for Indians, IHS is a nondefense, discretionary (NDD) line item in the budget. This creates a situation in which funding levels are inconsistent with no consideration of all the external factors that escalate the need for increased appropriations. Referred to as bureau budgeting, discretionary budgeting is extremely sensitive to the political environment—a way to provide oversight of bureau officials in the form of annual budgeting. "Government has not committed itself legally to a precise level of services. Rather, it has promised to provide a bureaucracy that it is to be hoped will provide an acceptable level" (White, 1998, p. 511). Authorization provides legislation for funding but appropriations deal directly with prioritization of programs within the budget constraints. White further describes how entitlements differ from bureau budgeting, describing social insurance programs (entitlements) as displacing uncertainty about the future from the individual to the government.

Given the treaty and trust obligations of the United States, why should access to health care for AI/ANs be uncertain, unreliable, or denied because of the misalignment of IHS funding within the federal budgeting system? The impact of not adjusting funding for population growth or inflation is noted as diminished purchasing power (see Figure 17.1).

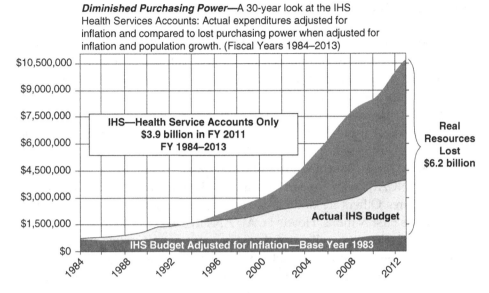

Diminished Purchasing Power—A 30-year look at the IHS Health Services Accounts: Actual expenditures adjusted for inflation and compared to lost purchasing power when adjusted for inflation and population growth. (Fiscal Years 1984–2013)

FIGURE 17.1 Indian health purchasing power 1984 to 2012.

Source: National Indian Health Board (2012).

Compounding the underfunding of IHS is the complex nature of how the funding is accessed, and whether tribes have a successful infrastructure to augment funding. In addition to economic development, tribes have different levels of capabilities to supplement the funding received. The Indian Health Care Improvement Act provides tribes with the ability to supplement funding through the vehicle of third-party billing at their health facilities (Indian Health Care Improvement Act, 2000). If the tribe has the capacity to successfully write and administer governmental grants, various grant programs may also supplement funding. Tribes widely criticize grant-funding vehicles, as they philosophically believe this mechanism does not uphold the federal government's trust and treaty responsibility for the provision of health care for tribal citizens. The competitive nature and nonrecurring format of funding cause tribal governments concern about the sustainability of these grant-funded services and programs, in some cases providing a disincentive to apply.

Additionally, multiple agencies within the federal system have appropriations intended for the health of all U.S. citizens, some with earmarks for AI/ANs and some inaccessible to tribal governments. It is virtually impossible for Indian tribes to easily find and access all the funding vehicles that could potentially improve their overall funding. A problem identified with grant-funding agencies is that the tribes with better grant-writing capabilities have better success in receiving funding although the need may be greater for those tribes that do not have those same capabilities. Unequal access to care translates into increasing health degradation. Tribes are reluctant to access grant programs that have an uncertain future-funding component, given that it would be problematic to stop offering a service once it has begun.

CURRENT DEMOGRAPHICS AND INDIAN HEALTH SERVICE PROFILE

The population served by the IHS represents 2.2 million citizens of the 566 federally recognized tribes throughout the United States (229 of which are in Alaska), excluding tribal members living outside a defined "service area" for a federally recognized tribe, citizens of state-recognized tribes, or other nonrecognized tribes (IHS, 2014). Reservation-based AI/ANs live in 37 states in the United States, residing on lands of approximately 100 million acres. Two thirds of this population live in 10 states: California, Oklahoma, Arizona, New Mexico, Texas, North Carolina, New York, Alaska, Washington, and South Dakota (National Congress of American Indians [NCAI] Policy Research Center, 2013). Some tribes have land bases in millions of acres. Others are landless as a result of the failed policies of the United States toward its First Nations. However, AI/ANs live in every state in the United States because of relocation policies and employment opportunities. Circumstances and economic conditions vary widely throughout Indian country. The statistics speak for themselves, with 40% of the AI/ANs on reservations living in poverty, 24.8% lacking complete plumbing, 20.5% lacking a complete kitchen, 18.9% with no telephone, and 27.2% living in overcrowded conditions (U. S. Census Bureau, 2011).

The 2010 population of the United States was 307,747,716 with an AI/AN population of 3,188,000, or 1.03% of the entire population (U. S. Census Bureau, 2011). This is a self-reported measure for the U.S. Census and is higher than the number served by IHS as a result of eligibility requirements for service. Therefore, many AI/ANs have unmet health care needs above and beyond what is reported to the Indian Health Service. The median age of the Native population is 26 years, contrasted with the median age of the U.S. population of 37 years. Roughly 42% of the population is under the age of 24, contrasted with 34% of the general U.S. population under 24 years (NCIA Policy Research Center, 2013). Only 8% of this population is over the age of 65 years.

The Indian Health Care System is comprised of the Indian Health Service, Tribal Health Programs, and Urban Programs (I/T/U). Provision of care and funding occurs in various ways: Direct services in which the IHS funds and provides care in tribal communities; tribal programs in which tribes contract or compact for the funding under the Indian Self-Determination and Education Assistance Act (P.L. 93-638 as amended) and through self-managed health care programs within their communities (Indian Health Care Improvement Act, 2000); and in urban programs for those citizens living in urban areas not associated with tribal communities. Approximately 45,907 inpatient and 13,180,745 outpatient visits were provided in the year 2013 across all these systems (IHS, 2014).

DIRECT CARE VERSUS CONTRACT CARE

Direct care is provided at various facilities in the I/T/U system, as noted in Table 17.1. Care in these facilities is limited, with no program offering tertiary care for medically intense needs such as open-heart surgery. Although 46

TABLE 17.1 Direct Care Facilities

	HOSPITALS	HEALTH CENTERS	ALASKA VILLAGE CLINICS	HEALTH STATIONS
IHS (Direct & Urban)	28	61	N/A	34
Tribal	17	249	164	70

Source: Indian Health Service (2014).

facilities offer emergency room and inpatient care, not every tribal citizen has access to those facilities. Those facilities typically operate with an average daily census of 45 or fewer patients, and only 20 have operating rooms (Oversight Hearing on Contract Health Services, 2009).

Contract care addresses the following circumstances:

1. For care that is not directly provided, there is a line item in the budget for "purchased and referred care," formerly known as Contract Health Services. Purchased and referred care is utilized in situations where no IHS direct care facility exists.
2. The existing IHS direct care element is incapable of providing required emergency and/or specialty care.
3. Utilization in the direct care element exceeds staffing.
4. Supplementation of alternate resources (i.e., Medicare, Medicaid, or private insurance) is required to provide comprehensive health care to eligible AI/ANs.

Purchased and referred services, including inpatient and outpatient care, routine ambulatory emergency care, transportation and medical support services, such as diagnostic imaging, physical therapy, laboratory, nutrition and pharmacy services, are prioritized on the basis of available funds (IHS, 2008). Owing to the underfunded nature of the program, many tribal health and IHS programs must use the urgent/emergent category ("life or limb") as limiters for the care of their people rather than the disease management and prevention categories. Additionally, coming from these funds are Catastrophic Health Emergency Funds (CHEF), which provide funding for high-cost cases over $25,000 such as traumas, cancer care, and so on. CHEF funds typically run out of money long before the fiscal year ends.

The effect of not receiving adequate and timely care is a decline in the overall health status of this population, an increase in the acuity caused by exacerbation of illness, entry into the system in a more acute state, resulting in higher cost of care. This perpetuates the crisis of unmet needs and rising budgetary needs without additional appropriations. Table 17.2 provides data on the level of unmet need, and the projected cost to provide for deferred and denied care. It is important to note that these data are likely incomplete.

TABLE 17.2 Indian Health Service Estimated Unmet Needs, Fiscal Year 2011

CATEGORY OF UNMET NEED REPORTED FOR 2011	NUMBER OF CASES REPORTED FOR 2011	ESTIMATED AMOUNT OF UNMET NEED ($)
Denied	68,215	351,362,529
Deferred	83,740	431.330.241
Unreimbursed CHEF	928	17,670,622
Total	152,883	800,363,392

Source: National Indian Health Board (2012).

PROBLEM

Although there have been notable gains during President Obama's adminis-tration (U.S. Government Accountability Office, 2012), Indian Health Services remains severely underfunded. The estimate for full funding is approximately $27.6 billion, contrasted with a fiscal year 2014 budget of $5.302 billion, or a $22.3 billion deficit.

Appropriations buy fewer health care services with each passing year. The gap between spending for a Medicare beneficiary (mandatory funding) and the discretionary spending on an American Indian has grown eight-fold between 1982 and 2002, with a difference of 250% of per capita appropriations for Medicare recipients as opposed to Indian Health Care per capita recipients (Westmoreland & Watson, 2006). Similarly, it has not kept pace with other benchmarks for health care spending, with $7,535 an average expenditure per person nationally and $2,896 for AI/ANs (see Figure 17.2).

IMPACT

The Indian Health Service has been chronically underfunded; it is currently at 56% of its level of need (National Congress of American Indians, 2014). Directly attributable to this chronic underfunding are the abysmal health statistics for the AI/AN population: a life expectancy 4.1 years shorter than that of the U.S. population (anecdotally, many tribal leaders share that their average life expec-tancy hovers around 50 years of age), and higher rates of mortality than other Americans resulting from alcoholism (552% higher), diabetes (182% higher), unintentional injuries (138% higher), and suicide (74% higher; IHS, 2013). Given the remoteness of some tribal communities, villages, pueblos, and reservations, the need to travel great distances to access care further strains an already over-taxed budget. Recruitment of health care personnel is difficult because of the remoteness and the instability of annual budgets.

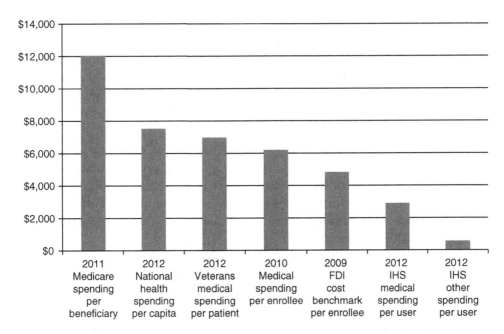

FIGURE 17.2 2012 Indian Health Service expenditures per capita and other federal health care expenditures per capita.

Source: National Indian Health Board (2014).

SEQUESTRATION AND THE INDIAN HEALTH SERVICE

Despite a historic increase of 29% in the past 4 years, funding levels remain dangerously low (National Congress of American Indians, 2014). Sequestration resulting from the "balanced budget act"—P.L. 112-25 Budget Control Act of 2011—decreased total funding by 5% during 2013 followed by a 0.2% rescission in the Consolidated and Further Continuing Appropriations Act (Native Care Act, 2013), which resulted in a decrease to the Indian Health Services budget of $220 million. The result was less available care to Indian country with an estimated elimination of 804,000 outpatient visits and 3,000 inpatient visits for a health care system struggling to provide even the most basic services to a population with striking health care inequalities.

Federal health programs specifically exempted from sequestration were entitlement (Medicare, Medicaid, and Children's Health Insurance Program) and discretionary (Veteran's health). The Congressional Budget Office estimated that discretionary spending for 2014 would have decreased by another 3% as a result of automatic spending cuts that lower the caps on discretionary funding (Congressional Budget Office, 2013), had the budget not been balanced. The Center for Budget and Policy Priorities notes: "Under the [2011 Budget

Control Act], Non Defense Discretionary spending will fall to its lowest level as a share of the gross domestic product (GDP) on record by 2016, with data going back to 1962 and will continue to fall thereafter" (Center on Budget and Policy Priorities, 2014, p. 5.).

The "PayGo" rule further complicates this contentious budget environment. This rule requires a financial offset elsewhere in the budget to fund any new entitlement program (Center on Budget and Policy Priorities, 2013). Estimates indicate that the trust fund that provides funding for Medicare will be depleted by 2024 (Geithner et al., 2012). Therefore, lacking political will to fundamentally change how the Indian Health Service is funded, how might the budget be improved, or, at the very least, stabilized to the extent that inadequate funding does not reduce the amount of care provided with each new budget year? It will require multiple strategies to correct this deficiency.

The following initiatives are currently advocated by tribal leaders: full funding of contract support costs without diminution of services, advanced appropriations, exemption from sequestration, the correction of the definition of *Indian* within the Affordable Care Act to ensure AI/ANs participate fully in any Indian-specific provisions within that Act, full funding of current services—including federal and tribal salary and benefit costs medical and nonmedical inflation and population growth—and Medicare-like rates for Contract Health Services (McCollum, 2014; Native Care Act,113th Congress, 2013–2014).

CONCLUSIONS

Without any formal representation in Congress, tribes and tribal organizations must work through their democratically elected representatives to ensure that the trust and treaty rights of our AI/ANs are upheld by the U.S. government using the vehicles of policy and legislation. An apt description of the long-standing problems facing Indian country, "wicked problems," are problems that are relentless or persistent, with temporary and imperfect solutions that involve multiple government and policy jurisdictions (Agranoff & McGuire, 2003; Roberts, 2000; Weber & Khademian, 2008). Tribes, tribal organizations, federal agencies, and legislators could be characterized as a governance network whose work involves agenda setting, legislative efforts, evaluation, consultation, coalition building, and implementation of policy (Ansell & Gash, 2008). "Collaborative governance" defines this process as "A governing arrangement where one or more public agencies directly engage non-state stakeholders in a collective decision-making process that is formal, consensus oriented and deliberative, and that aims to make or implement public policy or manage public programs or assets" (Ansell & Gash, 2008 p. 554).

Federal agency partners, legislative committee staff, White House policy experts, tribal leaders, tribal organizations, health economists, health policy experts, and technical advisors have committed to resolving this issue. A budget summit was held from October 12 to 13, 2014, to begin to work toward health equity through adequate health funding for Indian health. Although this work will take time, the results will be improved health.

STUDY QUESTIONS

♦ If you were to advise Congress at an Indian health care briefing, as a nurse, what would be your three most seminal points as to why and how funding needs to change?

♦ Discuss your greatest concerns about trends in Indian health.

♦ Why do you think funding structures in regard to Indian health have lagged behind all other federal health programs?

USEFUL WEBSITES

Indian Health Service—Newsroom, https://www.ihs.gov/newsroom/

Kappler, C.J. (Ed.). (1904). *Indian affairs: Laws and treaties. Vol. II (Treaties) in part.* Washington, DC: Government Printing Office. http://digital.library.okstate.edu/kappler/vol2/toc.htm

U.S. Code, Title 25-Indians, https://www.law.cornell.edu/uscode/text/25

REFERENCES

Act to Regulate Trade and Intercourse with the Indian Tribes, 1 Stat. 137 (1790).

Agranoff, R., & McGuire, M. (2003). *Collaborative public management: New strategies for local government.* Cambridge, MA: MIT Press.

Ansell, C., & Gash, A. (2008). Collaborative governance in theory and practice. *Journal of Public Administration Research and Theory, 18*(4), 543–571. doi:10.1093/jopart/mum032

Bergman, A. B. (1999). A political history of the Indian Health Service. *Milbank Quarterly, 77*(4), 571–604. doi:10.1111/1468-0009.00152

Budget Control Act, Pub. Law. No. 1 12-25 (2011).

Center on Budget and Policy Priorities. (2011). *Policy basics: Introduction to the federal budget process.* Washington, DC: Author.

Center on Budget and Policy Priorities. (2013). *Policy basics: Non-defense discretionary programs.* Washington, DC: Author.

Cherokee nation v. Georgia, 30. U.S. 1 (Supreme Court of the United States. 1831.

Committee on Indian Affairs United States Senate. (1928). *Survey of condition of the Indians in the United States: Indian Affairs, United States Senate 71st congress, 2nd session.* Washington, DC: U.S. Government Printing Office.

Congressional Budget Office. (2013). *The 2013 long term budget outlook.* Washington, DC: Author.

Consolidated Further Continuing Appropriations Act, Pub. L. No. 113-6 (2013).

Cornell S., Kalt J. P. (Eds.). (2008). *The state of native nations: Conditions under U.S. policies of self-determination* (The Harvard Project). New York, NY: Oxford University Press.

Deloria, V. J., & DeMallie, R. J. (Eds.). (1999). *Documents of American Indian diplomacy: Treaties, agreements and conventions, 1775–1979* (Vol. 1). Norman, OK: University of Oklahoma Press.

Geithner, T. F., Solis, H. L., Sebelius, K., Astrue, M., Blahous, C. P., Reischauer, R. D., & Tavenner, M. B. (2012). *2012 annual report of the boards of trustees of the federal hospital insurance and federal supplementary medical insurance trust funds.* Washington, DC: The Boards of Trustees of the Federal Hospital Insurance and Federal Supplementary Medical Insurance Trust Funds.

Indian Health Care Improvement Act, 25 U.S.C. §1601 (2000).

Indian Health Service. (2008). *Indian health manual (IHM)—Chapter 3—Contract health services*. Washington, DC: Department of Health and Human Services.

Indian Health Service. (2013). *IHS fact sheets: Indian health disparities*. Retrieved from https://www.ihs.gov/newsroom/factsheets/disparities

Indian Health Service. (2014, January). *IHS year 2014 profile*. Retrieved from http://www.ihs.gov/newsroom/index.cfm/factsheets/ihsyear2014/profile.

Indian Reorganization Act, Pub. L. No. 73-383 (1934).

Inouye, D. (1993). *Perspectives on Indian health care. Remarks to the national summit on Indian health care reform, Washington, DC*. Oakland, CA: American Indian Resources Institute.

Johnson v. M'intosh, 1. U.S. 543 (Supreme Court of the United States, 1823).

McCollum, B. (2014). *McCollum introduces bipartisan legislation to improve access to health care for Native Americans*. Retrieved from https://mccollum.house.gov/press-release/mccollum-introduces-bipartisan-legislation-improve-access-health-care-native-americans

National Indian Health Board. (2012). *Together building on our trust for the health of our people*. Washington, DC: Author.

National Congress of American Indians Policy Research Center. (2013). *Geographic & demographic profile of Indian country*. Retrieved from http://www.ncai.org/policy-research-center/initiatives/projects/cic

National Congress of American Indians. (2014). *FY 2015 Indian country budget request: An honorable budget for Indian country: Equitable funding for tribes*. Washington, DC: National Congress of American Indians.

National Indian Health Board. (2014). *National tribal budget recommendations to DHHS-2015*. Washington, DC: Author.

Native Care Act, H.R. 4843, 113th Congress (2013–2014) (2014).

Oversight hearing on contract health services: Committee on Indian Affairs, United States House of Representatives. (2009). (Testimony of Dr. Yvette Roubideaux, Director of Indian Health Services).

Patient Protection and Affordability Act, Part III Indian health, Pub. L. no 111-148, §10211 (2011).

Roberts, N. C. (2000). Wicked problems and network approaches to resolution. *International Public Management Review, 1*, 1–19.

Silvern, S. E. (1999). Scales of justice: Law, American Indian treaty rights and the political construction of scale. *Political Geography, 18*(6), 639–668. doi:10.1016/S0962-6298(99)00001-3

Snyder Act, 25 U.S.C. §13, 42 stat 208 (1921).

Staley, R. A. (2012). American Indian treaty diplomacy in the papers of the continental congress, 1774–1789. *Government Information Quarterly, 29*(2), 252–260. doi:10.1016/j.giq.2011.09.005

Stone, D. (2002). *Policy paradox: The art of political decision making*. New York, NY: W.W. Norton

U.S. Census Bureau. (2011). *American community survey 1 year estimates*. Washington, DC: Author.

U.S. Government Accountability Office. (2012). *Indian health service: Action needed to ensure equitable allocation of resources for the contract health program* (No. GAO-12-446). Washington, DC: Author.

United States Constitution art.1§ clause 3.

Weber, E. P., & Khademian, A. M. (2008). Wicked problems, knowledge challenges and collaborative capacity builders in network settings. *Public Administration Review, 68*, 334–349.

Westmoreland, T. M., & Watson, K. R. (2006). Redeeming hollow promises: The case for mandatory spending on health care for American Indians and Alaska natives. *American Journal of Public Health, 96*(4), 600–605. doi:10.2105/AJPH.2004.053793

White, J. (1998). Entitlement budgeting vs. bureau budgeting. *Public Administration Review, 58*(6), 510–521. Retrieved from http://search.proquest.com/docview/197166032?accountid=15172

Wilkins, D. E. (2009). *Documents of Native American political development: 1500's to 1933.* New York, NY: Oxford University Press.

Wilkinson, C. (1988). In The American Indian Resources Institute (Ed.), *Indian tribes as sovereign governments* (10th ed.). Oakland, CA: American Indian Lawyer Training Program. Part II. pp. 91–99.

Worcester v. Georgia, 31. U.S. 515 (Supreme Court of the United States, 1832).

EIGHTEEN

The Future of Nursing Report and American Indian Nursing Education

Margaret P. Moss

LEARNING OBJECTIVES

♦ To become familiar with the seminal Institute of Medicine (2010) report: *The Future of Nursing: Leading Change, Advancing Health* and the background organizations that wrote it
♦ To demonstrate understanding of the four key recommendations of *The Future of Nursing: Leading Change, Advancing Health* report and its "fit" with Indian Country
♦ To differentiate between challenges in obtaining nursing education in Indian Country and those in dominant culture settings

KEY TERMS

♦ Institute of Medicine
♦ Robert Wood Johnson Foundation

♦ Tribal College
♦ Violence Against Women Act (VAMA)

KEY CONCEPTS

♦ Leading change
♦ Maximizing education

♦ Shaping policy
♦ Structural barriers

In 2010, the Institute of Medicine (IOM) and the Robert Wood Johnson Foundation (RWJF) released the landmark report: *Future of Nursing: Leading Change, Advancing Health*. Within its first year of release, this report became the most downloaded report in IOM's history (IOM, 2011). The report offers key messages and recommendations to "guide the transformation of the nursing profession" (IOM, 2011, para. 1). In this chapter, we explore the "fit" of the *Future of Nursing* (FoN) report to American Indian health and nursing.

INSTITUTE OF MEDICINE

In 1863, the National Academy of Sciences (NAS) was chartered by President Lincoln as a nongovernmental body that provides "independent, objective advice to the nation on matters related to science and technology" (NAS, 2015, para. 2).

TABLE 18.1 List of Selected IOM Reports 2000 to 2015

YEAR	TITLE
	National Academies Press in Health and Medicine
2000	To Err Is Human: Building a Safer Health System
2001	Crossing the Quality Chasm: A New Health System for the 21st Century
2003	Veterans and Agent Orange: Update 2002
2004	Immunization Safety Review: Vaccines and Autism
2005	Making Better Drugs for Children with Cancer
2006	Evaluating the HRSA Traumatic Brain Injury Program
2008	Retooling for an Aging America: Building the Health Care Workforce
2009	Initial National Priorities for Comparative Effectiveness Research
2010	HIV Screening and Access to Care: Exploring Barriers and Facilitators to Expanded HIV Testing
2011	The Future of Nursing: Leading Change, Advancing Health
2012	Country-Level Decision Making for Control of Chronic Diseases: Workshop Summary
2014	Treatment for Posttraumatic Stress Disorder in Military and Veteran Populations: Final Assessment
2015	Vital Signs: Core Metrics for Health and Health Care Progress

The IOM, as an arm of the NAS, was created in 1970 to provide authoritative and unbiased health information to the public and to decision makers (IOM, 2015). Although it is widely regarded in academic medicine as the epitome of professional achievement to be inducted as a member of this august body of primarily physicians, but also some nurses and others in health-related professions, the IOM is not well known in nonacademic nursing circles. This is unfortunate as the IOM has been instrumental over many decades in informing the Congress, the public, and health professionals on important areas such as health disparities, quality, safety, and nursing. This has been accomplished through roundtables, workshops, and widely available reports on timely subjects (Table 18.1).

Many people have heard of hospital deaths in the United States over a year being compared to a jetliner crashing every day. But few would be able to point to these data coming from a 2000 IOM report—*To Err Is Human: Building a Safer Health System* (IOM, 2000). The reports are free on the IOM site to read online or download.

The IOM's effort with the RWJF on the FoN has been noticed by many, yet direct care nurses are largely unaware of the report. This author recently took an informal poll, talking with nurses in a 200-bed community hospital in 2014 to see whether they had heard of the report, and 90% said that they did not know what it was. The others had *heard* of it, but could not really say what it was about. This anecdotal finding is in line with that reported by Bleich (2012) a little over a year after the report was released, in which few direct care nurses knew of the report. Bleich was a member of the committee that worked on the report. The committee was made up largely of nurses and physicians, and although it is difficult to tell from a name or position, it does not appear that any American Indians or Alaska Natives (AI/ANs) were on this panel. As we get even further from its release date, readership and understanding does not appear to have increased in the bedside-nurse population.

THE ROBERT WOOD JOHNSON FOUNDATION

The RWJF is the largest philanthropic organization in the United States dedicated solely to health concerns of the nation with a focus on lasting, real change (RWJF, 2015). Its mission is "to improve the health and health care of all Americans" (RWJF, para. 2). The RWJF has a diversity statement acknowledging that inclusion in all domains of diversity can only help all Americans (RWJF, 2015). One of its areas of focus is in health leadership and the workforce.

The RWJF/IOM collaboration on the FoN report resulted in a partnership of RWJF and AARP through the Center to Champion Nursing in America (CCNA) to guide the implementation of the recommendations as a central advising body. One way this is done is through a network of state-based action coalitions that are working on recommendations of the report at the state level. Therefore, there is both national and state input on the FoN moving forward. RWJF's latest tagline is "A Culture of health."

But What Is Missing?

As the reader of this text has learned, AI/ANs are citizens not just of the United States, or their state of residence, but of their own indigenous nations. Yet, in perusing the committee members, attending fora on the FoN prior to the report's release, reading the report, visiting the CCNA, and, in fact, being a former RWJF Health Policy Fellow (2008–2009), this author does not see inclusion of these nations in any realm of the FoN. Therefore, it appears that key messages and recommendations were devised without this voice. But then, how do they fit with Indian Country?

KEY MESSAGES FROM THE FON REPORT

1. Nurses should practice to the full extent of their education and training.
2. Nurses should achieve higher levels of education and training through an improved education system that promotes seamless academic progression.
3. Nurses should be full partners, with physicians and other health care professionals, in redesigning health care in the United States.
4. Effective workforce planning and policy making require better data collection and information infrastructure.

SEMINAL RECOMMENDATIONS FROM THE FON REPORT

1. Remove scope-of-practice barriers.
2. Expand opportunities for nurses to lead and diffuse collaborative improvement efforts.
3. Implement nurse residency programs.
4. Increase the proportion of nurses with a baccalaureate degree to 80% by 2020.
5. Double the number of nurses with a doctorate by 2020.
6. Ensure that nurses engage in lifelong learning.
7. Prepare and enable nurses to lead change to advance health.
8. Build an infrastructure for the collection and analysis of interprofessional health care workforce data.

THE FON REPORT AND DIVERSITY

The first time diversity is addressed is on page 7, where under Key Message #2, it is noted that the workforce should become more diverse ethnically and racially as well as in other areas such as gender diversity. Then on page 12, under Recommendation #4, it states that there should be attention to increasing diverse students to achieve a diverse workplace. There do not seem to be any recommendations as to *how* to do this.

American Indians and Alaska Natives are only mentioned twice in the report—in reference to what percentage of nurses (3%) are AI/AN and a chart showing enrollment of diverse students in 2008 to 2009. Considering that AI/ANs often have a divergent route to nursing (often tribal schools), have a unique political/nation standing, and are subject to cultural and geographical challenges that are arguably some of the toughest, there should have been specific attention to this most underrepresented group in both education and health care.

You have learned many of the geographical issues faced by AI/ANs—for instance, in Arizona, distances and heat are a challenge; in Alaska, boats and planes may be the only form of transportation; in South Dakota, there may not be any phone reception; and in Montana, mountains, snow, and −40°F temperatures exist. There should, at the very least, have been attention to rural versus urban in the context of becoming a nurse, and then being the nurse imagined in this report.

There were fewer than 20 references to "rural," and all were in the context of the rural patient. By their own key messages and recommendations, there must first be diverse students and a diverse workforce to take care of the diverse patients within the culture. For American Indians wanting to provide care on reservations, this will mostly be a rural context as most reservations are west of the Mississippi river (see Figure 18.1). In *any* report on or for the nation, there should be federal, state, and tribal input and consideration. This becomes especially true when cultural consideration is key to stakeholders, in this case the workforce and the patient population. And, including the indigenous voice becomes more important still when there are such massive existing inequities in life, in academia, in health care, and in nursing.

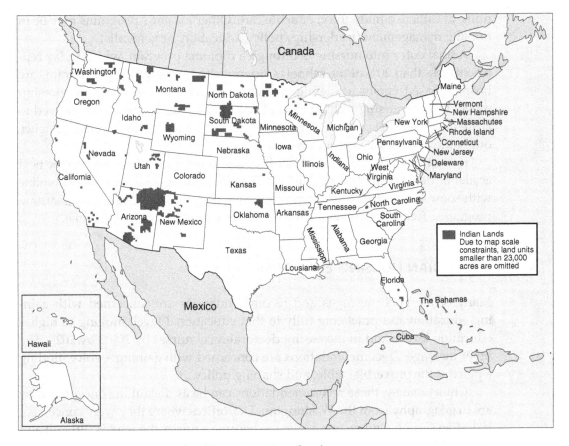

FIGURE 18.1 U.S. map of Indian reservations/lands.
Source: BIA (n.d.).

NURSING EDUCATION

Becoming a nurse in the United States includes many academic paths and entry points (Raines & Taglaireni, 2008). The nurse can first become a licensed practical or vocational nurse (LPN/LVN), usually through attendance at a community college, and then follow a completion program bridging into an associate's degree in nursing (ADN), associate of science in nursing (ASN), or bachelor of science in nursing (BSN). Alternately, the nurse can begin at either the ADN or BSN level without any previous licensure. The registered nurse (RN) is a license separate from the LPN and includes all professional nurses with an ADN or higher degree through master's and doctoral degrees. There are programs that lead from BSN directly to either an academic doctorate—the PhD—or the professional degree—doctor of nursing practice (DNP).

There are other programs where the would-be nurse could enter from a bachelor's in any discipline (e.g., history or English) to a master of science in nursing, earning the ability to sit for the basic licensure exam along the way. The master of science in nursing is often focused on advanced practice—family, pediatric, neonatal, or geriatric/adult nurse practitioner; certified registered nurse anesthetist; midwifery; or acute care. Other master's programs may be in nursing management/leadership/policy, education, or generalist.

A final entry into nursing is through a diploma program, which today represents less than 20% of the schools/programs for nursing. These programs are hospital based versus academic institution based, and use an apprenticeship model to gain nursing techniques and education. Nursing education moved to academia in the last century, with only a few diploma programs left in existence out of the around 1,000 programs today.

In today's world, once initial RN licensure is obtained, movement to the next academic degree can often be done via distance learning, online or hybrid (online with some face-to-face classroom time), as well as in face-to-face only learning programs. Technology plays a large role in the education of today's nurse.

AMERICAN INDIAN NURSING EDUCATION

Many of the FoN messages and recommendations are concerned with gaining education and practicing fully to that educational level, moving to higher education levels, and in increasing doctoral-level nurses by 200% by 2020. The other messages/recommendations are concerned with gaining a voice, finding a place at the proverbial table, and shaping policy.

Unfortunately, these recommendations can be as distant in concept as they are in geography from the Washington, DC, offices where they were conceived. In Indian Country, when one aspires to become a nurse, the road is difficult and filled with many obstacles. The road is difficult for most who aspire to this calling, but then add in multiple additional hindrances at every turn.

High School

This cannot be stressed enough: one must finish high school or its equivalent in order to apply to and gain admission and be successful in nursing school. For those living on the reservation, high school is usually in a remote area and/or is underfunded. There can be several scenarios. Students attend tribally run high schools, are bussed out to border towns for public school, or may attend parochial school if available—parochial schools require tuition or scholarships. There are issues with each of these scenarios around resources, perceived and real racism, role models and mentors, and available experiential opportunities—as in the health professions. Minority students are more likely to enter the health professions if they have had a role model, if they have "crossed the threshold" in some sort of mentored onsite experience, and if they are not the "lone wolf," that is, there is at least a cohort of three who will move through the same learning experience together. The high school graduation rate on the Pine Ridge Reservation in South Dakota in 2010 was 45% of the large public school (Maxwell, 2013). In Alaska, AI/AN students graduated at a rate of 42% (Sheehy, 2013).

And then there is coping with everyday life. In a recent *New York Times* article (Dunne, 2015), descriptions of the life some middle and high school students endure on the Pine Ridge reservation in South Dakota are at once stunning and devastating. It could just as easily have been describing issues in Barrow, Alaska; Red Lake, Minnesota; or Fort Berthold, North Dakota. It mentions the current tribally declared emergency created by an epidemic of students killing themselves in the face of racism—chants of "dirty Indian"; alcoholism consuming some families; methamphetamine abuse; sexual, emotional, and physical abuse. And there is hopelessness, isolation, abject poverty, and hunger, as far as the eye and mind can see.

Follow-up commentary from Pine Ridge residents included statements that 20% of students will have attempted suicide by the end of high school and, from a pediatrician on site, when he asked 5-year-olds, they could not come up with any what-do-you-want-to-be-when-you-grow-up dreams, let alone answering "nurse" (Dunne, 2015).

AI/AN Women

As it stands today, nursing is still largely dominated by women. There are some striking statistics that distinguish AI/AN women from American women, all races. And these statistics will impact who will be available for entering nursing school and any furtherance of nursing education. American Indian women are murdered at *a rate 10 times that* of all other Americans (Gilg, 2014; Williams, 2012). They are sexually assaulted at a rate four times that of other women, and 1 in 3 will have been raped in her lifetime (Gilg 2014; Williams 2012). In these instances, 86% of the crimes are perpetrated on Native women by non-Native men. They are not prosecuted as a result of limits of prosecution by tribes for violent crimes involving non-Native perpetrators (Monet, 2014).

Young Alaska Native women commit suicide at a rate *19* times that of other women, especially by age 24 (Woodard, 2012). Few perpetrators are ever prosecuted (Williams, 2012). Girls discuss what their strategies will be "when" they get raped, . . . not "if." Sex trafficking is exploding on the Plains. The Violence Against Women Act (VAWA, 2013) never covered Indian Country until the last authorization. In the last reauthorization, there was only a partial inclusion of reservation-based American Indian women, including only three tribes (out of 566), and even then only as a pilot. There are still laws on the books that do not allow an Indian tribe to prosecute a non-Indian, which is at the root of this problem. "For American Indian women, however, these facts are old news—really old news. It has been open season on American Indian women in this country for more than 200 years" (Pember, 2010, para. 3). If getting to the next day in one piece is the goal, then grades, graduation, and college applications become a distant second.

Recognizing these stark difficulties, whether reservation, rural, or urban, are nursing schools prepared to mentor and facilitate this population successfully through nursing school with each new level?

As much of this book has described, there are few resources in Indian Country, less than 0.3% of nurses are American Indian, and it is rare to have more than one AI/AN student in a nursing program that is not on or near a reservation. As this author alluded to in the Preface, there were never any other American Indian students or faculty in any of her three nursing programs. Although the author had no cohort, she did have role models, albeit not Native, and did enter hospitals and other health care environments throughout high school in a learning capacity.

Completing high school in urban areas can be just as difficult for the AI/AN student. And completing high school has to occur before entering a nursing program. High school graduation rates for urban AI/ANs are abysmal. For example, in Minneapolis, MN, a top-10 city with AI/AN population, the graduation rate was around 25% in 2012, and in 2014 purportedly moved to 33% (Minneapolis Public Schools, 2015). Let us repeat that—33%. This means almost 70% do not graduate high school, and this represents an improvement. Graduation rates for African Americans, although another atrocious percentage (43%), is 24% higher than that for AI/ANs. For Whites in the city, it is 72%. This is stunning on many levels. First, why has there not been a cry as to why this is happening and a demand for action? Second, if there are so few high school-graduate role models, how can there be nursing role models? Nationally, 15% of AI/ANs drop out of high school as opposed to 6% of White students (National Indian Education Association, 2015a).

For those who do graduate, they have passed a hurdle that 70% to 85% of their contemporaries found too difficult, not because of lack of intelligence or capability but as a result of formidable societal, familial, and structural barriers to success. If they have been able to finish high school and at such a level as to successfully apply to a nursing program, it will have been through an abundance of fortitude, sacrifice, and aspiration. However, this monumental effort will likely not be recognized by schools, their admissions committees, faculty, or other students. When they arrive, they are just another student, their context will remain unseen.

Tribal Nursing Schools

There are 36 tribal colleges and universities (TCU; National Indian Education Association, 2015b) that are found mostly in rural and reservation areas and that are largely underfunded (Bosman, 2013), just as with the Indian Health System. There are TCU nursing programs that include direct care workers, certified nursing assitants, certified medications aide (CMA), prenursing, LPN, RN, and/or RN completion programs. Most of these schools are 2-year community colleges. One school in Montana, the Salish Kootenai, has had a BSN program for years and was the first and only one in Indian Country (Table 18.2).

A quick look at the offerings reveals that there are only six RN programs currently accepting students at the associate's-degree level, and one BSN that is a completion program at Salish Kootenai University. Four TCU have prenursing programs that allow the student to transfer into nursing programs in affiliated state or private nursing programs. The maximum number of nursing programs offered are at the LPN (7) level.

Beyond this, reservation-based AI/AN students must go out of their nations, families, culture, and geography to complete their education. This takes a huge leap of faith. There likely have been no role models for this, no experiences assuring that the leap will be fine, or others to leap with.

TABLE 18.2 TCU Nursing/Prenursing Programs

SCHOOL/STATE	PROGRAMS OFFERED
Iḷisaġvik College, AK	CNA
Tohono O'odham Community College, AZ	Direct care worker
Fond du Lac Comtamunity College, MN	CNA, LPN, mobility nursing
Fort Peck Community College, MT	Prenursing
Salish Kootenai College, MT	ASN, RN-BSN
Stone Child College, MT	Prenursing
Navajo Technical University, NM	Preprofessional nursing, ASN (not accepting new students 2015)
Cankdeska Cikana (Little Hoop) Community College, ND	Prenursing
Fort Berthold Community College, ND	LPN, ADN
Sitting Bull College, ND	LPN
Turtle Mountain Community College, ND	ADN
United Tribes Technical College, ND	LPN
Oglala Lakota College, SD	Associate of arts in nursing
Sinte Gleska University, SD	CNA, CMA, LPN
Sisseton-Wahpeton College, SD	LPN
College of Menominee Nation, WI	LPN, LPN-ADN

FON RECOMMENDATIONS AND AI/AN NURSES

This section divides the FoN recommendations into two broad groups: (a) gaining education, practicing to its fullest scope, and pushing for more, including lifelong learning; and (b) shaping policy, being at the table as full partners in health care redesign, and leading change.

Education

So how does nursing education the fit with the FoN? The major impediments to further nursing education for most is time, cost, and family obligations. For AI/AN nurses graduating from TCU, the vast majority will have an associate's degree. Even those in urban areas will likely have entered a community college for their first professional licensure. It would seem unlikely that the TCU will be offering new BSN programs any time in the near future; therefore achieving this next level will require leaving their homes, or attempting distance or online programs. Either path will require financial assistance as the average BSN completion program costs $12,000 and $26,000 (Martin, 2013). National figures of poverty for AI/ANs are twice that of the U.S., all races (~30% vs. 15%; U.S. Census Bureau, 2011). Buying books requires an average of another $300. Then there is Internet service, computer, printer, and so on, which may have been available at the brick-and-mortar schools accessed for the associate's degree, but will not be available for online programs.

Additionally, wireless phone and data service is not always available, especially in Indian Country. A quick look at two large wireless providers in the 2015 market reveals that in the current Verizon Wireless coverage map, the Plains area is almost exclusively "uncovered" and AT&T has gaps throughout the west. Therefore, if one is a nurse in these areas, even everyday contact can be challenging, let alone keeping in contact with faculty, joining Skype or other Internet-based meeting, or completing forum work. This is not true on either coast or in major cities in the Midwest, where most of the recommending experts seem to have been based. It is mostly taken for granted that phones, data, the web, and so forth will be at one's fingertips (Box 18.1).

Box 18.1 24/7 Access to the World

During my time with the RWJF Health Policy Fellowship (2008–2009), I encouraged my co-fellows to visit the Pine Ridge reservation as one of our two state visits that year. The other was Boston, MA, as we were in the Health Reform era.

We were five MDs, one PhD nurse, and a kinesiologist. Most were from big-city areas, and most were from the East Coast, Texas, or Illinois.

All were in their suits, Senate-issued BlackBerries in hand. We got into the waiting van at the Rapid City, South Dakota, airport and headed out. Within minutes, no one's devices worked. Such panic, such consternation! Nothing! A couple of us knew this would happen, as one MD was a woman from New Mexico.

We would periodically dip in the road in a small valley, and all devices would suddenly bing, bing, bing, and/or vibrate. Then just as suddenly, all communication was lost again.

This went on for the several days we were there. What if this was your reality as a nurse? And you want to increase your level of education in this service-limited context?

Could you and would you do it?

At one time we were surrounded by buffalo on the road. That partially made up for it.

American Indian and Alaska Natives are also a younger population by about 6 years. There are more children under age 18 than there are in the United States at large. Many AI/AN nurses will have family duties and small children at home. The time factor for those working and serving their Native communities, the geographies, distance, as well as weather may be a factor. Those working as nurses in cities often maintain roles and expectations "back home." Vacation time may be eaten up by "doings" and responsibilities out of the city and, therefore, is not available for the visits needed for hybrid programs or other educational necessaries.

SHAPING POLICY

Another aspect of the IOM report is becoming a leader, being at the table, shoulder to shoulder with other professions, and shaping policy rather than being shaped by it. As this author has wandered throughout Indian Country for over two decades in a nurse's capacity (whether direct care, management, academic, or board member) and has spoken to AI/AN nurses on the ground, several things have become apparent. First, in terms of getting to the table, they do not even know "the table" exists.

Just as many direct-care nurses are not familiar with the FoN, many AI/AN nurses are unfamiliar with initiatives, opportunities, or developments in health care delivery. They are unaware of the American Academy of Nursing, the IOM, and other institutions of the health professions.

As one moves toward national and governmental bodies to inform and be informed, there will be overwhelmingly dominant culture members, chairs, and participants, who, in many cases, will be male when moving out of nursing-specific bodies. This author has made it a small, anecdotal "investigation" to note who the leaders in most hospitals are, and found they are largely male, usually of the dominant culture.

Therefore, given often an associate's degree education, having battled through poverty and isolation, dealt with non-Native male dominance with often dire results, and having little voice in educational and professional capacities, how will this nurse suddenly achieve the recommendations as written?

THE FUTURE OF NURSING AND THE AMERICAN INDIAN NURSE

Recognizing the overwhelming difficulties that many AI/ANs, women, nursing students, and nurses will have encountered in accessing the health professions, what, then, is a transforming outlook? What kinds of recommendations would include this unique segment of the U.S. population in health care? What is the future of nursing for: (a) this politically distinct group; (b) this most underrepresented of the racial minorities; (c) those entering the profession from the highest poverty rates, lowest high school-graduation rates, with exceptionally few role models; and (d) those surrounded by violence, especially on women, from either a rural/frontier or inner-city voice in transforming the profession?

There should be a key message and related recommendation specific to effectively adding diversity and inclusion to nursing. This should *not* only reside in descriptions but should also be as named messages and recommendations, as often, that is all that readers will see. There should be a key message and related recommendation of required collaboration among federal, state, and tribes toward the future of nursing, not between federal and state alone. There should be a key message and related recommendation in recognition of "other ways of knowing," such as indigenous knowledge specifically *not* reflected in higher and higher levels of Western education. And, finally, there should be a key message and related recommendation in terms of shaping policy—where stories are paramount. The gaps in care and the roots of health disparities lie in structural determinants of health. The AI/AN is already expert in most cases in terms of both an understanding of these structural barriers and the stories that accompany them. These nurses are uniquely ready to add to the transformation of nursing health care delivery success, and, therefore, to affect patient outcomes. But they are not sought out, not included, and not heard.

Unique Strengths

In one way, AI/AN nurses know what all other nurses know, *and* they know what they know. If they have been educated and have gained the clinical efficiency to pass in an accredited nursing program, be it at a TCU or otherwise, and then licensed by their state to practice, then objectively, they know what other nurses know.

In the context of Indian Country—rural, frontier, or urban (such as the Little Earth Community in Minneapolis, MN)—AI/AN nurses also know what only they know. They understand the histories recounted in this text, they have lived through difficulties often specific to AI/ANs, the knowledge is in their epigenetic expressions, and they transmit indigenous knowledge to the next generation. Storytelling is their gift (Moss 2009).

TCU and Other Program Successes

Although there are few schools with nursing programs in Indian Country, students who are there often have opportunities to learn indigenous languages and histories. Cultural programming is interwoven into every aspect of the schooling. Being successful in two worlds is often needed and honored, more so than achieving higher education in the Western world alone (Figure 18.2)

In a social location model stemming from the author's work on the Zuni reservation in 2000, this can be illustrated thus (Moss, 2000). If one is completely proficient in indigenous medicine and religion, one is likely not at the same level in academic medicine and health care. This is the result of the time needed on site for the indigenous proficiency along with one's many roles and responsibilities. The reverse is also true. If one has achieved the highest levels in academia, one may not have been able to become the most proficient and knowledgeable in the indigenous practices. There are, of course, those with knowledge and proficiency in both, so much so as to become a bridge of sorts.

However, that is not to say there cannot be successes in Western education in Indian Country. At the author's reservation, in the Fort Berthold Community College Nursing ADN program, 24 out of 25 students sitting for licensure since 2008 passed, a 96% passing rate (FBCC, 2015). This means there were several cohorts in which 100% passed.

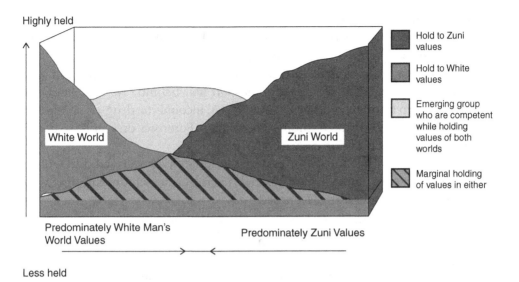

FIGURE 18.2 Social location of American Indians living in two worlds.
Source: Moss (2000).

There are several programs in universities as well with a focus on nursing that are targeted toward either AI/AN students or those wishing to work in Indian Country. The Recruitment/Retention of American Indians into Nursing (RAIN) Program at the University of North Dakota stemming from the Indian Health Care Improvement Act (1988 amendment) seeks to increase the number of nurses, nurse midwives, and nurse practitioners and has been highly successful; the former Indian Health Service/Health Resources and Services Administration-funded-and-administered Native Nurse Career Opportunity Program at the University of Minnesota offered funding and support for those seeking a master's degree in nursing, with most successfully graduating; and the American Indian Students United for Nursing (ASUN) Project at Arizona State University has been ongoing. These programs usually relieve, in part or whole, the tuition burden for students and provide cultural connections for students who arrived at the university, away from their families, roles, and nations.

Indigenous Knowledge and Health Decisions

The idea that there are other ways of knowing that can add to the nursing narrative must be widely embraced by the larger profession and health care delivery. Chapter 6 touched on some of the plants, methods, and ideas of indigenous knowledge; however, there are whole networks of healers, healing knowledge, and environmental understanding that could be of use in nursing, as seen in Chapter 4.

There was a hantavirus outbreak in New Mexico and surrounding regions in 1993 that was killing people rapidly, their lungs filled with fluid almost overnight. American Indians elders (mostly Diné) said the cause was mice resulting from effects of weather and rain. This knowledge was passed down through oral history and lore. It took the Centers for Disease Control and Prevention, the Indian Health Service (IHS) and the National Institutes of Health much investigation to come to the same conclusions.

Hair has been said to hold information; the person's spirit can act as a portal of vulnerability for one who has left hair behind. We now know that in fact hair can be analyzed. It can show DNA, alcohol- or drug-use patterns, and environmental exposures among other things. Forensics on hair have been used to convict individuals of crimes.

Although indigenous and Western thought may be derived differently, they often come to the same findings. Each is useful, each includes differing perspectives. Neither should be discounted.

Shaping Health Policy With the Indigenous Voice

As nurses, we often pay attention to health outcomes. In the United States, health outcomes are largely a result of genetics, environment, and circumstances that include access to Western health care. Some of these environmental and circumstantial issues are called "social determinants of health" (Marmot, Friel, Bell, Houweling, & Taylor, 2008). As nurses, we seem to pay a little less attention to the social determinants of health for our patients, such as whether they have access to good nutrition, food security, housing and safety, transportation, education, and the ability and opportunity to exercise. We pay more attention to the health issues that were presented acutely. However, as stated at the beginning of the text, it is part of nurses' basic education to take a holistic look at the patient, community, and environment. If these social determinants of health are not positively in place and reliable access to health care is unavailable, there are likely to be dire consequences, such as those described throughout this text; diversifying the workforce can only help (Williams et al., 2014).

Some of the experts in the social determinants of health are nurses, advocates, and residents in Indian Country. The numbers for poor nutrition, education, transportation, and so forth are far below those for all other Americans. But beyond even these determinants are what are called structural determinants of health. Structural determinants of health, as defined here, are those that put social determinants of health into place. An example is transportation as a social determinant of health. Any lack of transportation that blocks access to food, health care, appointments, education, and associated activities will produce considerable health effects.

Transportation is often the number one issue for AI/AN elderly. But it was policies and law—state and federal—that limited transportation. Policies removed AI/ANs from original lands, put reservations in place, and then offered limited or no services to transportation. Great distances can be involved in just getting to banks (if they have an account), full-service groceries, clinics and hospitals, and cities. The problem, then, in this scenario is missed appointments, aggravated physical conditions, falls, no medications, and on and on. This is one reason why AI/ANs have more abridged lives than the U.S. average for all races (Figure 18.3). The percentage of elderly in AI/AN populations is shockingly low (The National Congress of American Indian [NCAI], 2013).

Transportation is but one issue. Nutrition is big, safety is monumental, especially for women and children. In shaping policy, should food, transportation, and safety funding be cut in order to pay for hospital and clinic care, and insurance? It has been estimated that the social determinants of health make up 75% of one's health.

There are major age distribution differences between AI/ANs and the U.S. total population. These lie at either end of the life span. Although, as expressed previously, there are far fewer elderly AI/ANs than in the general population, there are many more young AI/ANs by percentage of population (Figure 18.4; National Congress of American Indians [NCAI], 2013).

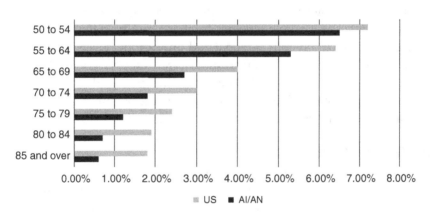

FIGURE 18.3 Age distribution of AI/AN elderly versus U.S. total population.

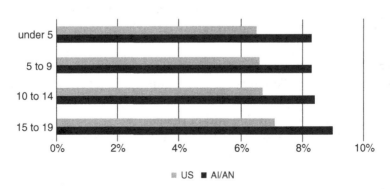

FIGURE 18.4 Age distribution of AI/AN youth to U.S. total population.

Because the AI/AN population is younger, there are more workers available to support the elderly. This is in direct contrast to the U.S. population as a whole, in which it has long been recognized that there are not enough younger people to add to the economy, Medicare, Social Security, or work in elder services to support the "gray tsunami" of the baby boomers. The nursing profession would be wise to recognize this and use it in planning for the health care and elder care education and workforce arenas for this and other populations.

CONCLUSIONS

Nurses in Indian Country understand social determinants of health and the associated structural determinants as written about throughout this text. Some of the most stunning of these disparities in poverty, housing, food, and education, for example (outlined in Chapter 3), are in many cases the result of federal laws and policies on removal, reservations, assimilation and tribal termination. They also know the histories, geographies, and policies that have impacted their achievement of obtaining a Western nursing education, patient outcomes, and factors affecting Indian Country as a whole whether from the county, state, regional, or national levels. Their voices on both personal and professional levels will be important in the future of nursing as it is transformed, as few others have this knowledge.

The stories of nurses and patients are unending, the range is 566+ tribes wide, and the depth is 500 years postcontact. These nurses and others who have committed to American Indian health hold several keys to doors yet unopened.

CRITICAL-THINKING EXERCISES

◆ You work with a university program that wants to recruit more AI/AN nursing students. Pick the educational level and cultural area(s) you will be targeting. What understandings must you have prior to such an endeavor. Describe needed personnel, activities, supplies, community resources, and academic resources that you will need for success.
◆ You want to take some ideas about social and structural determinants of health to the state legislature. Create a story to describe an AI/AN patient's circumstances and issues. What would be your question?

STUDY QUESTIONS

◆ Discuss why American Indian nurse and community voices should add to the future of nursing.
◆ What recommendations would you add or delete?
◆ What are the most important social or structural determinants of health in your view, and why?

USEFUL WEBSITES

◆ American Academy of Nursing, http://www.aannet.org/
◆ Future of Nursing online report, http://www.iom.edu/Reports/2010/The-Future-of-Nursing-Leading-Change-Advancing-Health.aspx

◆ National Academy of Sciences, http://nationalacademyofsciences.org/?referrer= https://www.google.com/
◆ Tribal Colleges, http://www.niea.org/students/tribal-colleges-and-universities.aspx
◆ *Winds of Change* magazine of the American Indian Science and Engineering Society, http://www.aises.org/news/woc

REFERENCES

BIA (n.d.) Indian Lands. http://nationalmap.gov/small_scale/printable/images/pdf/fedlands/BIA_2.pdf. accessed Nov 13, 2015.

Bleich, M. R. (2012). The future of nursing report and direct care nurses. *American Journal of Nursing, 112*(2), 11. doi:10.1097/01.NAJ.0000411157.87879.8a

Bosman, J. (2013). Leveling the playing field for tribal colleges. *Minority Nurse.* Retrieved June 8, 2015, from http://minoritynurse.com/leveling-the-playing-field-for-tribal-colleges/

Dunne, M. (2015). Suicides on an Indian reservation. *The New York Times.* Retrieved June 8, 2015, from http://www.nytimes.com/2015/05/11/opinion/suicides-on-an-indian-reservation.html?_r=0

Fort Berthold Community College. (2015). *Licensure—Nursing.* Retrieved June 15, 2015, from http://nhsc.edu/wp-content/uploads/2015/08/Licensure_-_Nursing.pdf

Gilg, D. (2014). *Prosecutions in Indian Country violence against women.* U.S. Attorneys Office—Department of Justice. Retrieved June 13, 2015, from http://www.justice.gov/usao/priority-areas/indian-country/violence-against-women

Institute of Medicine. (2000). *To err is human: Building a safer health system.* Retrieved June 4, 2015, from http://www.nap.edu/openbook.php?record_id=9728&page=26

Institute of Medicine. (2011). *The future of nursing: Leading change, advancing health.* Committee on the Robert Wood Johnson Foundation: Initiative on the future of nursing. Washington, DC: National Academies Press.

Institute of Medicine. (2015). *About the IOM.* Retrieved June 4, 2015, from http://www.iom.edu/About-IOM.aspx

Marmot, M., Friel, S., Bell, R., Houweling, T. A., & Taylor, S. (2008). Closing the gap in a generation: Health equity through action on the social determinants of health. *The Lancet, 372,* 1661–1669.

Martin, D. (2013). BSN degree completion: Why, what and how much. Retrieved from http://www.nursetogether.com/bsn-degree-completion-why-what-and-how-much

Maxwell, L. (2013). *Education in Indian Country: Running in place—Education week.* Retrieved June 12, 2015, from http://www.edweek.org/ew/projects/2013/native-american-education/running-in-place.html

Minneapolis Public Schools. (2015). *Graduation rates up 7 percent over two years in MPS.* Retrieved June 8, 2015, from http://www.mpls.k12.mn.us/uploads/mps_grad_rates_press_release_2-19-14.pdf

Monet, J. (2014). Prosecuting non–Native Americans. *Al Jazeera America.* Retrieved June 13, 2015, from http://america.aljazeera.com/articles/2014/2/22/prosecuting-non-nativeamericans.html

Moss, M. P. (2000). *Zuni elders: Ethnography of American Indian aging* (Unpublished doctoral dissertation) Texas Medical Center, Houston, TX.

Moss, M. P. (2009). Storytelling. In R. Lindquist, M. Snyder, & M. F. Tracy (Eds.), *Complementary and alternative therapies in nursing* (pp. 183–196). New York, NY: Springer Publishing Company.

National Academy of Sciences. (2015) *Overview: NAS mission.* Retrieved June 4, 2015, from http://www.nasonline.org/about-nas/mission/

The National Congress of American Indians. (2013). *Native American heritage month.* Retrieved June 20, 2015, from http://www.aianheritagemonth.org/

National Indian Education Association. (2015a). *Statistics on native students.* Retrieved from http://www.niea.org/Research/Statistics.aspx

National Indian Education Association. (2015b). *Tribal colleges and universities.* Retrieved June 9, 2015, from http://www.niea.org/Students/Tribal-Colleges-and-Universities.aspx

Pember, M. (2010, August 30). Silent No More. *The Progressive.* Retrieved on November 30, 2015, from http://progressive.org/news/2010/08/147687/silent-no-more

Raines, C. F., & Taglaireni, M. E. (2008). Career pathways in nursing: Entry points and academic progression. *Online Journal of Issues in Nursing, 13*(3), 3.

Robert Wood Johnson Foundation. (2015) *RWJF and diversity.* Retrieved June, 8, 2015, from http://www.rwjf.org/content/dam/files/rwjf-web-files/Policies/RWJF_diversity.pdf

Sheehy, K. (2013, June 6). Graduation rates dropping among Native American students. *U.S. News & World Report.* Retrieved June 12, 2015, from http://www.usnews.com/education/high-schools/articles/2013/06/06/graduation-rates-dropping-among-native-american-students

U.S. Census Bureau. (2011). *American Indian and Alaska Native heritage month: November 2011.* https://www.census.gov/newsroom/releases/archives/facts_for_features_special_editions/cb11-ff22.html

Violence Against Women Reauthorization Act of 2013, Pub. Law No: 113–4 (2013).

Williams, T. (2012, February 20). On Indian reservations, higher crime and fewer prosecutions. *The New York Times.* Retrieved from http://www.nytimes.com/2012/02/21/us/on-indian-reservations-higher-crime-and-fewer-prosecutions.html?_r=0

Woodard, S. (2012). *Suicide is epidemic for American Indian youth: What more can be done?—Investigations.* Retrieved June 13, 2015, from http://investigations.nbcnews.com/_news/2012/10/10/14340090-suicide-is-epidemic-for-american-indian-youth-what-more-can-be-done?lite

List of Federally Recognized Tribes

TABLE A.1 566 Indian Entities Recognized and Eligible to Receive Services From the U.S. Bureau of Indian Affairs

(*Note:* Due to the large number of tribes, tribes in the state of Alaska have been broken out and may be found in Table A.2)

1	Absentee–Shawnee Tribe of Indians of Oklahoma
2	Agua Caliente Band of Cahuilla Indians of the Agua Caliente Indian Reservation, California
3	Ak Chin Indian Community of the Maricopa (Ak Chin) Indian Reservation Arizona
4	Alabama–Coushatta Tribe of Texas (previously listed as the Alabama Coushatta Tribes of Texas)
5	Alabama–Quassarte Tribal Town Alturas Indian Rancheria, California
6	Apache Tribe of Oklahoma
7	Arapaho Tribe of the Wind River Reservation, Wyoming
8	Aroostook Band of Micmacs (previously listed as the Aroostook Band of Micmac Indians)
9	Assiniboine and Sioux Tribes of the Fort Peck Indian Reservation, Montana
10	Augustine Band of Cahuilla Indians, California (previously listed as the Augustine Band of Cahuilla Mission Indians of the Augustine Reservation)
11	Bad River Band of the Lake Superior Tribe of Chippewa Indians of the Bad River Reservation, Wisconsin
12	Bay Mills Indian Community, Michigan
13	Bear River Band of the Rohnerville Rancheria, California
14	Berry Creek Rancheria of Maidu Indians of California
15	Big Lagoon Rancheria, California
16	Big Pine Paiute Tribe of the Owens Valley (previously listed as the Big Pine Band of Owens Valley Paiute Shoshone Indians of the Big Pine Reservation, California)
17	Big Sandy Rancheria of Western Mono Indians of California (previously listed as the Big Sandy Rancheria of Mono Indians of California)
18	Big Valley Band of Pomo Indians of the Big Valley Rancheria, California

(continued)

TABLE A.1 566 Indian Entities Recognized and Eligible to Receive Services From the U.S. Bureau of Indian Affairs (*continued*)

19	Bishop Paiute Tribe (previously listed as the Paiute–Shoshone Indians of the Bishop Community of the Bishop Colony, California)
20	Blackfeet Tribe of the Blackfeet Indian Reservation of Montana
21	Blue Lake Rancheria, California
22	Bridgeport Indian Colony (previously listed as the Bridgeport Paiute Indian Colony of California)
23	Buena Vista Rancheria of Me-Wuk Indians of California
24	Burns Paiute Tribe (previously listed as the Burns Paiute Tribe of the Burns Paiute Indian Colony of Oregon)
25	Cabazon Band of Mission Indians, California
26	Cachil DeHe Band of Wintun Indians of the Colusa Indian Community of the Colusa Rancheria, California
27	Caddo Nation of Oklahoma
28	Cahto Tribe of the Laytonville Rancheria
29	Cahuilla Band of Mission Indians of the Cahuilla Reservation, California
30	California Valley Miwok Tribe, California
31	Campo Band of Diegueno Mission Indians of the Campo Indian Reservation, California
32	Capitan Grande Band of Diegueno Mission Indians of California: Barona Group of Capitan Grande Band of Mission Indians of the Barona Reservation, California
33	Viejas (Baron Long) Group of Capitan Grande Band of Mission Indians of the Viejas Reservation, California
34	Catawba Indian Nation (aka Catawba Tribe of South Carolina)
35	Cayuga Nation Cedarville Rancheria, California
36	Chemehuevi Indian Tribe of the Chemehuevi Reservation, California
37	Cher-Ae Heights Indian Community of the Trinidad Rancheria, California
38	Cherokee Nation Cheyenne and Arapaho Tribes, Oklahoma (previously listed as the Cheyenne–Arapaho Tribes of Oklahoma)
39	Cheyenne River Sioux Tribe of the Cheyenne River Reservation, South Dakota
40	Chicken Ranch Rancheria of Me-Wuk Indians of California
41	Chippewa Cree Indians of the Rocky Boy's Reservation, Montana (previously listed as the Chippewa Cree Indians of the Rocky Boy's Reservation, Montana)
42	Chitimacha Tribe of Louisiana
43	Citizen Potawatomi Nation, Oklahoma
44	Cloverdale Rancheria of Pomo Indians of California
45	Cocopah Tribe of Arizona

(continued)

TABLE A.1 566 Indian Entities Recognized and Eligible to Receive Services From the U.S. Bureau of Indian Affairs (*continued*)

46	Coeur D'Alene Tribe (previously listed as the Coeur D'Alene Tribe of the Coeur D'Alene Reservation, Idaho)
47	Cold Springs Rancheria of Mono Indians of California
48	Colorado River Indian Tribes of the Colorado River Indian Reservation, Arizona and California
49	Comanche Nation, Oklahoma
50	Confederated Salish and Kootenai Tribes of the Flathead Reservation
51	Confederated Tribes and Bands of the Yakama Nation
52	Confederated Tribes of Siletz Indians of Oregon (previously listed as the Confederated Tribes of the Siletz Reservation)
53	Confederated Tribes of the Chehalis Reservation
54	Confederated Tribes of the Colville Reservation
55	Confederated Tribes of the Coos, Lower Umpqua and Siuslaw Indians
56	Confederated Tribes of the Goshute Reservation, Nevada and Utah
57	Confederated Tribes of the Grand Ronde Community of Oregon
58	Confederated Tribes of the Umatilla Indian Reservation (previously listed as the Confederated Tribes of the Umatilla Reservation, Oregon)
59	Confederated Tribes of the Warm Springs Reservation of Oregon
60	Coquille Indian Tribe (previously listed as the Coquille Tribe of Oregon)
61	Cortina Indian Rancheria (previously listed as the Cortina Indian Rancheria of Wintun Indians of California)
62	Coushatta Tribe of Louisiana
63	Cow Creek Band of Umpqua Tribe of Indians (previously listed as the Cow Creek Band of Umpqua Indians of Oregon)
64	Cowlitz Indian Tribe Coyote Valley Band of Pomo Indians of California
65	Crow Creek Sioux Tribe of the Crow Creek Reservation, South Dakota
66	Crow Tribe of Montana
67	Death Valley Timbi-sha Shoshone Tribe (previously listed as the Death Valley Timbi-Sha Shoshone Band of California)
68	Delaware Nation, Oklahoma
69	Delaware Tribe of Indians
70	Dry Creek Rancheria Band of Pomo Indians, California (previously listed as the Dry Creek Rancheria of Pomo Indians of California)
71	Duckwater Shoshone Tribe of the Duckwater Reservation, Nevada

(continued)

TABLE A.1 566 Indian Entities Recognized and Eligible to Receive Services From the U.S. Bureau of Indian Affairs (*continued*)

72	Eastern Band of Cherokee Indians Eastern Shawnee Tribe of Oklahoma
73	Elem Indian Colony of Pomo Indians of the Sulphur Bank Rancheria, California
74	Elk Valley Rancheria, California
75	Ely Shoshone Tribe of Nevada
76	Enterprise Rancheria of Maidu Indians of California
77	Ewiiaapaayp Band of Kumeyaay Indians, California
78	Federated Indians of Graton Rancheria, California
79	Flandreau Santee Sioux Tribe of South Dakota
80	Forest County Potawatomi Community, Wisconsin
81	Fort Belknap Indian Community of the Fort Belknap Reservation of Montana
82	Fort Bidwell Indian Community of the Fort Bidwell Reservation of California
83	Fort Independence Indian Community of Paiute Indians of the Fort Independence Reservation, California
84	Fort McDermitt Paiute and Shoshone Tribes of the Fort McDermitt Indian Reservation, Nevada and Oregon
85	Fort McDowell Yavapai Nation, Arizona
86	Fort Mojave Indian Tribe of Arizona, California & Nevada
87	Fort Sill Apache Tribe of Oklahoma
88	Gila River Indian Community of the Gila River Indian Reservation, Arizona
89	Grand Traverse Band of Ottawa and Chippewa Indians, Michigan
90	Greenville Rancheria (previously listed as the Greenville Rancheria of Maidu Indians of California)
91	Grindstone Indian Rancheria of Wintun Wailaki Indians of California
92	Guidiville Rancheria of California
93	Habematolel Pomo of Upper Lake, California
94	Hannahville Indian Community, Michigan
95	Havasupai Tribe of the Havasupai Reservation, Arizona
96	Ho-Chunk Nation of Wisconsin
97	Hoh Indian Tribe (previously listed as the Hoh Indian Tribe of the Hoh Indian Reservation, Washington)
98	Hoopa Valley Tribe, California

(continued)

TABLE A.1 566 Indian Entities Recognized and Eligible to Receive Services From the U.S. Bureau of Indian Affairs (*continued*)

99	Hopi Tribe of Arizona
100	Hopland Band of Pomo Indians, California (formerly Hopland Band of Pomo Indians of the Hopland Rancheria, California)
101	Houlton Band of Maliseet Indians
102	Hualapai Indian Tribe of the Hualapai Indian Reservation, Arizona
103	Iipay Nation of Santa Ysabel, California (previously listed as the Santa Ysabel Band of Diegueno Mission Indians of the Santa Ysabel Reservation)
104	Inaja Band of Diegueno Mission Indians of the Inaja and Cosmit Reservation, California
105	Ione Band of Miwok Indians of California
106	Iowa Tribe of Kansas and Nebraska
107	Iowa Tribe of Oklahoma
108	Jackson Band of Miwuk Indians (previously listed as the Jackson Rancheria of Me-Wuk Indians of California)
109	Jamestown S'Klallam Tribe Jamul Indian Village of California
110	Jena Band of Choctaw Indians
111	Jicarilla Apache Nation, New Mexico
112	Kaibab Band of Paiute Indians of the Kaibab Indian Reservation, Arizona
113	Kalispel Indian Community of the Kalispel Reservation Karuk Tribe (previously listed as the Karuk Tribe of California)
114	Kashia Band of Pomo Indians of the Stewarts Point Rancheria, California
115	Kaw Nation, Oklahoma
116	Kewa Pueblo, New Mexico (previously listed as the Pueblo of Santo Domingo)
117	Keweenaw Bay Indian Community, Michigan
118	Kialegee Tribal Town Kickapoo Traditional Tribe of Texas
119	Kickapoo Tribe of Indians of the Kickapoo Reservation in Kansas
120	Kickapoo Tribe of Oklahoma
121	Kiowa Indian Tribe of Oklahoma
122	Klamath Tribes Koi Nation of Northern California (previously listed as the Lower Lake Rancheria, California)
123	Kootenai Tribe of Idaho
124	La Jolla Band of Luiseno Indians, California (previously listed as the La Jolla Band of Luiseno Mission Indians of the La Jolla Reservation)
125	La Posta Band of Diegueno Mission Indians of the La Posta Indian Reservation, California

(continued)

TABLE A.1 566 Indian Entities Recognized and Eligible to Receive Services From the U.S. Bureau of Indian Affairs (*continued*)

126	Lac Courte Oreilles Band of Lake Superior Chippewa Indians of Wisconsin
127	Lac du Flambeau Band of Lake Superior Chippewa Indians of the Lac du Flambeau Reservation of Wisconsin
128	Lac Vieux Desert Band of Lake Superior Chippewa Indians of Michigan
129	Las Vegas Tribe of Paiute Indians of the Las Vegas Indian Colony, Nevada
130	Little River Band of Ottawa Indians, Michigan
131	Little Traverse Bay Bands of Odawa Indians, Michigan
132	Lone Pine Paiute-Shoshone Tribe (previously listed as the Paiute Shoshone Indians of the Lone Pine Community of the Lone Pine Reservation, California)
133	Los Coyotes Band of Cahuilla and Cupeno Indians, California (previously listed as the Los Coyotes Band of Cahuilla & Cupeno Indians of the Los Coyotes Reservation)
134	Lovelock Paiute Tribe of the Lovelock Indian Colony, Nevada
135	Lower Brule Sioux Tribe of the Lower Brule Reservation, South Dakota
136	Lower Elwha Tribal Community (previously listed as the Lower Elwha Tribal Community of the Lower Elwha Reservation, Washington)
137	Lower Sioux Indian Community in the State of Minnesota
138	Lummi Tribe of the Lummi Reservation
139	Lytton Rancheria of California
140	Makah Indian Tribe of the Makah Indian Reservation
141	Manchester Band of Pomo Indians of the Manchester Rancheria, California (previously listed as the Manchester Band of Pomo Indians of the Manchester-Point Arena Rancheria, California)
142	Manzanita Band of Diegueno Mission Indians of the Manzanita Reservation, California
143	Mashantucket Pequot Indian Tribe (previously listed as the Mashantucket Pequot Tribe of Connecticut)
144	Mashpee Wampanoag Tribe (previously listed as the Mashpee Wampanoag Indian Tribal Council, Inc.)
145	Match-e-be-nash-she-wish Band of Pottawatomi Indians of Michigan
146	Mechoopda Indian Tribe of Chico Rancheria, California
147	Menominee Indian Tribe of Wisconsin
148	Mesa Grande Band of Diegueno Mission Indians of the Mesa Grande Reservation, California
149	Mescalero Apache Tribe of the Mescalero Reservation, New Mexico
150	Miami Tribe of Oklahoma

(continued)

TABLE A.1 566 Indian Entities Recognized and Eligible to Receive Services From the U.S. Bureau of Indian Affairs (*continued*)

151	Miccosukee Tribe of Indians Middletown Rancheria of Pomo Indians of California
152	Minnesota Chippewa Tribe, Minnesota (Six component reservations: Bois Forte Band (Nett Lake), Fond du Lac Band, Grand Portage Band, Leech Lake Band, Mille Lacs Band, White Earth Band)
153	Mississippi Band of Choctaw Indians
154	Moapa Band of Paiute Indians of the Moapa River Indian Reservation, Nevada
155	Mohegan Tribe of Indians of Connecticut (previously listed as Mohegan Indian Tribe of Connecticut)
156	Mooretown Rancheria of Maidu Indians of California
157	Morongo Band of Mission Indians, California (previously listed as the Morongo Band of Cahuilla Mission Indians of the Morongo Reservation)
158	Muckleshoot Indian Tribe (previously listed as the Muckleshoot Indian Tribe of the Muckleshoot Reservation, Washington)
159	Narragansett Indian Tribe Navajo Nation, Arizona, New Mexico, & Utah
160	Nez Perce Tribe (previously listed as the Nez Perce Tribe of Idaho)
161	Nisqually Indian Tribe (previously listed as the Nisqually Indian Tribe of the Nisqually Reservation, Washington)
162	Nooksack Indian Tribe
163	Northern Cheyenne Tribe of the Northern Cheyenne Indian Reservation, Montana
164	Northfork Rancheria of Mono Indians of California
165	Northwestern Band of Shoshoni Nation (previously listed as the Northwestern Band of Shoshoni Nation of Utah (Washakie)
166	Nottawaseppi Huron Band of the Potawatomi, Michigan (previously listed as the Huron Potawatomi, Inc.)
167	Oglala Sioux Tribe (previously listed as the Oglala Sioux Tribe of the Pine Ridge Reservation, South Dakota)
168	Ohkay Owingeh, New Mexico (previously listed as the Pueblo of San Juan)
169	Omaha Tribe of Nebraska Oneida Nation of New York
170	Oneida Tribe of Indians of Wisconsin
171	Onondaga Nation Otoe-Missouria Tribe of Indians, Oklahoma
172	Ottawa Tribe of Oklahoma
173	Paiute Indian Tribe of Utah (Cedar Band of Paiutes, Kanosh Band of Paiutes, Koosharem Band of Paiutes, Indian Peaks Band of Paiutes, and Shivwits Band of Paiutes) (formerly Paiute Indian Tribe of Utah [Cedar City Band of Paiutes, Kanosh Band of Paiutes, Koosharem Band of Paiutes, Indian Peaks Band of Paiutes, and Shivwits Band of Paiutes])

(continued)

TABLE A.1 566 Indian Entities Recognized and Eligible to Receive Services From the U.S. Bureau of Indian Affairs (*continued*)

174	Paiute-Shoshone Tribe of the Fallon Reservation and Colony, Nevada
175	Pala Band of Luiseno Mission Indians of the Pala Reservation, California
176	Pascua Yaqui Tribe of Arizona
177	Paskenta Band of Nomlaki Indians of California
178	Passamaquoddy Tribe Pauma Band of Luiseno Mission Indians of the Pauma & Yuima Reservation, California
179	Pawnee Nation of Oklahoma
180	Pechanga Band of Luiseno Mission Indians of the Pechanga Reservation, California
181	Penobscot Nation (previously listed as the Penobscot Tribe of Maine)
182	Peoria Tribe of Indians of Oklahoma
183	Picayune Rancheria of Chukchansi Indians of California
184	Pinoleville Pomo Nation, California (previously listed as the Pinoleville Rancheria of Pomo Indians of California)
185	Pit River Tribe, California (includes XL Ranch, Big Bend, Likely, Lookout, Montgomery Creek and Roaring Creek Rancherias)
186	Poarch Band of Creeks (previously listed as the Poarch Band of Creek Indians of Alabama)
187	Pokagon Band of Potawatomi Indians, Michigan and Indiana
188	Ponca Tribe of Indians of Oklahoma
189	Ponca Tribe of Nebraska
190	Port Gamble S'Klallam Tribe (previously listed as the Port Gamble Band of S'Klallam Indians)
191	Potter Valley Tribe, California
192	Prairie Band Potawatomi Nation (previously listed as the Prairie Band of Potawatomi Nation, Kansas)
193	Prairie Island Indian Community in the State of Minnesota
194	Pueblo of Acoma, New Mexico
195	Pueblo of Cochiti, New Mexico
196	Pueblo of Isleta, New Mexico
197	Pueblo of Jemez, New Mexico
198	Pueblo of Laguna, New Mexico
199	Pueblo of Nambe, New Mexico
200	Pueblo of Picuris, New Mexico

(continued)

TABLE A.1 566 Indian Entities Recognized and Eligible to Receive Services From the U.S. Bureau of Indian Affairs (*continued*)

201	Pueblo of Pojoaque, New Mexico
202	Pueblo of San Felipe, New Mexico
203	Pueblo of San Ildefonso, New Mexico
204	Pueblo of Sandia, New Mexico
205	Pueblo of Santa Ana, New Mexico
206	Pueblo of Santa Clara, New Mexico
207	Pueblo of Taos, New Mexico
208	Pueblo of Tesuque, New Mexico
209	Pueblo of Zia, New Mexico
210	Puyallup Tribe of the Puyallup Reservation
211	Pyramid Lake Paiute Tribe of the Pyramid Lake Reservation, Nevada
212	Quartz Valley Indian Community of the Quartz Valley Reservation of California Quechan Tribe of the Fort Yuma Indian Reservation, California & Arizona
213	Quileute Tribe of the Quileute Reservation
214	Quinault Indian Nation (previously listed as the Quinault Tribe of the Quinault Reservation, Washington)
215	Ramona Band of Cahuilla, California (previously listed as the Ramona Band or Village of Cahuilla Mission Indians of California)
216	Red Cliff Band of Lake Superior Chippewa Indians of Wisconsin
217	Red Lake Band of Chippewa Indians, Minnesota
218	Redding Rancheria, California
219	Redwood Valley or Little River Band of Pomo Indians of the Redwood Valley Rancheria California (previously listed as the Redwood Valley Rancheria of Pomo Indians of California)
220	Reno–Sparks Indian Colony, Nevada
221	Resighini Rancheria, California Rincon Band of Luiseno Mission Indians of the Rincon Reservation, California
222	Robinson Rancheria (previously listed as the Robinson Rancheria Band of Pomo Indians, California and the Robinson Rancheria of Pomo Indians of California)
223	Rosebud Sioux Tribe of the Rosebud Indian Reservation, South Dakota
224	Round Valley Indian Tribes, Round Valley Reservation, California (previously listed as the Round Valley Indian Tribes of the Round Valley Reservation, California)
225	Sac & Fox Nation of Missouri in Kansas and Nebraska

(continued)

TABLE A.1 566 Indian Entities Recognized and Eligible to Receive Services From the U.S. Bureau of Indian Affairs (*continued*)

226	Sac & Fox Nation, Oklahoma
227	Sac & Fox Tribe of the Mississippi in Iowa
228	Saginaw Chippewa Indian Tribe of Michigan Saint Regis Mohawk Tribe (previously listed as the St. Regis Band of Mohawk Indians of New York)
229	Salt River Pima–Maricopa Indian Community of the Salt River Reservation, Arizona
230	Samish Indian Nation (previously listed as the Samish Indian Tribe, Washington)
231	San Carlos Apache Tribe of the San Carlos Reservation, Arizona
232	San Juan Southern Paiute Tribe of Arizona
233	San Manuel Band of Mission Indians, California (previously listed as the San Manual Band of Serrano Mission Indians of the San Manual Reservation)
234	San Pasqual Band of Diegueno Mission Indians of California
235	Santa Rosa Band of Cahuilla Indians, California (previously listed as the Santa Rosa Band of Cahuilla Mission Indians of the Santa Rosa Reservation)
236	Santa Rosa Indian Community of the Santa Rosa Rancheria, California
237	Santa Ynez Band of Chumash Mission Indians of the Santa Ynez Reservation, California
238	Santee Sioux Nation, Nebraska
239	Sauk-Suiattle Indian Tribe Sault Ste. Marie Tribe of Chippewa Indians, Michigan Scotts Valley Band of Pomo Indians of California
240	Seminole Tribe of Florida (previously listed as the Seminole Tribe of Florida [Dania, Big Cypress, Brighton, Hollywood & Tampa Reservations])
241	Seneca Nation of Indians (previously listed as the Seneca Nation of New York)
242	Seneca–Cayuga Nation (previously listed as the Seneca-Cayuga Tribe of Oklahoma)
243	Shakopee Mdewakanton Sioux Community of Minnesota
244	Shawnee Tribe Sherwood Valley Rancheria of Pomo Indians of California
245	Shingle Springs Band of Miwok Indians, Shingle Springs Rancheria (Verona Tract), California
246	Shinnecock Indian Nation
247	Shoalwater Bay Indian Tribe of the Shoalwater Bay Indian Reservation (previously listed as the Shoalwater Bay Tribe of the Shoalwater Bay Indian Reservation, Washington)
248	Shoshone Tribe of the Wind River Reservation, Wyoming
249	Shoshone–Bannock Tribes of the Fort Hall Reservation
250	Shoshone–Paiute Tribes of the Duck Valley Reservation, Nevada
251	Sisseton–Wahpeton Oyate of the Lake Traverse Reservation, South Dakota

(*continued*)

TABLE A.1 566 Indian Entities Recognized and Eligible to Receive Services From the U.S. Bureau of Indian Affairs (*continued*)

252	Skokomish Indian Tribe (previously listed as the Skokomish Indian Tribe of the Skokomish Reservation, Washington)
253	Skull Valley Band of Goshute Indians of Utah
254	Smith River Rancheria, California
255	Snoqualmie Indian Tribe (previously listed as the Snoqualmie Tribe, Washington) Soboba Band of Luiseno Indians, California
256	Sokaogon Chippewa Community, Wisconsin
257	Southern Ute Indian Tribe of the Southern Ute Reservation, Colorado
258	Spirit Lake Tribe, North Dakota
259	Spokane Tribe of the Spokane Reservation
260	Squaxin Island Tribe of the Squaxin Island Reservation
261	St. Croix Chippewa Indians of Wisconsin
262	Standing Rock Sioux Tribe of North & South Dakota
263	Stillaguamish Tribe of Indians of Washington (previously listed as the Stillaguamish Tribe of Washington)
264	Stockbridge Munsee Community, Wisconsin
265	Summit Lake Paiute Tribe of Nevada
266	Suquamish Indian Tribe of the Port Madison Reservation
267	Susanville Indian Rancheria, California
268	Swinomish Indian Tribal Community (previously listed as the Swinomish Indians of the Swinomish Reservation of Washington)
269	Sycuan Band of the Kumeyaay Nation
270	Table Mountain Rancheria of California
271	Tejon Indian Tribe
272	Te-Moak Tribe of Western Shoshone Indians of Nevada (Four constituent bands: Battle Mountain Band, Elko Band, South Fork Band, and Wells Band)
273	The Chickasaw Nation
274	The Choctaw Nation of Oklahoma
275	The Modoc Tribe of Oklahoma
276	The Muscogee (Creek) Nation
277	The Osage Nation (previously listed as the Osage Tribe)
278	The Quapaw Tribe of Indians

(continued)

TABLE A.1 566 Indian Entities Recognized and Eligible to Receive Services From the U.S. Bureau of Indian Affairs (*continued*)

279	The Seminole Nation of Oklahoma
280	Thlopthlocco Tribal Town
281	Three Affiliated Tribes of the Fort Berthold Reservation, North Dakota
282	Tohono O'odham Nation of Arizona
283	Tonawanda Band of Seneca (previously listed as the Tonawanda Band of Seneca Indians of New York)
284	Tonkawa Tribe of Indians of Oklahoma
285	Tonto Apache Tribe of Arizona
286	Torres Martinez Desert Cahuilla Indians, California (previously listed as the Torres-Martinez Band of Cahuilla Mission Indians of California)
287	Tulalip Tribes of Washington (previously listed as the Tulalip Tribes of the Tulalip Reservation, Washington)
288	Tule River Indian Tribe of the Tule River Reservation, California
289	Tunica-Biloxi Indian Tribe Tuolumne Band of Me-Wuk Indians of the Tuolumne Rancheria of California
290	Turtle Mountain Band of Chippewa Indians of North Dakota
291	Tuscarora Nation
292	Twenty-Nine Palms Band of Mission Indians of California
293	United Auburn Indian Community of the Auburn Rancheria of California
294	United Keetoowah Band of Cherokee Indians in Oklahoma
295	Upper Sioux Community, Minnesota
296	Upper Skagit Indian Tribe
297	Ute Indian Tribe of the Uintah & Ouray Reservation, Utah
298	Ute Mountain Tribe of the Ute Mountain Reservation, Colorado, New Mexico & Utah
299	Utu Utu Gwaitu Paiute Tribe of the Benton Paiute Reservation, California
300	Walker River Paiute Tribe of the Walker River Reservation, Nevada
301	Wampanoag Tribe of Gay Head (Aquinnah)
302	Washoe Tribe of Nevada & California (Carson Colony, Dresslerville Colony, Woodfords Community, Stewart Community, & Washoe Ranches)
303	White Mountain Apache Tribe of the Fort Apache Reservation, Arizona
304	Wichita and Affiliated Tribes (Wichita, Keechi, Waco & Tawakonie), Oklahoma
305	Wilton Rancheria, California Winnebago Tribe of Nebraska

(continued)

TABLE A.1 566 Indian Entities Recognized and Eligible to Receive Services From the U.S. Bureau of Indian Affairs (*continued*)

306	Winnemucca Indian Colony of Nevada
307	Wiyot Tribe, California (previously listed as the Table Bluff Reservation— Wiyot Tribe)
308	Wyandotte Nation Yankton Sioux Tribe of South Dakota
309	Yavapai–Apache Nation of the Camp Verde Indian Reservation, Arizona
310	Yavapai–Prescott Indian Tribe (previously listed as the YavapaiPrescott Tribe of the Yavapai Reservation, Arizona)
311	Yerington Paiute Tribe of the Yerington Colony & Campbell Ranch, Nevada
312	Yocha Dehe Wintun Nation, California (previously listed as the Rumsey Indian Rancheria of Wintun Indians of California)
313	Yomba Shoshone Tribe of the Yomba Reservation, Nevada
314	Ysleta del Sur Pueblo (previously listed as the Ysleta Del Sur Pueblo of Texas)
315	Yurok Tribe of the Yurok Reservation, California
316	Zuni Tribe of the Zuni Reservation, New Mexico

Note: Some listings include multiple tribes.
Author's note: In July 2015, during production of this book, the 567th tribe, the Pamunkey Tribe of Virginia gained federal recognition. For more information see http://indiancountrytodaymedianetwork.com/2015/07/07/federal-recognition-virginias-pamunkey-tribe-long-time-coming-160981

TABLE A.2 Native Entities Within the State of Alaska Recognized and Eligible to Receive Services From the U.S. Bureau of Indian Affairs

1	Agdaagux Tribe of King Cove
2	Akiachak Native Community
3	Akiak Native Community
4	Alatna Village
5	Algaaciq Native Village (St. Mary's)
6	Allakaket Village Angoon Community Association
7	Anvik Village
8	Arctic Village (See Native Village of Venetie Tribal Government)
9	Asa'carsarmiut Tribe
10	Atqasuk Village (Atkasook)
11	Beaver Village
12	Birch Creek Tribe
13	Central Council of the Tlingit & Haida Indian Tribes
14	Chalkyitsik Village
15	Cheesh-Na Tribe (previously listed as the Native Village of Chistochina)

TABLE A.2 Native Entities Within the State of Alaska Recognized and Eligible to Receive Services From the U.S. Bureau of Indian Affairs (*continued*)

16	Chevak Native Village
17	Chickaloon Native Village
18	Chignik Bay Tribal Council (previously listed as the Native Village of Chignik) Chignik Lake Village
19	Chilkat Indian Village (Klukwan)
20	Chilkoot Indian Association (Haines)
21	Chinik Eskimo Community (Golovin)
22	Chuloonawick Native Village
23	Circle Native Community
24	Craig Tribal Association (previously listed as the Craig Community Association)
25	Curyung Tribal Council
26	Douglas Indian Association
27	Egegik Village
28	Eklutna Native Village
29	Emmonak Village
30	Evansville Village (aka Bettles Field)
31	Galena Village (aka Louden Village)
32	Gulkana Village
33	Healy Lake Village
34	Holy Cross Village
35	Hoonah Indian Association
36	Hughes Village
37	Huslia Village
38	Hydaburg Cooperative Association
39	Igiugig Village
40	Inupiat Community of the Arctic Slope
41	Iqurmuit Traditional Council
42	Ivanoff Bay Village
43	Kaguyak Village
44	Kaktovik Village (aka Barter Island)

(continued)

TABLE A.2 Native Entities Within the State of Alaska Recognized and Eligible to Receive Services From the U.S. Bureau of Indian Affairs (*continued*)

45	Kasigluk Traditional Elders Council
46	Kenaitze Indian Tribe
47	Ketchikan Indian Corporation
48	King Island Native Community
49	King Salmon Tribe
50	Klawock Cooperative Association
51	Knik Tribe
52	Kokhanok Village
53	Koyukuk Native Village
54	Levelock Village
55	Lime Village
56	Manley Hot Springs Village
57	Manokotak Village
58	McGrath Native Village
59	Mentasta Traditional Council
60	Metlakatla Indian Community, Annette Island Reserve
61	Naknek Native Village
62	Native Village of Afognak
63	Native Village of Akhiok
64	Native Village of Akutan
65	Native Village of Aleknagik
66	Native Village of Ambler
67	Native Village of Atka
68	Native Village of Barrow Inupiat Traditional Government
69	Native Village of Belkofski
70	Native Village of Brevig Mission
71	Native Village of Buckland
72	Native Village of Cantwell
73	Native Village of Chenega (aka Chanega)

(continued)

TABLE A.2 Native Entities Within the State of Alaska Recognized and Eligible to Receive Services From the U.S. Bureau of Indian Affairs (*continued*)

74	Native Village of Chignik Lagoon
75	Native Village of Chitina
76	Native Village of Chuathbaluk (Russian Mission, Kuskokwim)
77	Native Village of Council
78	Native Village of Deering
79	Native Village of Diomede (aka Inalik)
80	Native Village of Eagle
81	Native Village of Eek
82	Native Village of Ekuk
83	Native Village of Ekwok (previously listed as Ekwok Village)
84	Native Village of Elim
85	Native Village of Eyak (Cordova)
86	Native Village of False Pass
87	Native Village of Fort Yukon
88	Native Village of Gakona
89	Native Village of Gambell
90	Native Village of Georgetown
91	Native Village of Goodnews Bay
92	Native Village of Hamilton
93	Native Village of Hooper Bay
94	Native Village of Kanatak
95	Native Village of Karluk
96	Native Village of Kiana
97	Native Village of Kipnuk
98	Native Village of Kivalina
99	Native Village of Kluti Kaah (aka Copper Center)
100	Native Village of Kobuk
101	Native Village of Kongiganak
102	Native Village of Kotzebue
103	Native Village of Koyuk

(continued)

TABLE A.2 Native Entities Within the State of Alaska Recognized and Eligible to Receive Services From the U.S. Bureau of Indian Affairs (*continued*)

104	Native Village of Kwigillingok
105	Native Village of Kwinhagak (aka Quinhagak)
106	Native Village of Larsen Bay
107	Native Village of Marshall (aka Fortuna Ledge)
108	Native Village of Mary's Igloo
109	Native Village of Mekoryuk
110	Native Village of Minto
111	Native Village of Nanwalek (aka English Bay)
112	Native Village of Napaimute
113	Native Village of Napakiak
114	Native Village of Napaskiak
115	Native Village of Nelson Lagoon
116	Native Village of Nightmute
117	Native Village of Nikolski
118	Native Village of Noatak
119	Native Village of Nuiqsut (aka Nooiksut)
120	Native Village of Nunam Iqua (previously listed as the Native Village of Sheldon's Point)
121	Native Village of Nunapitchuk
122	Native Village of Old Harbor (previously listed as Village of Old Harbor)
123	Native Village of Ouzinkie
124	Native Village of Paimiut
125	Native Village of Perryville
126	Native Village of Pilot Point
127	Native Village of Pitka's Point
128	Native Village of Point Hope
129	Native Village of Point Lay
130	Native Village of Port Graham
131	Native Village of Port Heiden
132	Native Village of Port Lions

(*continued*)

TABLE A.2 Native Entities Within the State of Alaska Recognized and Eligible to Receive Services From the U.S. Bureau of Indian Affairs (*continued*)

133	Native Village of Ruby
134	Native Village of Saint Michael
135	Native Village of Savoonga
136	Native Village of Scammon Bay
137	Native Village of Selawik
138	Native Village of Shaktoolik
139	Native Village of Shishmaref
140	Native Village of Shungnak
141	Native Village of Stevens
142	Native Village of Tanacross
143	Native Village of Tanana
144	Native Village of Tatitlek
145	Native Village of Tazlina
146	Native Village of Teller
147	Native Village of Tetlin
148	Native Village of Tuntutuliak
149	Native Village of Tununak
150	Native Village of Tyonek
151	Native Village of Unalakleet
152	Native Village of Unga
153	Native Village of Venetie Tribal Government (Arctic Village and Village of Venetie)
154	Native Village of Wales
155	Native Village of White Mountain
156	Nenana Native Association
157	New Koliganek Village Council
158	New Stuyahok Village
159	Newhalen Village
160	Newtok Village
161	Nikolai Village
162	Ninilchik Village

(continued)

TABLE A.2 Native Entities Within the State of Alaska Recognized and Eligible to Receive Services From the U.S. Bureau of Indian Affairs (*continued*)

163	Nome Eskimo Community
164	Nondalton Village
165	Noorvik Native Community
166	Northway Village
167	Nulato Village
168	Nunakauyarmiut Tribe Organized Village of Grayling (aka Holikachuk)
169	Organized Village of Kake
170	Organized Village of Kasaan
171	Organized Village of Kwethluk
172	Organized Village of Saxman
173	Orutsararmiut Traditional Native Council (previously listed as Orutsararmuit Native Village (aka Bethel))
174	Oscarville Traditional Village
175	Pauloff Harbor Village
176	Pedro Bay Village
177	Petersburg Indian Association
178	Pilot Station Traditional Village
179	Platinum Traditional Village
180	Portage Creek Village (aka Ohgsenakale)
181	Pribilof Islands Aleut Communities of St. Paul & St. George Islands
182	Qagan Tayagungin Tribe of Sand Point Village
183	Qawalangin Tribe of Unalaska Rampart Village
184	Saint George Island (See Pribilof Islands Aleut Communities of St. Paul & St. George Islands)
185	Saint Paul Island (See Pribilof Islands Aleut Communities of St. Paul & St. George Islands)
186	Seldovia Village Tribe
187	Shageluk Native Village
188	Sitka Tribe of Alaska
189	Skagway Village
190	South Naknek Village

(continued)

TABLE A.2 Native Entities Within the State of Alaska Recognized and Eligible to Receive Services From the U.S. Bureau of Indian Affairs (*continued*)

191	Stebbins Community Association
192	Sun'aq Tribe of Kodiak (previously listed as the Shoonaq' Tribe of Kodiak)
193	Takotna Village
194	Tangirnaq Native Village (formerly Lesnoi Village (aka Woody Island))
195	Telida Village
196	Traditional Village of Togiak
197	Tuluksak Native Community
198	Twin Hills Village
199	Ugashik Village
200	Umkumiut Native Village (previously listed as Umkumiute Native Village)
201	Village of Alakanuk
202	Village of Anaktuvuk Pass
203	Village of Aniak
204	Village of Atmautluak
205	Village of Bill Moore's Slough
206	Village of Chefornak
207	Village of Clarks Point
208	Village of Crooked Creek
209	Village of Dot Lake
210	Village of Iliamna
211	Village of Kalskag
212	Village of Kaltag
213	Village of Kotlik
214	Village of Lower Kalskag
215	Village of Ohogamiut
216	Village of Old Harbor
217	Village of Red Devil
218	Village of Salamatoff
219	Village of Sleetmute

(continued)

TABLE A.2 Native Entities Within the State of Alaska Recognized and Eligible to Receive Services From the U.S. Bureau of Indian Affairs (*continued*)

220	Village of Solomon
221	Village of Stony River
222	Village of Venetie (see Native Village of Venetie Tribal Government)
223	Village of Wainwright
224	Wrangell Cooperative Association
225	Yakutat Tlingit Tribe
226	Yupiit of Andreafski

66 State-Recognized Tribes

Alabama
Cher-O-Creek Intra Tribal Indians
Cherokee Tribe of Northeast Alabama
Cherokees of Southeast Alabama
Echota Cherokee Tribe of Alabama
Ma-Chis Lower Creek Indian Tribe of Alabama
Mowa Band of Choctaw Indians
Piqua Shawnee Tribe
Star Clan of Muscogee Creeks
United Cherokee Ani-Yun-Wiya Nation

Connecticut
Eastern Pequot Tribal Nation
Schaghticoke Tribal Nation

Delaware
Lenape Indian Tribe of Delaware
Nanticoke Indian Association, Inc.

Georgia
Cherokee of Georgia Tribal Council
Georgia Tribe of Eastern Cherokee
Lower Muskogee Creek Tribe

Louisiana
Addai Caddo Tribe
Biloxi–Chitimacha Confederation of Muskogee
Choctaw–Apache Community of Ebarb
Clifton Choctaw
Four Winds Tribe Louisiana Cherokee Confederacy
Grand Caillou/Dulac Band
Isle de Jean Charles Band
Louisiana Choctaw Tribe
Pointe-Au-Chien Indian Tribe
United Houma Nation

Maryland
Piscataway Indian Nation
Piscataway Conoy Tribe

Massachusetts
Nipmuc Nation

Montana
Little Shell Tribe of Chippewa Indians

New Jersey
Nanticoke Lenni-Lenape Tribal Nation
Powhatan Renape Nation
Ramapough Lunaape Nation

New York
Tonawada Band of Seneca
Tuscarora Nation
Unkechaug Nation

North Carolina
Cohaire Intra-Tribal Council, Inc.
Haliwa–Saponi Indian Tribe
Lumbee Tribe
Meherrin Nation
Occaneechi Band of the Saponi Nation
Sappony
Waccamaw-Siouan Tribe

South Carolina
Beaver Creek Indians
Edisto Natchez Kusso Tribe of South Carolina
Pee Dee Nation of Upper South Carolina
Pee Dee Indian Tribe of South Carolina
Santee Indian Organization
The Waccamaw Indian People
Wassamasaw Tribe of Varnertown Indians

Texas
Lipan Apache Tribe

Vermont
Elnu Abenaki Tribe
Nulhegan Band of the Coosuk Abenaki Nation
Koasek Abenaki Tribe
Mississquoi Abenaki Tribe

Virginia
Cheroenhaka (Nottoway)
Chickahominy Tribe
Eastern Chickahominy Tribe
Mattaponi
Monacan Nation
Nansemond
Nottoway of Virginia
Pamunkey
Pattawomeck
Rappahannock
Upper Mattaponi Tribe

Source: National Conference of State Legislatures—State Recognized Tribes (see http://www.ncsl
.org/research/state-tribal-institute/list-of-federal-and-state-recognized-tribes.aspx#s-ny)

About the Authors

Because this is a unique addition to the American Indian and nursing literature, we highlight in this section the equally unique contributors who we hope will be resources for the readers/learners. All but two are American Indian. These two are nurses who work(ed) in the population. All but another two are nurses, three are male, and one is the chief of a federally recognized tribe; they offer an inimitable mix of experiences and perspectives. The contributors are presented in alphabetical order:

Nicolle L. Gonzales
Donna M. Grandbois
S. Neyooxet Greymorning
Bette Jacobs
Marilynn Malerba
Lisa Martin
Ruth E. Meilstrup
Margaret P. Moss
Christopher M. Nelson
Lee Anne Nichols
C. June Strickland
Lillian Tom-Orme
Theodore C. Van Alst, Jr.

Nicolle L. Gonzales, MSN RN, CNM (Chapter 10), is Diné, and a member of the Navajo Nation. She grew up in Waterflow, New Mexico, and resides on San Ildefonso Pueblo reservation with her husband and three children. She completed her midwifery education at the University of New Mexico, and is working to develop a birthing center for Native American families that will ultimately provide access to culturally safe prenatal care using indigenous Native American medicines and methodologies. She has participated on several educational panels on cultural safety and 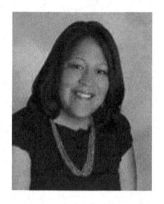 on the revitalization of indigenous Native American cultural knowledge surrounding women's health and traditional birth practices. She has served as a mentor for Native American nursing and midwifery students and is also working toward developing a Native American Midwifery organization.

Donna M. Grandbois, PhD, MSN, RN (Chapter 15), is an enrolled member of the Turtle Mountain Chippewa tribe of North Dakota. As a Native nurse educator, it is not inconceivable that Donna was the first Native American nurse in her college to become a clinical instructor after graduating with a master's degree in nursing. By 1997, few Native nurses had gone on to receive a master's degree and only 16 or 17 had received doctoral degrees nationwide in 2008 when Dr. Grandbois earned her doctoral degree in gerontology. To go from student to colleague is usually somewhat challenging, but in retrospect, 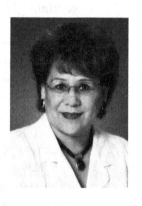 Dr. Grandbois realized she really was not seen as a colleague, given the hierarchical culture of academia. Rather, she was free to enjoy sharing her practice experiences and expertise with the mental health nursing students who were assigned to her clinical groups. Is it not interesting that the top causes of death for Native people are heart disease, cancer, unintentional injuries, diabetes, and stroke? All are amenable to prevention, treatment, and recovery with a change of heart and proper guidance to make lifestyle changes and to have equitable access to the resources necessary to live healthy, holistic lives. Perhaps the time has come to include Indigenous People in the dialogue if we are really determined to end health disparities.

S. Neyooxet Greymorning, PhD (Chapter 6), received his doctorate from the University of Oklahoma in 1992, where he was trained in political, linguistic, and ethnomedical anthropology. He currently holds joint positions in anthropology and Native American studies at the University of Montana. His research interests have focused on language and political issues among Indigenous Peoples of Australia, Canada, New Zealand, E. Timor, and the United States. Professor Greymorning has lectured as a visiting scholar at universities throughout the United States, Australia, 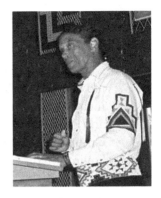 Canada, New Zealand, and, during the 2001–2002 academic year, served as the acting director of the Indigenous Governance Programs at the University of Victoria in British Columbia, Canada. In his work toward developing strategies for Native language restoration, since 1995 he has served, as the executive director of Hinono'eitiit Ho'oowu' (Arapaho Language Lodge) in Wyoming—a position that has been instrumental in his development of a breakthrough method for second language instruction and acquisition called accelerated second language acquisition. Professor Greymorning has published numerous articles on Native political and language issues, and has been named four times to Who's *Who Among American College and University Professors*—1999, 2004, 2005, 2009.

Bette Jacobs, PhD, RN, FAAN (Chapter 12), is professor, health systems administration; distinguished scholar and cofounder at the O'Neill Institute for Global and National Health Law; and a fellow and visiting professor at Campion Hall, University of Oxford. A Native American whose body of work spans community, academic, service, and corporate leadership, she is recognized for contributions in successful start-ups, financial integrity, and interdisciplinary innovations. She served with distinction as dean of the Georgetown University School of Nursing and Health Studies for 11 years, overseeing unprecedented program 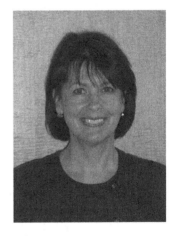 growth within the university. Previous executive experience includes vice presidency for Honda of America Manufacturing; founding faculty member and associate director of applied research at the Civitan International Research Center; and acting dean of graduate studies and research at California State University. Dr. Jacobs's extraordinary cross-disciplinary and cross-sector leadership has fostered innovation and improved systems. Her personal and professional activities emanate from crossing childhood cultural boundaries triangulating a colonized, missionized tribal history through pathways in education, business, and service. Strong cultural roots anchor and animate her work to advance the common good with practical abilities to do so.

She has mentored students and fellows in many fields in places as representative as Wyoming, Texas, England, China, and Japan. Dr. Jacobs is a long-time member of organizations such as the Society for the Advancement of Chicanos and Native Americans into Science, work groups such as the International Group on Indigenous Health Measurement, and served on boards ranging from environmental health and safety to Reading is Fundamental.

Dr. Jacobs has been involved with social entrepreneurship throughout her career. Her current scholarship and teaching on nonprofit governance incorporates the entire scope of a diverse and unique experience. Since her sabbatical at Oxford University, this body of work reflects a deeper understanding of the British charity model that shaped the foundation used for U.S. and international aid. She has pursued areas where harmony across nonprofit, public, and commercial sectors contributes to improving the human condition. In addition, her research is informed by political theory, Jesuit Catholic values, and the Honda philosophy, and focuses on the nonprofit sector as a primary vehicle for the common good.

Chief Mutáwi Mutáhash (Many Hearts) Marilynn "Lynn" Malerba, DNP, RN (Chapters 8 and 17), became the 18th chief of the Mohegan Tribe on August 15, 2010, and is the first female chief in the tribe's modern history. The position is a lifetime appointment made by the Tribe's Council of Elders. Dr. Malerba follows in the footsteps of many strong female role models in the Mohegan Tribe, including her mother, Loretta Roberge, who holds the position of Tribal Nonner (elder female of respect), as well as her great-grandfather, Chief Matagha (Burrill Fielding). Prior to becoming chief, she served as chairwoman 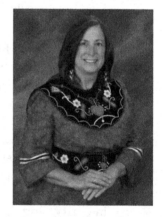 of the Tribal Council, and also worked in tribal government as executive director of Health and Human Services. Preceding her work for the Mohegan Tribe, Dr. Malerba had a long career as a registered nurse, and ultimately as the director of cardiology and pulmonary services at Lawrence & Memorial Hospital. She holds a master's degree in public administration from the University of Connecticut and an honorary doctorate from the University of St. Joseph in Hartford, and earned a doctor of nursing practice at Yale University.

She is chairwoman of the Tribal Self-Governance Advisory Committee of the federal Indian Health Service (IHS), and one of fourteen tribal leaders serving on the Justice Department's Tribal Nations Leadership Council. She is also a member of the board of directors for the Center for National Policy.

Locally, she serves as a trustee for Chelsea Groton Bank, board of trustees for the University of St. Joseph in West Hartford, and as advisory committee member for the Harvard University Native American Program, and served on the board of directors for Lawrence Memorial Hospital for 11 years. She lives in Uncasville with her husband, Paul, and has two adult daughters, Elizabeth and Angela.

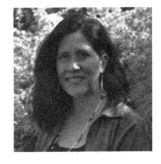

Lisa Martin, PhD, RN, PHN (Chapter 16), is an assistant professor of nursing at St. Catherine's University in St. Paul, Minnesota, and has several years of experience teaching in graduate and undergraduate programs. She holds a BS from Augsburg College in Minneapolis, Minnesota, and an MS in nursing administration and a PhD in nursing from the University of Minnesota. Lisa began her academic career at the University of Minnesota as a research assistant with the Center for Adolescent Nursing, and as a science administrator with the American Indian Alaska Native MS to PhD Nursing Science Bridge Project, which was established to double the number of American Indian nurses with PhDs in the United States. Prior to serving at the University of Minnesota, Lisa worked as a public health nurse in Minneapolis/St. Paul with low-income families and as a clinical educator, nursing supervisor, and project manager with several interdisciplinary public health programs. She has extensive experience building research collaboratives with reservation and urban-based American Indian communities and with community-based participatory research. Her doctoral dissertation "The Lived Experience of Urban-Based American Indian Adolescents with Type 2 Diabetes," presented a phenomenological view of diabetes in adolescents that led to her current research efforts with youth and obesity in low-income, rural, and American Indian communities. Lisa's areas of interest include diabetes prevention in American Indian youth; American Indian health care and research; cultural competency; nursing education; nursing workforce diversity, equity, and inclusivity; and conflict resolution. Lisa is Ojibwe and a member of the Lac Du Flambeau Band of Chippewa Indians, Lac Du Flambeau, Wisconsin.

Ruth E. Meilstrup, RN (Chapter 5), earned a diploma in nursing at Blodgett Memorial Hospital School of Nursing, Grand Rapids, Michigan. For the first 20 years of her career, she worked in private sector hospitals, and gained experience in psychiatric, pediatric, obstetric, and medical–surgical nursing. After moving to Santa Fe, New Mexico, in 1990, Ms. Meilstrup joined the staff at the Santa Fe Indian Hospital, where she continued until her retirement in 2014. While there, she worked on the medical–surgical unit, where she was a pediatric

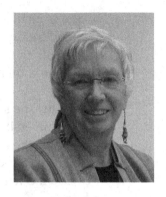

nursing specialist. For 10 years as house supervisor, she was responsible for several quality-improvement projects, the Point of Care Testing program, and Staffing Effectiveness Standard compliance for The Joint Commission.

Ms. Meilstrup is married and has raised two sons. Retirement allows her to pursue her love of travel and camping.

Margaret P. Moss, PhD, JD, RN, FAAN, is an enrolled member of the Three Affiliated Tribes of North Dakota—the Mandan, Hidatsa, and Arikara Nation. Dr. Moss is the Assistant Dean of Diversity and Inclusion and Associate Professor at the University at Buffalo, School of Nursing. She was formerly an associate professor and coordinator of the Nursing Management, Policy, and Leadership Specialty at the Yale University School of Nursing, and was the first director of Yale School of Nursing's doctor of nursing practice program. Dr. Moss received her PhD in nursing from the University of Texas at Houston, Health Sciences Center in 2000—her dissertation was an ethnography on aging in the Zuni tribe of New Mexico.

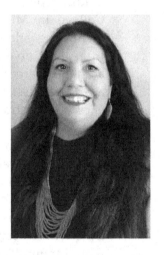

She subsequently received a distinguished alumni award. Dr. Moss completed a 2-year postdoctorate fellowship at the Native Elder Research Center, a National Institutes of Health–funded Resource Center for Minority Aging Research based at the University of Colorado, and concurrently entered and completed law school, focusing on federal Indian law, elder law, and health law. She is one of only 20 doctorally prepared American Indian nurses in the United States, and is the first and only American Indian to hold both nursing and juris doctorates. Dr. Moss was a 2008–2009 Robert Wood Johnson Health Policy Fellow, and staffed the Senate Special Committee on Aging under Senators Martinez and Corker. Also in 2008, she was inducted as a fellow of the American Academy of Nursing. Dr. Moss has just completed a Fulbright Canada (2014) experience at McGill University in Montreal, Quebec, Canada, as the visiting research chair in indigenous/Aboriginal life across the North American context. Dr. Moss is often sought out to speak, teach, and advocate on American Indian health and policy issues.

Christopher M. Nelson, MPH, BSN, RN (Chapter 14), is a public health nurse in Alaska with a research focus on circumpolar health and well-being. His current project involves Arctic environmental toxicology with an interest in contaminants and zoonotic agents in subsistence hunting and fishing game animals of the Alaska Native and American Indian populations of Alaska, the First Nations peoples of Nunavut and Nunavik, Canada, and the North, West, and East Greenlandic peoples.

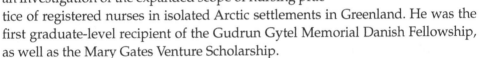

He recently completed the first public health Fulbright Fellowship in Greenland (and Denmark) with an investigation of the expanded scope of nursing practice of registered nurses in isolated Arctic settlements in Greenland. He was the first graduate-level recipient of the Gudrun Gytel Memorial Danish Fellowship, as well as the Mary Gates Venture Scholarship.

He will begin pursuing a PhD in nursing science in 2015, and hopes to become a professor of nursing with an Arctic health research practice.

Lee Anne Nichols, PhD, RN (Chapter 9), is currently at the University of Tulsa School of Nursing in Oklahoma. She is an associate professor in community health nursing. Dr. Nichols is a citizen (tribal member) of Cherokee Nation of Oklahoma. Dr. Nichols received her PhD in clinical nursing research from the University of Arizona College of Nursing in 1994. She completed a 2-year postdoctoral fellowship in developmental disability research at the University of Alabama at Birmingham Civitan International Research Center in 1996. During her postdoctoral fellowship, she served as the project director for the American Indian Families Project. She has worked in collaboration with several Indian tribes in the southeastern part of the United States. Her program of research is with American Indian families with developmental disabilities.

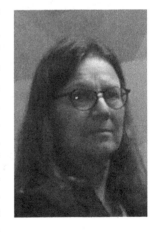

Currently, she is refining her conceptual model, The Pattern of American Indians: Harmony Ethos. She uses the model with American Indian families in her program of research.

Nationally, she has made several presentations on American Indian family research, and has published in several research journals. Dr. Nichols has also developed an American Indian nurse leadership curriculum in collaboration with a team of Indian nurse leaders at Arizona State University and the Indian Health Service. She has presented several week-long workshops on the American Indian nurse leadership curriculum. She has served as a consultant to nursing programs regarding the recruitment and retention of American Indian nursing students.

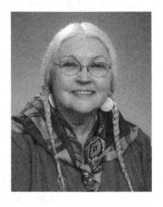

C. June Strickland, PhD, RN (Chapter 13), (Cherokee) is a professor of psychosocial and community health nursing at the University of Washington School of Nursing in Seattle. She earned her MS and PhD degrees at the University of Washington. Her nursing research focus is on health behavior change with Pacific Northwest American Indians. In this respect, she has conducted research in suicide prevention and American Indian/Alaska Native research community capacity building with National Institute of Nursing research funding. She has provided proposal development training for American Indian/Alaska Native tribes in the United States through the Spirit of Eagles National Cancer Institute Community Networks funding, and developed a training manual for the Association of American Indian Physicians. She has received awards for excellence in graduate teaching from the University of Washington, and the Dr. Frank Dukepoo Senior Native Research award from the Native Research Network. She is committed to developing culturally appropriate instruments, examining the cultural appropriateness of research methods with American Indians, and assuring community engagement. She is a member of the National Cancer Institute Native Research Network, serves on the Food and Drug Administration Risk Communications Advisory Committee, and supervises community health field sites for both undergraduate and graduate students in rural American Indian reservations in Washington State.

Lillian Tom-Orme, PhD, MPH, RN, FAAN (Chapter 11), is a research assistant professor in the division of epidemiology and adjunct assistant professor and diversity coordinator for the College of Nursing—University of Utah. Her research interests include health disparity issues, transcultural health, and cancer and diabetes care in Native Americans.

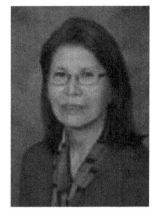

She currently has membership in the American Public Health Association, American Diabetes Association, Native Research Network, Network for Cancer Researchers among American Indian and Alaska Native Populations, National Coalition of Ethnic Minority Nurses Associations, and the Transcultural Nursing Society.

She serves on the Minority Women's Health Panel of Experts (Department of Health and Human Services), and has served on the advisory board for the National Institute of Minority Health Disparities, and as Native American research liaison for the National Cancer Institute.

Theodore C. Van Alst, Jr. (Chapter 2), is an assistant professor of Native American studies at the University of Montana, and former assistant dean and director of the Native American Cultural Center at Yale University. Recent work includes his edited volume *The Faster, Redder, Road: The Best UnAmerican Stories of Stephen Graham Jones,* released in April 2015, as well as "Expectations and Preferences for Counseling and Psychotherapy in Native Americans," in the *Journal of Indigenous Research*. He has worked as a consultant on multiple projects for the Disney Channel as well as on National Public Radio's *All Things Considered*, and has recently appeared in multiple segments of the

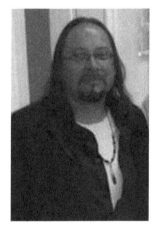

History Channel series *Mankind the Story of All of Us*. He has been interviewed by *The Washington Post*, Canadian Broadcast Corporation, *Native America Calling, Smithsonian Magazine*, and Al-Jazeera America on a variety of subjects, from Native representation and Tonto to spaghetti westerns, headdresses, and *Twilight*.

Index

Printed in the United States
By Bookmasters